Clinical Utility of Optical Coherence Tomography in Ophthalmology

Clinical Utility of Optical Coherence Tomography in Ophthalmology

Editor

Jose Ignacio Fernandez-Vigo

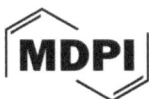

Basel • Beijing • Wuhan • Barcelona • Belgrade • Novi Sad • Cluj • Manchester

Editor
Jose Ignacio Fernandez-Vigo
Hospital Clínico San Carlos (IdISSC)
Madrid
Spain

Editorial Office
MDPI AG
Grosspeteranlage 5
4052 Basel, Switzerland

This is a reprint of articles from the Special Issue published online in the open access journal *Journal of Clinical Medicine* (ISSN 2077-0383) (available at: https://www.mdpi.com/journal/jcm/special_issues/C92CVM3742).

For citation purposes, cite each article independently as indicated on the article page online and as indicated below:

Lastname, A.A.; Lastname, B.B. Article Title. *Journal Name* **Year**, *Volume Number*, Page Range.

ISBN 978-3-7258-2539-4 (Hbk)
ISBN 978-3-7258-2540-0 (PDF)
doi.org/10.3390/books978-3-7258-2540-0

Cover image courtesy of Jose Ignacio Fernandez-Vigo

© 2024 by the authors. Articles in this book are Open Access and distributed under the Creative Commons Attribution (CC BY) license. The book as a whole is distributed by MDPI under the terms and conditions of the Creative Commons Attribution-NonCommercial-NoDerivs (CC BY-NC-ND) license.

Contents

About the Editor vii

Preface ix

José Ignacio Fernández-Vigo, Daniela Rego-Lorca, Francisco Javier Moreno-Morillo, Bárbara Burgos-Blasco, Alicia Valverde-Megías, Carmen Méndez-Hernández, et al.
Intervortex Venous Anastomosis in the Macula in Central Serous Chorioretinopathy Imaged by En Face Optical Coherence Tomography
Reprinted from: *J. Clin. Med.* **2023**, *12*, 2088, doi:10.3390/jcm12062088 1

José Ignacio Fernández-Vigo, Bárbara Burgos-Blasco, Lucía De-Pablo-Gómez-de-Liaño, Inés Sánchez-Guillén, Virginia Albitre-Barca, Susana Fernández-Aragón, et al.
Objective Classification of Glistening in Implanted Intraocular Lenses Using Optical Coherence Tomography: Proposal for a New Classification and Grading System
Reprinted from: *J. Clin. Med.* **2023**, *12*, 2351, doi:10.3390/jcm12062351 12

Bachar Kudsieh, José Ignacio Fernández-Vigo, Ignacio Flores-Moreno, Jorge Ruiz-Medrano, Maria Garcia-Zamora, Muhsen Samaan and Jose Maria Ruiz-Moreno
Update on the Utility of Optical Coherence Tomography in the Analysis of the Optic Nerve Head in Highly Myopic Eyes with and without Glaucoma
Reprinted from: *J. Clin. Med.* **2023**, *12*, 2592, doi:10.3390/jcm12072592 22

Juan Queiruga-Piñeiro, Alberto Barros, Javier Lozano-Sanroma, Andrés Fernández-Vega Cueto, Ignacio Rodríguez-Uña and Jesús Merayo-LLoves
Assessment by Optical Coherence Tomography of Short-Term Changes in IOP-Related Structures Caused by Wearing Scleral Lenses
Reprinted from: *J. Clin. Med.* **2023**, *12*, 4792, doi:10.3390/jcm12144792 38

Cecilia Czakó, Dóra Gerencsér, Kitti Kormányos, Klaudia Kéki-Kovács, Orsolya Németh, Gábor Tóth, et al.
Evaluation of Retinal Blood Flow in Patients with Monoclonal Gammopathy Using OCT Angiography
Reprinted from: *J. Clin. Med.* **2023**, *12*, 5227, doi:10.3390/jcm12165227 55

Carolina Arruabarrena, Antonio Rodríguez-Miguel, Fernando de Aragón-Gómez, Purificación Escámez, Ingrid Rosado and Miguel A. Teus
Normative Data for Macular Thickness and Volume for Optical Coherence Tomography in a Diabetic Population without Maculopathies
Reprinted from: *J. Clin. Med.* **2023**, *12*, 5232, doi:10.3390/jcm12165232 63

Gustavo Espinoza, Katheriene Iglesias, Juan C. Parra, Ignacio Rodriguez-Una, Sergio Serrano-Gomez, Angelica M. Prada and Virgilio Galvis
Agreement and Reproducibility of Anterior Chamber Angle Measurements between CASIA2 Built-In Software and Human Graders
Reprinted from: *J. Clin. Med.* **2023**, *12*, 6381, doi:10.3390/jcm12196381 78

Ana Palazon-Cabanes, Begoña Palazon-Cabanes, Jose Javier Garcia-Medina, Aurora Alvarez-Sarrion and Monica del-Rio-Vellosillo
Normative Database of the Superior–Inferior Thickness Asymmetry for All Inner and Outer Macular Layers of Adults for the Posterior Pole Algorithm of the Spectralis SD-OCT
Reprinted from: *J. Clin. Med.* **2023**, *12*, 7609, doi:10.3390/jcm12247609 89

Linbo Bian, Wenlong Li, Rui Qin, Zhengze Sun, Lu Zhao, Yifan Zhou, et al.
Ocular Biometry Features and Their Relationship with Anterior and Posterior Segment Lengths among a Myopia Population in Northern China
Reprinted from: *J. Clin. Med.* **2024**, *13*, 1001, doi:10.3390/jcm13041001 . . . . **99**

Aurora Alvarez-Sarrion, Jose Javier Garcia-Medina, Ana Palazon-Cabanes, Maria Dolores Pinazo-Duran and Monica Del-Rio-Vellosillo
Evaluation of the Diagnostic Capability of Spectralis SD-OCT 8 × 8 Posterior Pole Software with the Grid Tilted at 7 Degrees and Horizontalized in Glaucoma
Reprinted from: *J. Clin. Med.* **2024**, *13*, 1016, doi:10.3390/jcm13041016 . . . . **110**

Giuseppe Covello, Maria Novella Maglionico, Michele Figus, Chiara Busoni, Maria Sole Sartini, Marco Lupidi and Chiara Posarelli
Evaluation of Anatomical and Tomographic Biomarkers as Predictive Visual Acuity Factors in Eyes with Retinal Vein Occlusion Treated with Dexamethasone Implant
Reprinted from: *J. Clin. Med.* **2024**, *13*, 4533, doi:10.3390/jcm13154533 . . . . **124**

Luca Lucchino, Elvia Mastrogiuseppe, Francesca Giovannetti, Alice Bruscolini, Marco Marenco and Alessandro Lambiase
Anterior Segment Optical Coherence Tomography for the Tailored Treatment of Mooren's Ulcer: A Case Report
Reprinted from: *J. Clin. Med.* **2024**, *13*, 5384, doi:10.3390/jcm13185384 . . . . **135**

Tiffany Tse, Hoyoung Jung, Mohammad Shahidul Islam, Jun Song, Grace Soo, Khaldon Abbas, et al.
Single-Shot Ultra-Widefield Polarization-Diversity Optical Coherence Tomography for Assessing Retinal and Choroidal Pathologies
Reprinted from: *J. Clin. Med.* **2024**, *13*, 5415, doi:10.3390/jcm13185415 . . . . **143**

About the Editor

Jose Ignacio Fernandez-Vigo

Dr. Jose Ignacio Fernandez-Vigo is currently affiliated with the Retina Department at Hospital Clínico San Carlos, Madrid, and the Centro Internacional de Oftalmología Avanzada in Madrid. He is an accomplished Ophthalmologist, whose research mainly focuses on retinal diseases, and he is recognized for his expertise in optical coherence tomography (OCT) and ocular imaging. Dr. Fernandez-Vigo is also an Associate Professor of Medicine in the Department of Immunology, Ophthalmology, and ENT at the Complutense University of Madrid (UCM).

His scientific interests center on OCT, retinal diseases, vitreoretinal surgery, macular degeneration, retinal imaging and glaucoma. Among his numerous accolades, Dr. Fernandez-Vigo was awarded the prestigious Arruga Award in 2023 by the Spanish Society of Ophthalmology for being the best ophthalmologist in Spain under 40, recognizing his outstanding scientific trajectory. He has authored more than 150 indexed publications in PubMed and written 28 book chapters on ophthalmology.

His dedication to academia and research extends to mentoring, having directed five doctoral theses and supervised numerous graduate and master's theses. Dr. Fernandez-Vigo is also involved in clinical research, having participated in 35 clinical trials, and he is additionally a reviewer for 27 high-impact journals, acting as the Retina Section Editor for the Archives of the Spanish Society of Ophthalmology. Moreover, he is a member of several esteemed societies, serving as a board member for the Madrid division of the Spanish Society of Retina and Vitreous (SERV), and has been recognized with 37 awards from various ophthalmological societies and research institutes.

Preface

We are pleased to present this Special Issue reprint, "Clinical Utility of Optical Coherence Tomography in Ophthalmology", which brings together a collection of cutting-edge research articles and reviews pertaining to rapid advancements in optical coherence tomography (OCT) technology. OCT has transformed ophthalmology by improving our ability to visualize and assess both the posterior and anterior segments of the eye, leading to more accurate diagnoses and treatments across various subspecialties, including the retina, cornea, and glaucoma.

This reprint aims to highlight the latest innovations in OCT, such as intraoperative OCT, en face OCT, and wide-field OCT, and their clinical impact in enhancing surgical precision and postoperative care. The scope of this work is to provide vital insights into the ongoing evolution of this technology and its significant role in improving patient outcomes.

We hope this collection serves as a resource for clinicians, researchers, and healthcare professionals interested in the advancements of OCT and its application in ophthalmological practice. We are grateful to the authors who contributed their expertise to this Special Issue and to the peer reviewers whose insights helped improve the quality of the submissions. We would also like to extend our sincere thanks to the editorial team for their invaluable support throughout this process.

Jose Ignacio Fernandez-Vigo
Editor

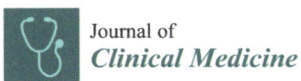

Article

Intervortex Venous Anastomosis in the Macula in Central Serous Chorioretinopathy Imaged by En Face Optical Coherence Tomography

José Ignacio Fernández-Vigo [1,2,*], Daniela Rego-Lorca [1], Francisco Javier Moreno-Morillo [1,3], Bárbara Burgos-Blasco [1], Alicia Valverde-Megías [1], Carmen Méndez-Hernández [1], Lorenzo López-Guajardo [1] and Juan Donate-López [1]

1. Ophthalmology Department, Hospital Clínico San Carlos, Institute of Health Research (IdISSC), 28040 Madrid, Spain
2. Centro Internacional de Oftalmología Avanzada, 28010 Madrid, Spain
3. Ophthalmology Department, Hospital Infanta Sofía, San Sebastián de los Reyes, 19171 Madrid, Spain
* Correspondence: jfvigo@hotmail.com; Tel.: +34-913303132

Abstract: Purpose: To assess the presence of macular intervortex venous anastomosis in central serous chorioretinopathy (CSCR) patients using en face optical coherence tomography (EF-OCT). Methods: A cross-sectional study where EF-OCT 6 × 6 and 12 × 12 mm macular scans of patients with unilateral chronic CSCR were evaluated for anastomosis between vortex vein systems in the central macula. The presence of prominent anastomoses was defined as a connection with a diameter ≥150 µm between the inferotemporal and superotemporal vortex vein systems which crossed the temporal raphe. Three groups were studied: CSCR eyes (with an active disease with the presence of neurosensorial detachment; n = 135), fellow unaffected eyes (n = 135), and healthy eyes as controls (n = 110). Asymmetries, abrupt termination, sausaging, bulbosities and corkscrew appearance were also assessed. Results: In 79.2% of the CSCR eyes there were prominent anastomoses in the central macula between the inferotemporal and superotemporal vortex vein systems, being more frequent than in fellow eyes and controls (51.8% and 58.2% respectively). The number of anastomotic connections was higher in the affected eye group (2.9 ± 1.8) than in the unaffected fellow eye group (2.1 ± 1.7) and the controls (1.5 ± 1.6) ($p < 0.001$). Asymmetry, abrupt terminations and the corkscrew appearance of the choroidal vessels were more frequent in the affected eyes, although no differences in sausaging or bulbosities were observed. Conclusions: Intervortex venous anastomoses in the macula were common in CSCR, being more frequently observed in affected eyes than in fellow unaffected eyes and healthy controls. This anatomical variation could have important implications concerning the pathogenesis and classification of the disease.

Keywords: central serous chorioretinopathy; choroidal vessels; en face optical coherence tomography; intervortex veins anastomosis; pachychoroid disease

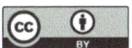

1. Introduction

Central serous chorioretinopathy (CSCR) is one of the main causes of visual function impairment in working age patients. It is characterized by the presence of subretinal fluid (SRF) and could be associated with serous retinal pigment epithelium (RPE) detachment in the macula and the posterior pole [1].

The exact cause of CSCR is not fully understood, but it is believed to be related to choroidal vessel dilation and hyperpermeability, hence CSCR is included among the newly described pachychoroid diseases [2–4]. In this group of conditions, the abnormally dilated choroidal vessels produce direct compression of the overlying choriocapillaris (CC) [5,6]. This compression can alter the normal barrier function of the complex between the CC–RPE, leading to the accumulation of fluid. Abnormalities in the flow patterns, such as impaired or irregular flow of the CC and choroid, have been observed in CSCR patients corresponding to indocyanine green angiography (ICGA) anomalies [7–13].

Recently developed, en face optical coherence tomography (EF-OCT) is a rapid and non-invasive high-resolution imaging technique that allows for the obtaining of coronal images of the retina and choroid (C-Scans). Dansingani et al., using this technology, described common morphological features in the choroidal vessels of eyes with pachychoroid spectrum-related disorders, including the presence of dilated vessels with a distinctive morphology [14]. In addition, different characteristics and the appearance of the choroidal vessels have been described to be associated with CSCR eyes, such as an asymmetry of the choroidal vessel [15], an abrupt termination [14], or the presence of sausaging and bulbosities [16].

Accumulating evidence suggests that the presence of pachychoroid is possibly caused by vortex vein congestion leading to a remodeling to create new choroidal drainages routes via intervortex venous anastomosis [11,17–19]. Spaide et al. reported that intervortex venous anastomoses are common in pachychoroid eyes, including those with CSCR [20]. However, to date, there are no studies evaluating the presence of macular choroidal anastomoses in a large population of CSCR patients by means of EF-OCT.

Hence, the objective of the present study is to assess the presence of intervortex venous anastomosis in the macula in CSCR patients by EF-OCT, as well as other characteristics of the choroidal vessels, comparing affected CSCR with the fellow unaffected eyes and with healthy controls.

2. Materials and Methods

A cross-sectional study including 135 patients with unilateral chronic CSCR recruited among those who were attended over the period from January 2020 to May 2022, in Hospital Clínico San Carlos, Madrid (Spain) was conducted.

To participate in the study, individuals had to meet all of the inclusion criteria and none of the exclusion criteria, and to provide written informed consent. The study was approved by the Center's Institutional Review Board, and the study protocol adhered to the tenets of the Declaration of Helsinki. The CSCR diagnosis was conducted in a multimodal imaging exploration based on the newly proposed criteria [1].

Both eyes of each patient were included for the assessment of the presence of macular anastomosis of the intervortex veins. Three groups were studied: CSCR eyes (n = 135), unaffected fellow eyes (n = 135), and eyes of healthy controls (n = 110).

Inclusion criteria for the chronic CSCR eyes was the persistence of SRF for ≥4 months and no previous treatments. For the unaffected fellow eyes, no SRF or retinal pigment epithelium detachment could be present, or previously detected, in order to be included.

Concerning the control group, the inclusion criteria were: age 18 years or older, healthy Caucasian subjects, a refractive error between +3.0 and −3.0 diopters, and an intraocular pressure (IOP) of less than 21 mmHg in both eyes.

Exclusion criteria for all eyes included were: any other ocular pathology, systemic pathology that typically affects the vessels such as diabetes, arterial hypertension or cardiac disorders, significant opacity of the lens or cornea that hinders obtaining good quality images, any previous ocular surgery or ocular treatment in the previous three months.

On the same day, recruited subjects underwent a medical history and a comprehensive ophthalmological examination, including OCTA imaging after pupil dilation. The examination included visual acuity (VA), refraction, slit-lamp biomicroscopy, and posterior segment ophthalmoscopy. The sex and age of each participant were recorded.

2.1. OCT and OCTA Examination

The device employed for the scans was a Plex Elite (Zeiss Meditec, Dublin, CA, USA) using the AngioPlex Elite 9000 algorithm (AngioPlex Elite 9000, Zeiss, Germany). This device is based on swept-source OCTA (SS-OCTA) technology and uses a central wavelength between 1060 nm and 1040 nm with scanning speed of 200,000 A-scans per second that offers a transverse resolution of 20 µm and an axial resolution of 6.3 µm.

The OCTA images were obtained by two experienced examiners (JIFV and DRL). Only images of good quality, as determined by a signal quality > 7/10, were included in the study, being analyzed after applying the device's software projections removal algorithm and checking for appropriate segmentation.

The 6 × 6 mm and 12 × 12 mm scans centered on the macula were performed, and the SS-OCTA device was used to obtain the EF-OCT images (Figure 1). The small scan was used to measure the anastomosis with higher precision. For analysis, the image that corresponded to the choroid segmentation and was focused on the pachyvessels mainly in Haller's layer was selected. The automatic segmentation of the software by default, selecting the legacy mode, produced a slab 100 µm beneath the RPE and a thickness slab of 100 µm. This was used as a reference. However, due to the individual variability of the choroidal thickness and Haller's layer position in each subject, segmentation was individualized.

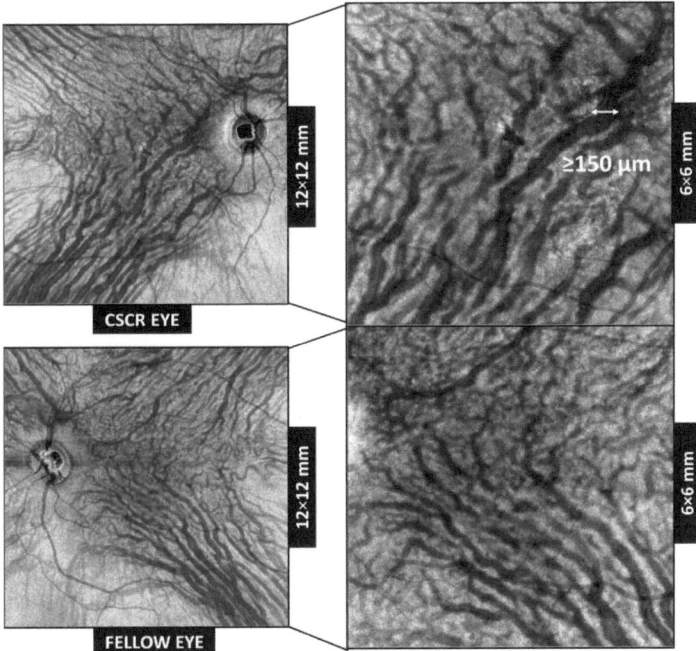

Figure 1. En face optical coherence tomography of the macular region used to analyze the presence of intervortex veins anastomosis in a cube scan of 6 × 6 mm and 12 × 12 mm in central serous chorioretinopathy (CSCR) eyes (upper row) and fellow unaffected eyes (bottom row).

The main variable was the presence of prominent anastomoses in the central macula, which was defined as a connection between the supero-temporal and infero-temporal vortex vein systems, with a diameter ≥150 µm, which crosses the temporal raphe (Figures 1 and 2). As previously defined by Spaide et al., anastomoses was considered to be present if there were two or more anastomotic vessels connecting the adjacent quadrants of vortex veins [20].

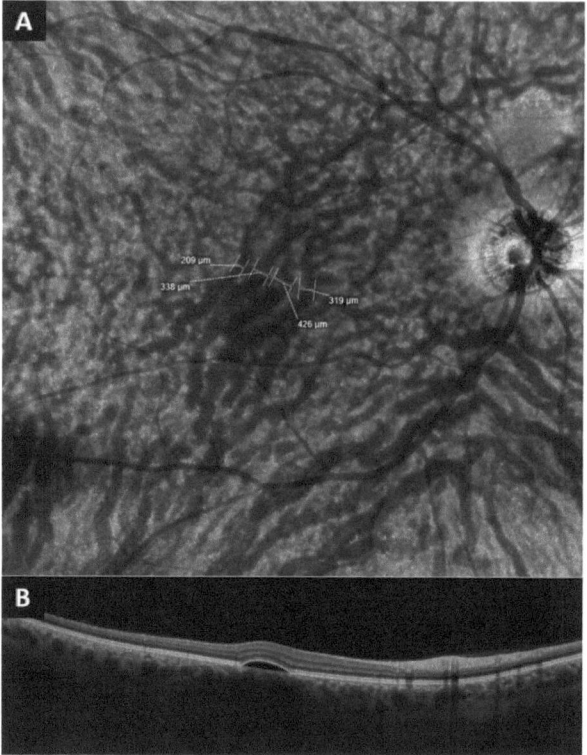

Figure 2. (**A**) En face optical coherence tomography of the macular region showing large anastomoses in a patient affected by central serous chorioretinopathy (CSCR). (**B**) B-scan showing the pachyvessels on the choroid in the central area.

In addition, the presence of asymmetries in the running pattern of the choroidal vessels relative to a horizontal line across the fovea was assessed. An asymmetry was defined as a predominance in the number or caliber of the supero-temporal or infero-temporal choroidal vessels that cross more than 1000 µm the medial raphe of the macula [15]. The presence of abrupt terminations in the pachyvessels on the EF-OCT images was also assessed (Figure 3) [14].

Lastly, the presence of sausaging, defined by Spaide as three or more contiguous fusiform dilations that vary by at least 50% from the narrowest to largest diameters, and bulbosities, defined as a focal 2× dilation of a blood vessel as compared with the diameter of the surrounding host vessel, were registered [16]. The presence of vessels twisted into a spiral shape, known as corkscrew vessels, was also noted (Figure 3) [21].

EF-OCT images were reviewed in a masked fashion by two independent and experienced readers (LLG and DRL), and the agreement between them was analyzed in the first 77 consecutive CSCR and control eyes. Two more readers were advised in case of disagreement (JIFV and FJMM).

2.2. Statistical Analysis

The software package SPSS® (Statistical Package for Social Sciences, v25.0; SPSS Inc., Chicago, IL, USA) was used to perform all statistical tests. Quantitative parameters were provided as the mean and standard deviation. Qualitative values were expressed as their frequency distributions. To assess the inter-rater reliability, the kappa statistic was calculated. Analysis of variance (ANOVA) was applied among the three groups to determine if there were differences. Furthermore, differences between groups were assessed by *t*-test for independent samples and a chi-square test for qualitative variables for paired comparison. The significance level was set at $p < 0.05$.

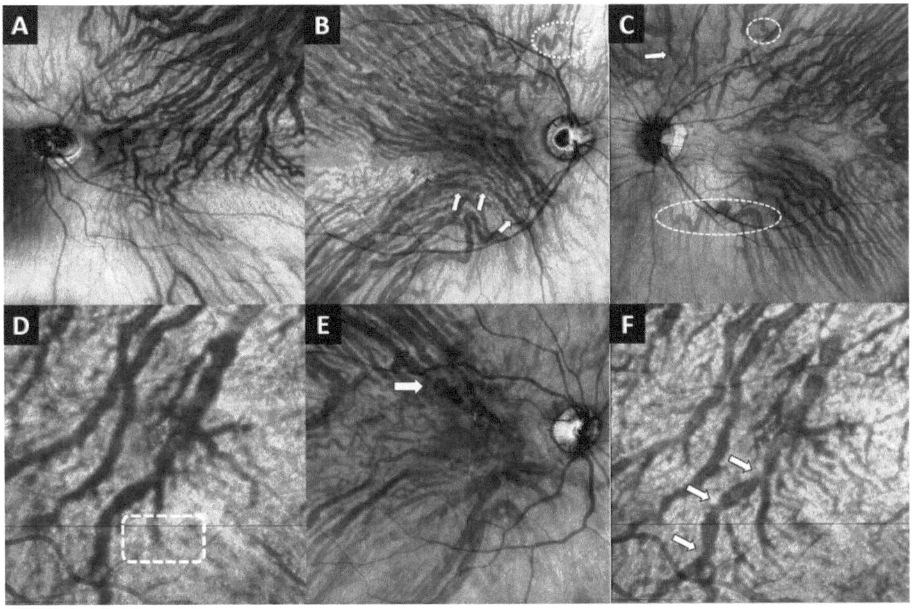

Figure 3. Examples of en face optical coherence tomography images of the choroidal vessel characteristics assessed. (**A**) Asymmetry with predominance of the superotemporal vessels. (**B**) Sausaging of the choroidal vessels (arrow) and corkscrew vessel (dotted circle). (**C**) Corkscrew vessels (dotted circles) and bulbosity (arrow). (**D**) Abrupt termination of a choroidal vessel. (**E**) Bulbosity of a choroidal vessel (arrow). (**F**) Sausaging of a choroidal vessel (arrows).

3. Results

The mean age of CSCR patients was 51 ± 10.7 years with 72.2% males, with the mean age of controls being 49.5 ± 14.2 years with 69.5% males ($p \geq 0.315$).

Among the 135 eyes with unilateral chronic CSCR (with persistent SRF), 79.2% (107 eyes) showed prominent anastomoses in the central macula between the inferotemporal and supero-temporal vortex vein systems, being more frequent than in the unaffected fellow eyes, in which 51.8% of these patients had anastomoses (defined as two or more) ($p < 0.001$). However, no differences were observed between the eyes of CSCR patients and the control group (58.2%; $p = 0.068$) (Table 1).

Regarding the number of macular anastomoses, anastomotic connections were more common in the affected CSCR group (2.9 ± 1.8) than in the unaffected fellow eye group (2.1 ± 1.7; $p < 0.001$) and in controls (1.5 ± 1.6 respectively; $p < 0.001$) (Table 1, Figure 4).

Good inter-rater agreement to determine the presence and number of the macular anastomoses was observed, with a kappa index ≥ 0.84 for CSCR and control eyes (Table 2).

An asymmetry in the distribution of the choroidal vessels was more frequent in 17% of the CSCR eyes than in the unaffected fellow eyes (8.9%) and controls (1.8%) ($p < 0.001$), observing a similar predominance between the supero-temporal and infero-temporal vessels in 11 and 12 CSCR eyes, respectively (Table 3, Figure 3).

Table 1. Results of the presence and number of choroidal anastomosis assessed by En Face optical coherence tomography in the three groups studied.

Group	% Patients with Anastomosis	N° Macular Anastomosis
1. Chronic unilateral CSCR (persistent SRF) (N = 135)	79.2% (107/135)	2.9 ± 1.8 (0 to 8)
2. Fellow unaffected eye (N = 135)	51.8% (70/135)	2.1 ± 1.7 (0 to 8)
3. Controls (N = 110 eyes, 57 patients)	58.2% (64/110)	1.5 ± 1.6 (0 to 6)
p-value ANOVA	<0.01 *	<0.01 *
p-value (paired comparison)	1 vs. 2: <0.01 *	1 vs. 2: <0.01 *
	1 vs. 3: <0.01 *	1 vs. 3: <0.01 *
	2 vs. 3: 0.068	2 vs. 3: <0.01 *

*: statistically significant.

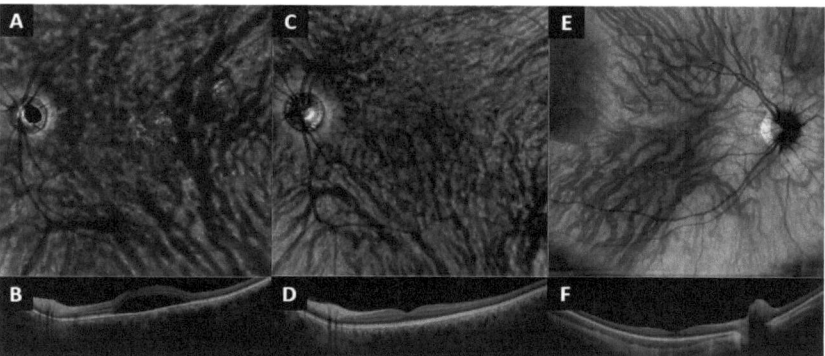

Figure 4. En face optical coherence tomography and the corresponding B scan of the macular region to analyze the presence of intervortex venous anastomosis. (**A**,**B**): example of an eye affected by central serous chorioretinopathy (CSCR). (**C**,**D**): Fellow unaffected CSCR eye. (**E**,**F**): example of a healthy control.

Table 2. Results of the kappa value for the inter-rater macular anastomoses assessment.

Parameter	Group Studied (n = 77 Eyes)	Kappa Value
Qualitative assessment: presence or absence of anastomoses	CSCR eyes	0.847
	Control eyes	0.860
Quantitative assessment: number of anastomoses	CSCR eyes	0.922
	Control eyes	0.848

An abrupt termination of the pachyvessels on the EF-OCT images was observed in 7.4% of the CSCR eyes, being more frequent than in the unaffected fellow eyes (2.9%) and in healthy subjects (1%) ($p < 0.001$), while observing no differences between fellow eyes and controls ($p = 0.864$) (Figure 3).

Table 3. Summary of the main characteristics of the choroidal vessels assessed by En Face optical coherence tomography.

Group	Asymmetries (%)	Abrupt Choroidal Vessels (%)	Sausaging (%)	BULBOSITIES (%)	Corkscrew Vessels (%)
1. Chronic unilateral CSCR (persistent SRF) (N = 135)	17% (23/135) 11 superior and 12 inferior predominance	7.4% (10/135)	23.7% (32/135)	22.9% (31/135)	15.5% (21/135)
2. Fellow unaffected eye (N = 135)	8.9% (12/135) 9 superior and 3 inferior predominance	2.9% (4/135)	7.4% (10/135)	14.8% (20/135)	6.6% (9/135)
3. Controls (N = 110 eyes, 57 patients)	1.8% (2/110) 1 superior and 1 inferior predominance	1% (1/110)	8.1% (9/110)	7.3% (8/110)	4.5% (5/110)
p-value ANOVA	<0.001 *	0.028	0.073	0.105	0.03
p-value (paired comparison)	1 vs 2: <0.001 *	1 vs 2: <0.001 *	1 vs 2: 0.206	1 vs 2: 0.195	1 vs 2: 0.015 *
	1 vs 3: <0.001 *	1 vs 3: <0.001 *	1 vs 3: 0.311	1 vs 3: 0.129	1 vs 3: 0.293
	2 vs 3: <0.001 *	2 vs 3: 0.864	2 vs 3: 0.434	2 vs 3: 0.591	2 vs 3: 0.547

*: statistically significant.

Sausaging and bulbosities were present in 23.7% and 22.9% of the CSCR eyes, 7.4% and 14.8% of the unaffected fellow eyes, and 8.1% and 7.3% of the controls, observing no differences among groups ($p \geq 0.129$). However, corkscrew choroidal vessels were more frequent in CSCR eyes than in the other groups ($p \leq 0.033$) (Figure 3).

4. Discussion

New hypotheses on the physiopathology of the choroidal changes in CSCR patients have been described in recent years, these being the presence of pachyvessels and macular choroidal anastomoses that are remarkably characteristic. In a recent study, Spaide et al. found good agreement between the pachyvessels on B-scan and EF-OCT images, and affirmed that the large anastomosis observed crossing the horizontal raphe in the macula in their study might have been considered as pachyvessels in previous reports [20].

In the present study, intervortex venous anastomosis in the macular area were common in CSCR patients using EF-OCT. This anatomical variation was more frequently observed in the affected eyes of CSCR patients than in the fellow unaffected eyes and healthy controls. Dansingani et al., using EF-OCT, stated that there were pachyvessels traversing the focus of disease in eyes with what they termed pachychoroid spectrum disorders [14]. Nonetheless, they did not specifically mention if this was in the macula or across a watershed zone, and they did not mention anastomoses.

Our findings are also in line with those reported by Spaide et al., who reviewed the ICGA images of 24 eyes with CSCR and found that macular anastomotic connections were more common in these patients compared to healthy controls ($p < 0.001$). The authors also described that, while patients with CSCR showed prominent anastomotic connections primarily centered in the macular region, patients with peripapillary pachychoroid syndrome presented them along the peripapillary region [20]. Interestingly, Ramtohul et al. have observed that the identification of pachyvessels crossing the choroidal watershed zones showed an excellent correlation between en face ultra-widefield (UWF) and OCT UWF ICGA images, showing distinctive features of choroidal venous insufficiency or choroidal congestion with both techniques [22].

Spaide et al. proposed that these anastomoses should be considered as present if there were two or more vessels connecting adjacent quadrants of vortex veins [20]. Our results support this consideration, as 45.4% of healthy controls showed one anastomotic vessel in one of their eyes, or in other words, 28.2% of healthy eyes have at least one anastomosis. Shiihara et al. used EF-OCT images, as in the present study, to quantitatively assess the diameter and running pattern of choroidal vessels in 41 eyes with CSCR, 41 fellow eyes, and 41 healthy controls [15]. In agreement with our results, Shiihara et al. observed the presence of pachyvessels in 31.7% of the normal eyes, as compared to 82.9% in CSCR eyes.

Regarding the definition criteria of anastomoses and pachyvessels, Spaide et al. proposed that these connecting vessels had to have a diameter equal to or greater than that of the retinal arcade vein at the border of the optic disc, which has been described to be around 120 µm [20]. Shiihara et al., determined a cut-off mean vessel diameter value between CSCR and normal eyes of 153 µm, having a sensitivity and specificity of 82.9% and 68.3%, respectively. In fact, they observed that eyes with CSCR had larger dilated choroidal vessels as compared with both the fellow eyes of CSCR patients and with healthy controls, the mean vessel diameter being 185 ± 39 µm in CSCR eyes, 171 ± 38 µm in fellow eyes, and 144 ± 20 µm in controls, with significant differences among groups ($p \leq 0.042$). For this reason, we only considered those anastomotic vessels with a diameter greater than 150 µm.

On the other hand, Spaide et al. proposed that there may be a subpopulation of patients with pachychoroid-related abnormalities that do not have venous intervortex anastomoses [20]. The results in the present study are in accordance with this idea, because a fifth of the chronic CSCR patients (20.8%) did not have any macular choroidal anastomosis.

Furthermore, asymmetries in choroidal anastomoses were evaluated. The presence of asymmetrical vessels running in Haller's layer was more frequently detected in CSCR eyes and fellow eyes than in controls (17% versus 8.9% versus 1.8%), observing no predominance of the supero-temporal or infero-temporal vessels in CSCR eyes. In Shiihara et al.'s study, which had a highly refined automatic method, the symmetry index was 59.4 ± 5.8% in controls, 55.3 ± 7.2% in fellow eyes, and 53.7 ± 6.0% in CSCR eyes. No differences between the CSCR eyes and its fellow eye were noted ($p = 0.568$), although it was significantly smaller in the CSCR and fellow eyes compared to normal eyes (≤ 0.007). The authors suggested that the existence of a watershed zone in the subfoveal region in CSCR and its fellow eye is less likely than in normal eyes. Differences between Shiihara et al.'s study and the present one includes a smaller number of CSCR patients (41 vs. 135), and all included subjects were Japanese, which is in contrast with ours, in which all subjects were Caucasian. Furthermore, they used a 7 × 7 mm exploration field instead of a 12 × 12 mm one, and the scanning speed was 100,000, while it was 200,000 scans/sec in the present one. Recently, Terao et al. described, using also en face OCT, that the asymmetric dilated vortex vein is a common finding in patients with CSC, being associated with certain biometric factors such as short axial length [23].

Abrupted terminations were also investigated, as Dansingani et al. stated that unlike physiologic vessels, pachyvessels do not narrow at their distal extent, but appear to terminate abruptly [14]. We observed that abrupted termination of the pachyvessels on the EF-OCT images was more frequently observed in the CSCR eyes (7.4%), than in the unaffected fellow eyes (2.9%) and in healthy subjects 1%. On the contrary, Spaide et al. did not observe an abrupt termination of any large vein in any eye using ICGA (20). In our study, when we analyzed the scan cube of the choroidal vessels with an abrupt termination and followed its direction and course, we could observe that these vessels at some point changed to a vertical trajectory. We hypothesize that this could be the actual reason for the apparent abrupt termination, this probably being an artefact, since any vessel in the body becomes thinner at its terminal end unless there is an obstruction.

Recently, variations in the venous caliber, such as sausaging and bulbosities, have been described in eyes with CSCR using widefield ICGA, and could be associated with pathophysiologic alterations related to increased pressure within and remodeling of the larger choroidal veins [16]. In a study including 73 eyes of 41 patients, the sausaging of vessels was seen in three quadrants per eye, the use of corticosteroids being the only significant risk factor. They also described a total of 39 bulbosities in 26 eyes (35.6%), preferentially involving intervortex venous anastomoses. In the present study, sausaging and bulbosities were frequent in CSCR eyes (23.7 and 22.9%), but this vessel appearance was also observed in the fellow and control eyes, with no differences between groups ($p \geq 0.129$), but with a greater tendency to the existence of the latter in CSC eyes than in fellow eyes and controls. However, one explanation for the lower number of bulbosities in our study could be the limited macular area scanned in contrast with the evaluation of the four quadrants by ICGA done by Spaide et al. Moreover, it should be highlighted that the presence of corkscrew vessels was significantly higher in CSCR eyes than in fellow eyes and controls, this possibly being related to an impaired or altered vascular flow, which subsequently resulted in the appearance of this abnormality.

This is the first study to employ EF-OCT in a large population of CSCR patients to study choroidal macular anastomoses, as well as other choroidal vessel characteristics such as asymmetries, abrupt terminations, vascular caliber variations like sausaging and bulbosities, or a corkscrew appearance. These findings could have important implications in the understanding of pachychoroid disease. Nevertheless, future studies are warranted to analyze whether changes in these anastomotic vessels occur over time, trying to detect thickening and evolution along with the chronicity of the disease, and to evaluate if these anastomoses are formed in the conversion from acute to chronic forms or are already present and to what degree. In this regard, Shiihara et al. have described that it was difficult to determine whether the choroidal vessels were enlarged or congenitally large in CSCR eyes. Hosoda et al. have previously described that genetic factors, specifically CFH and VIPR2 genes, could be associated with the larger vessel choroidal diameter Haller's layer since birth and after the presence of CSCR [24]. Matsumoto et al. performed a very interesting study creating a monkey model of vortex vein congestion by ligating two vortex veins, and they could observe pachychoroid-related findings, indicating that vortex vein congestion is involved in the pathogenesis of the pachychoroid. Nevertheless, the authors noted that the remodeling of the choroidal drainage route via intervortex venous anastomosis appeared to compensate for the vortex vein congestion created in this model [25]. In the future, it would also be interesting to observe if the cut-off value of 153 μm proposed by Shiihara et al. can predict the likelihood of developing CSC. Finally, as Spaide et al. posited, the detection of anastomosis may offer a method to classify subtypes of pachyvessels and their associated diseases [20].

The present study has several limitations. First, the initial approach to these images is a manual quantification of the number of anastomoses or the presence of vessel abnormalities. However, good inter-rater agreement was observed (kappa index ≥ 0.84). In addition, it is sometimes difficult to achieve a correct segmentation of Haller's layer and that the segmentation often needs to be manually adjusted. Therefore, algorithms to perform an automated segmentation of en face scans such as the one described by Shiihara et al. are needed to assess the large choroidal vessels [26]. However, algorithms should be improved to reliably analyze the high variability appearance of pathological choroids, as well as to analyze and quantify new features, including variations in the venous caliber, such as sausaging and bulbosities, or the presence of corkscrew vessels [16]. In addition, it should be noted that the entire vortex vein drainage area as well as the number or asymmetries in the latter were not assessed in the present study due to the limited scan size of the OCT device. Lastly, ICGA images of sausaging and bulbosities were not available for all the patients to compare the findings between this technique and en face OCT.

5. Conclusions

Choroidal anastomoses between the vortex veins in the macular area were common in CSCR. This anatomical variation was observed more frequently in the affected eyes of patients with CSCR than in the unaffected fellow eyes and in healthy controls. This finding could have important implications regarding the etiopathogenesis and classification or severity of the disease, and could even lead to new therapeutic proposals to reduce choroidal stasis.

Author Contributions: Concept and study design, J.I.F.-V.; study supervision, D.R.-L., F.J.M.-M., L.L.-G., J.D.-L.; data collection, J.I.F-V, D.R.-L., F.J.M.-M., B.B.-B., A.V.-M. and C.M.-H.; data interpretation, analysis and statistics, J.I.F.-V., D.R.-L., F.J.M.-M.; original draft preparation, J.I.F.-V.; reviewing and editing, J.I.F.-V., D.R.-L., F.J.M.-M., B.B.-B., A.V.-M., C.M.-H., L.L.-G. and J.D.-L. All authors have read and agreed to the published version of the manuscript.

Funding: This research received no external funding.

Institutional Review Board Statement: This observational study was approved by the Ethics Committee of San Carlos Clinical Hospital and conducted in accordance with the Declaration of Helsinki.

Informed Consent Statement: Informed consent to use the participants' medical information was obtained from all subjects involved in the study.

Data Availability Statement: Data used to support the findings presented in this study are available on request from the corresponding author.

Conflicts of Interest: The authors declare that they have no conflict of interest.

References

1. Chhablani, J.; Cohen, F.B.; Aymard, P.; Beydoun, T.; Bousquet, E.; Daruich-Matet, A.; Matet, A.; Zhao, M.; Cheung, C.M.G.; Freund, K.B.; et al. Multimodal Imaging-Based Central Serous Chorioretinopathy Classification. *Ophthalmol. Retin.* **2020**, *4*, 1043–1046. [CrossRef] [PubMed]
2. Kaye, R.; Chandra, S.; Sheth, J.; Boon, C.J.F.; Sivaprasad, S.; Lotery, A. Central serous chorioretinopathy: An update on risk factors, pathophysiology and imaging modalities. *Prog. Retin. Eye Res.* **2020**, *79*, 100865. [CrossRef] [PubMed]
3. Spaide, R.F.; Rochepeau, C.; Kodjikian, L.; Garcia, M.A.; Coulon, C.; Burillon, C.; Denis, P.; Delaunay, B.; Mathis, T.; Matet, A.; et al. Choriocapillaris Flow Features Follow a Power Law Distribution: Implications for Characterization and Mechanisms of Disease Progression. *Graefe's Arch. Clin. Exp. Ophthalmol.* **2019**, *257*, 905–912. [CrossRef]
4. Daruich, A.; Matet, A.; Dirani, A.; Bousquet, E.; Zhao, M.; Farman, N.; Jaisser, F.; Behar-Cohen, F. Central serous chorioretinopathy: Recent findings and new physiopathology hypothesis. *Prog. Retin. Eye Res.* **2015**, *48*, 82–118. [CrossRef]
5. Cheung, C.M.G.; Lee, W.K.; Koizumi, H.; Dansingani, K.; Lai, T.Y.Y.; Freund, K.B. Pachychoroid disease. *Eye* **2019**, *33*, 14–33. [CrossRef] [PubMed]
6. Ho, M.; Ho, M.; Lai, F.H.P.; Ng, D.S.C.; Iu, L.P.L.; Iu, L.P.L.; Chen, L.J.; Chen, L.J.; Mak, A.C.Y.; Mak, A.C.Y.; et al. Analysis of choriocapillaris perfusion and choroidal layer changes in patients with chronic central serous chorioretinopathy randomised to micropulse laser or photodynamic therapy. *Br. J. Ophthalmol.* **2020**, *33*, 14–33. [CrossRef]
7. Teussink, M.M.; Breukink, M.B.; Van Grinsven, M.J.J.P.; Hoyng, C.B.; Jeroen Klevering, B.; Boon, C.J.F.; De Jong, E.K.; Theelen, T. Oct angiography compared to fluorescein and indocyanine green angiography in chronic central serous chorioretinopathy. *Investig. Ophthalmol. Vis. Sci.* **2015**, *56*, 5229–5237. [CrossRef]
8. Iacono, P.; Tedeschi, M.; Boccassini, B.; Chiaravalloti, A.; Varano, M.; Parravano, M. Chronic Central Serous Chorioretinopathy: Early and Late Morphological and Functional Changes After Verteporfin Photodynamic Therapy. *Retina* **2019**, *39*, 980–987. [CrossRef] [PubMed]
9. Xu, Y.; Su, Y.; Li, L.; Qi, H.; Zheng, H.; Chen, C. Effect of photodynamic therapy on optical coherence tomography angiography in eyes with chronic central serous chorioretinopathy. *Ophthalmologica* **2017**, *237*, 167–172. [CrossRef]
10. Matet, A.; Daruich, A.; Hardy, S.; Behar-Cohen, F. Patterns of Choriocapillaris Flow Signal Voids in Central Serous Chorioretinopathy. *Retina* **2019**, *39*, 2178–2188. [CrossRef]
11. Spaide, R.F.; Gemmy Cheung, C.M.; Matsumoto, H.; Kishi, S.; Boon, C.J.F.; van Dijk, E.H.C.; Mauget-Faÿsse, M.; Behar-Cohen, F.; Hartnett, M.E.; Sivaprasad, S.; et al. Venous overload choroidopathy: A hypothetical framework for central serous chorioretinopathy and allied disorders. *Prog. Retin. Eye Res.* **2022**, *86*, 100973. [CrossRef] [PubMed]
12. Battista, M.; Borrelli, E.; Parravano, M.; Gelormini, F.; Tedeschi, M.; De Geronimo, D.; Sacconi, R.; Querques, L.; Bandello, F.; Querques, G. OCTA characterisation of microvascular retinal alterations in patients with central serous chorioretinopathy. *Br. J. Ophthalmol.* **2020**, *104*, 1453–1457. [CrossRef] [PubMed]
13. Rochepeau, C.; Kodjikian, L.; Garcia, M.A.; Coulon, C.; Burillon, C.; Denis, P.; Delaunay, B.; Mathis, T. Optical Coherence Tomography Angiography Quantitative Assessment of Choriocapillaris Blood Flow in Central Serous Chorioretinopathy. *Am. J. Ophthalmol.* **2018**, *194*, 26–34. [CrossRef]
14. Dansingani, K.K.; Balaratnasingam, C.; Naysan, J.; Freund, K.B. En Face Imaging of Pachychoroid Spectrum Disorders with Swept-Source Optical Coherence Tomography. *Retina* **2016**, *36*, 499–516. [CrossRef]

15. Shiihara, H.; Sonoda, S.; Terasaki, H.; Kakiuchi, N.; Yamashita, T.; Uchino, E.; Murao, F.; Sano, H.; Mitamura, Y.; Sakamoto, T. Quantitative analyses of diameter and running pattern of choroidal vessels in central serous chorioretinopathy by en face images. *Sci. Rep.* **2020**, *10*, 9591. [CrossRef]
16. Spaide, R.F.; Ngo, W.K.; Barbazetto, I.; Sorenson, J.A. Sausaging and Bulbosities of the Choroidal Veins in Central Serous Chorioretinopathy. *Retina* **2022**, *42*, 1638–1644. [CrossRef] [PubMed]
17. Kishi, S.; Matsumoto, H. A new insight into pachychoroid diseases: Remodeling of choroidal vasculature. *Graefe's Arch. Clin. Exp. Ophthalmol. = Albr. von Graefes Arch. fur Klin. und Exp. Ophthalmol.* **2022**, *42*, 3405–3417. [CrossRef]
18. Matsumoto, H.; Hoshino, J.; Mukai, R.; Nakamura, K.; Kikuchi, Y.; Kishi, S.; Akiyama, H. Vortex Vein Anastomosis at the Watershed in Pachychoroid Spectrum Diseases. *Ophthalmol. Retin.* **2020**, *4*, 938–945. [CrossRef] [PubMed]
19. Matsumoto, H.; Hoshino, J.; Mukai, R.; Nakamura, K.; Kishi, S.; Akiyama, H. Pulsation of anastomotic vortex veins in pachychoroid spectrum diseases. *Sci. Rep.* **2021**, *11*, 14942. [CrossRef]
20. Spaide, R.F.; Ledesma-Gil, G.; Gemmy Cheung, C.M. Intervortex Venous Anastomosis in Pachychoroid-Related Disorders. *Retina Publish Ah.* **2020**, *11*, 14942. [CrossRef]
21. Moreno-Morillo, F.J.; Fernández-Vigo, J.I.; Burgos-Blasco, B.; Llorente-La Orden, C.; Vidal-Villegas, B.; Santos-Bueso, E. Optical coherence tomography angiography of choroidal nodules in neurofibromatosis type-1: A case series. *Eur. J. Ophthalmol.* **2022**, *32*, NP91–NP94. [CrossRef] [PubMed]
22. Ramtohul, P.; Cabral, D.; Oh, D.; Galhoz, D.; Freund, K.B. En face Ultrawidefield OCT of the Vortex Vein System in Central Serous Chorioretinopathy. *Ophthalmol. Retin.* **2022**. [CrossRef]
23. Terao, N.; Imanaga, N.; Wakugawa, S.; Sawaguchi, S.; Tamashiro, T.; Yamauchi, Y.; Koizumi, H. Short Axial Length Is Related to Asymmetric Vortex Veins in Central Serous Chorioretinopathy. *Ophthalmol. Sci.* **2021**, *1*, 100071. [CrossRef] [PubMed]
24. Hosoda, Y.; Yoshikawa, M.; Miyake, M.; Tabara, Y.; Ahn, J.; Woo, S.J.; Honda, S.; Sakurada, Y.; Shiragami, C.; Nakanishi, H.; et al. CFH and VIPR2 as susceptibility loci in choroidal thickness and pachychoroid disease central serous chorioretinopathy. *Proc. Natl. Acad. Sci. USA* **2018**, *115*, 6261–6266. [CrossRef] [PubMed]
25. Matsumoto, H.; Mukai, R.; Saito, K.; Hoshino, J.; Kishi, S.; Akiyama, H. Vortex vein congestion in the monkey eye: A possible animal model of pachychoroid. *PLoS ONE* **2022**, *17*, e0274137. [CrossRef]
26. Shiihara, H.; Sonoda, S.; Terasaki, H.; Kakiuchi, N.; Shinohara, Y.; Tomita, M.; Sakamoto, T. Automated segmentation of en face choroidal images obtained by optical coherent tomography by machine learning. *Jpn. J. Ophthalmol.* **2018**, *62*, 643–651. [CrossRef]

Disclaimer/Publisher's Note: The statements, opinions and data contained in all publications are solely those of the individual author(s) and contributor(s) and not of MDPI and/or the editor(s). MDPI and/or the editor(s) disclaim responsibility for any injury to people or property resulting from any ideas, methods, instructions or products referred to in the content.

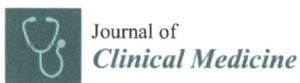 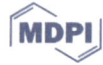

Article

Objective Classification of Glistening in Implanted Intraocular Lenses Using Optical Coherence Tomography: Proposal for a New Classification and Grading System

José Ignacio Fernández-Vigo [1,2,*], Bárbara Burgos-Blasco [2], Lucía De-Pablo-Gómez-de-Liaño [1,3], Inés Sánchez-Guillén [4,5], Virginia Albitre-Barca [1], Susana Fernández-Aragón [1], José Ángel Fernández-Vigo [1,5,6] and Ana Macarro-Merino [1,5]

1. Centro Internacional de Oftalmología Avanzada, 28010 Madrid, Spain
2. Department of Ophthalmology, Hospital Clínico San Carlos, Instituto de Investigación Sanitaria (IdISSC), 28040 Madrid, Spain
3. Department of Ophthalmology, Hospital Universitario 12 de Octubre, 28041 Madrid, Spain
4. Department of Ophthalmology, Hospital Perpetuo Socorro, 06010 Badajoz, Spain
5. Centro Internacional de Oftalmología Avanzada, 06011 Badajoz, Spain
6. Department of Ophthalmology, Universidad de Extremadura, 06006 Badajoz, Spain
* Correspondence: jfvigo@hotmail.com; Tel.: +34-917020826

Abstract: Purpose: To propose a classification of the glistening in intraocular lenses (IOL) using swept-source optical coherence tomography (SS-OCT) by means of a simple, objective and reproducible method that allows the quantification of the presence and severity of glistening. Methods: A cross-sectional study on a sample of 150 eyes of 150 patients who underwent cataract surgery in at least 600 days before the exam and attended a routine examination. Each subject was examined by SS-OCT after pupil dilation, identifying the presence of glistening or hyperreflective foci (HRF) in the central area of the IOL. The degree of glistening was classified into four categories: 0: ≤ 5 HRF; 1: 6 to 15 HRF; 2: 16 to 30 HRF; and 3: >30 HRF. The intra and interobserver reproducibility (intraclass correlation coefficient, ICC) in the quantification and classification of the glistening were calculated. The correlation between the horizontal and vertical scan of the IOL was also assessed. Results: Glistening was present in the IOL in 42.7% of the patients. The mean number of HRF or glistening microvacuoles was 10.4 ± 26.2 (range 0 to 239). In total, 63.3% of the IOLs had a grade 0, 20% grade a 1, 6.7% grade a 2 and 10% a grade 3. The intraobserver and interobserver reproducibility were very high, both for the absolute quantification of the glistening (ICC ≥ 0.994) and for the severity scale (ICC ≥ 0.967). There was an excellent correlation in the quantification of the IOL glistening between the horizontal and vertical scans (R ≥ 0.834; $p < 0.001$). Conclusions: The use of SS-OCT makes it possible to identify, quantify and classify IOL glistening in a simple, objective and reproducible way. This technique could provide relevant information for the study of the glistening on IOLs.

Keywords: glistening; intraocular lens; opacification; optical coherence tomography

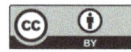

1. Introduction

Cataract surgery with an intraocular lens (IOL) implant is one of the most frequent surgeries performed worldwide [1]. There are two major complications specifically related to IOL. The first is serious but infrequent and consists in the opacification of the IOL, while the second, which is the glistening of the lens, is more frequent but generally described as less important [2–5].

Intraocular lens glistening is the presence of small (1 to 20 µm), shiny, white or yellow spots, which are fluid-filled microvacuoles (MVs), within the IOL after its implantation [2,6]. In the proposed mechanism in its formation, the IOL polymer absorbs water, which forms

MV with the IOL material. The difference in the refractive index between the water and the IOL polymer results in their characteristic appearance on the slit-lamp exam [7]. According to various authors, IOL glistening is influenced by the manufacturing process, the packaging system, the changes in temperature, the equilibrium water content, the IOL model, the IOL power, the breakdown of the blood–retina or blood–water barrier and the postoperative inflammation, especially in combined surgeries [3,6,8,9]. This glistening, or hydration-related phenomenon, has been observed in a variety of materials, including silicone, hydrogel and poly methyl methacrylate (PMMA) IOLs, but it is particularly common in hydrophobic acrylic IOLs [1,6,10,11].

The symptoms of glistening may include a decrease in vision, halos or glare, or a decrease in contrast sensitivity, although most studies cite no apparent effect of IOL glistening on visual acuity [2,6,12]. For these reasons, along with others, IOL explant has rarely been reported in the literature on IOL glistening [13]. However, the full impact of IOL glistening on postoperative visual function and its changes in the long term after surgery remain to be fully elucidated.

The first observations of this phenomenon of glistening formation on IOL materials were performed in vitro and in clinical practice after slit-lamp examinations [7,14–18]. However, the latter presents two main difficulties: it is a time-consuming technique and great photographic skill is required by an expert examiner to obtain valuable images of the glistening. Furthermore, this process usually requires the post-processing of the images. For these reasons, most authors detect IOL glistening using a slit-lamp examination and quantify them subjectively, based on a rating scale. Currently, one of the most popular glistening-classification systems is the Miyata scale, which is used to classify glistening in IOL, ranging from grade 0 (no glistening) to grade 3 (severe glistening) [19]. The lack of an objective, examiner-independent and reproducible method for in vivo glistening evaluation is a common problem [8].

Recently, different authors proposed the use of Scheimpflug-camera-based devices to assess and classify the glistening in IOLs. However, this technology does not provide images with sufficient resolution to perform an automated glistening count and classification. Optical coherence tomography (OCT) is a noninvasive imaging technique that has revolutionized ophthalmological diagnoses in several areas and could be a helpful tool in this area.

To date, no objective, fast and reproducible method for the assessment of IOL glistening in clinical practice has been described. In addition, no studies have focused on the utility of OCT in the assessment of IOL glistening in vivo, and only one clinical study has reported an OCT analysis of IOL glistening [20].

Therefore, the main objectives of the present study are to assess the utility of the OCT to identify and classify the severity of the glistening, as well as assessing the reproducibility of this classification system.

2. Methods

2.1. Patients

A cross-sectional study was conducted on 150 patients recruited consecutively from those attending the Centro Internacional de Oftalmologia Avanzada (Madrid, Spain) for a routine ophthalmological examination over the period of 1 November 2022, to 1 December 2022.

Subjects were invited to participate if they met all the inclusion criteria and none of the exclusion criteria after giving their written informed consent. The study protocol adhered to the tenets of the Declaration of Helsinki and was approved by the Center's Review Board.

Inclusion criteria were patients who underwent cataract surgery at least 600 days before the recruitment process began, with the SN60WF IOL models made of Acrysof hydrophobic acrylic material (Alcon, Fort Worth, TX, USA), and who were consulted for a routine examination. Exclusion criteria were complications during cataract surgery and postoperative uveitis. Furthermore, images of insufficient quality, determined as a signal strength intensity (SSI) ≤ 2, or with artefacts, were excluded.

One eye from each patient was randomly included in the general study, while both eyes from the same patient were included in the reproducibility study.

2.2. Study Protocol

The subjects enrolled provided their medical history and underwent a complete ophthalmological examination, including anterior-segment OCT (SS-OCT). The ophthalmological exam included visual acuity and cycloplegic refractive error, slit-lamp biomicroscopy, tonometry with Canon TX 10® pneumotonometer (Canon Inc., Tokyo, Japan) and posterior-segment ophthalmoscopy. The IOL model and the time since the surgery were registered. All the examinations were performed on the same day.

For the assessment of the IOL, the SS-OCT device employed was a DRI-Triton® (Topcon Corporation, Tokyo, Japan), which uses a central wavelength of 1050 nm with an axial resolution of 8 μm, a transverse resolution of 20 μm and a scanning speed of 100,000 A-scans per second. To obtain cross-sectional images of the IOL, we employed the anterior-segment lens of the device using the "line" anterior-segment capture mode of a 6 mm exploration field on the horizontal axis. Furthermore, a radial scan, which consisted in 12 scans centered on the pupil, was conducted. This type of scan was intentionally performed to study the vertical scan of the IOL in order to analyze the correlation between the severity of the glistening and the horizontal scan. All OCT images were acquired after pupil dilation by a well-trained examiner (JIFV), with the subjects sitting up. Only images of sufficient quality, defined as a signal-strength intensity (SSI) above 3, were accepted.

2.3. Assessment of the IOL Glistening by OCT

The presence of glistening was identified as hyperreflective foci (HRF) or MVs inside the optic of the IOL, between the anterior surface and posterior surface of the lens (Figure 1).

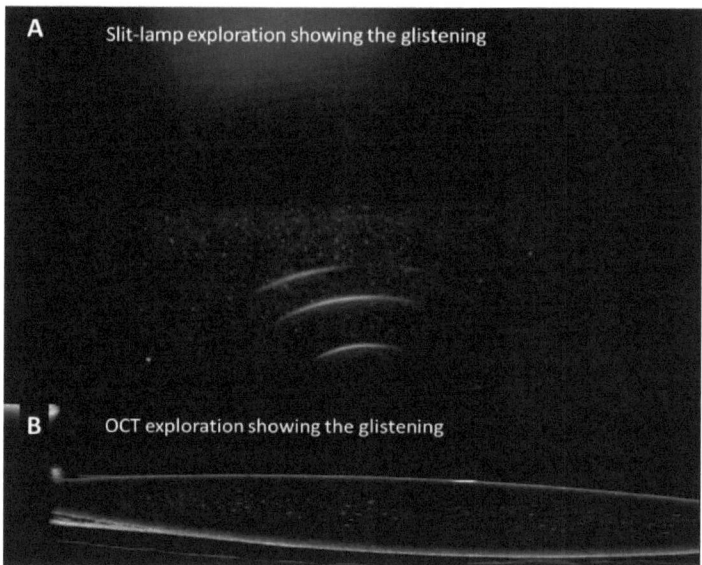

Figure 1. Example of an intraocular lens (IOL) with a high number of hyperreflective foci or microvacuoles in the optic of the lens viewed through slit-lamp photography (**A**) and optical coherence tomography (OCT) (**B**).

Based on a pilot study, the degree of glistening was classified into four categories: 0: ≤ 5 HRF; 1: 6 to 15 HRF; 2: 16 to 30 HRF; and 3: >30 HRF. Therefore, the glistening was described as the absolute number of HRF and as the severity grading (Figure 2). The evaluation of the OCT images was performed by two experienced examiners (JIFV and JAFV).

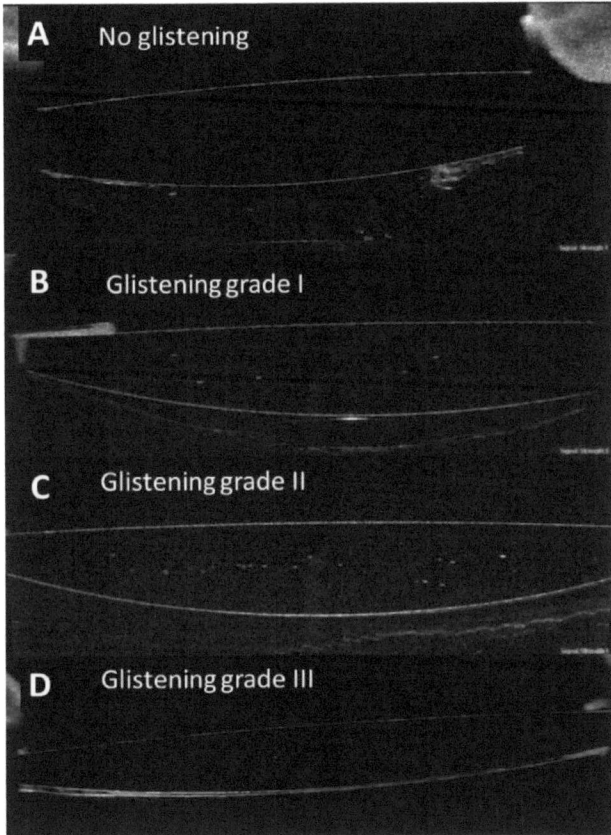

Figure 2. Optical coherence tomography of the optic of the intraocular lens (IOL) assessing the glistening and categorized into 4 groups based on the severity in the amount of hyperreflective foci or microvacuoles.

In a subgroup of 50 eyes from 25 patients, which were randomly selected, two OCT scans of the IOL were performed on the same day, separated by an interval of 2 min, to assess the repeatability of the images. It should be noted that no eye-tracking on the IOL was applied because it is not an available option in the device's software.

For intra and interobserver reproducibility, a different group of 50 eyes from 25 patients was assessed and examined once. Measurements were masked and independently conducted on the images by two observers (JIFV and JAFV) for interobserver reproducibility. To determine intraobserver reproducibility, one of the observers (JAFV) also took measurements of the same images one week after the first measurements.

2.4. Statistical Analysis

All statistical tests were performed using the software package, SPSS® (Statistical Package for Social Sciences, v25.0; SPSS Inc., Chicago, IL, USA). Quantitative data are provided as the mean and standard deviation. Qualitative data are expressed as their frequency distributions. Correlations were assessed through Pearson's correlation coefficients. In the reproducibility analysis, for each measurement, the intraclass correlation coefficient (ICC;

two-way mixed effects, absolute agreement, single measurement) was calculated for the two consecutive scans or measurements. Significance was set at $p < 0.05$.

3. Results

Demographics of the 150 patients included in the present study are presented in Table 1.

Table 1. Demographics of the patients and intraocular lenses (IOL) included in the present study. Mean ± standard deviation (range).

Parameter	Value
Age (years)	70.2 ± 11.3 (55–92)
Sex (female/male, %)	54/46
Eye (right/left)	51.5/48.5
Time since surgery (days)	1843 ± 843 (603–3617)
IOL power (diopters)	20.3 ± 4.1 (8–27)
IOL model and material	SN60WF (acrylic hydrophobic)

Intraocular lens glistening was detected in 42.7% of the patients included. The mean number of HRF or glistening dots was 10.4 ± 26.2, with a range from 0 to 239.

Regarding the severity of the glistening in the IOL, 63.3% of the eyes (95/150) had a grade of 0, 20% (30/150) had a grade of 1, 6.7% (10/150) had a grade of 2 and 10% (15/150) had a grade of 3. The numbers of MVs or HRF were as follows: in grade 0, 1.0 ± 1.4 (0 to 5); in grade 1, 9.6 ± 2.5 (6 to 15); in grade 2, 20.7 ± 4.6 (16 to 30); and in grade 3, 74.5 ± 46.2 (31 to 239).

The intraobserver and interobserver reproducibility were very high, both for the absolute quantification of the glistening (ICC ≥ 0.994) and for the severity scale (ICC ≥ 0.967). The repeatability for the absolute quantification and for the severity was also very high (ICC ≥ 0.955; Table 2).

Table 2. Reproducibility of OCT glistening measurements on the IOL (mean ± standard deviation) (N = 50 eyes).

	Parameter	Values	Parameter	Values
Intraobserver reproducibility	Measurement 1	11.62 ± 20.01 (0–90)	Severity scale 1	0.82 ± 0.94 (0–3)
	Measurement 2	11.32 ± 19.30 (0–85)	Severity scale 2	0.82 ± 0.94 (0–3)
	ICC	0.994 (0.990–0.997)	ICC	0.977 (0.961–0.987)
Interobserver reproducibility	Observer 1	11.62 ± 20.01 (0–90)	Severity scale observer 1	0.82 ± 0.94 (0–3)
	Observer 2	11.54 ± 18.87 (0–87)	Severity scale observer 2	0.84 ± 0.98 (0–3)
	ICC	0.996 (0.993–0.998)	ICC	0.967 (0.943–0.981)
Repeatability	Exploration 1	11.10 ± 18.5 (0–82)	Exploration 1	0.78 ± 1.07
	Exploration 2	9.63 ± 17.11 (0–87)	Exploration 2	0.75 ± 1.06
	ICC	0.958 (0.927–0.975)	ICC	0.955 (0.926–0.973)

There was an excellent correlation in the quantification of the IOL glistening between the horizontal and vertical scan, for both the right and the left eyes (R = 0.921 and R = 0.834 respectively; $p < 0.001$; Figure 3). However, the correlation in the vertical scans between the right and left eyes was moderate (R = 0.566; $p < 0.001$), and very similar to that in the horizontal scans between the right and left eyes (R = 0.582; $p < 0.001$).

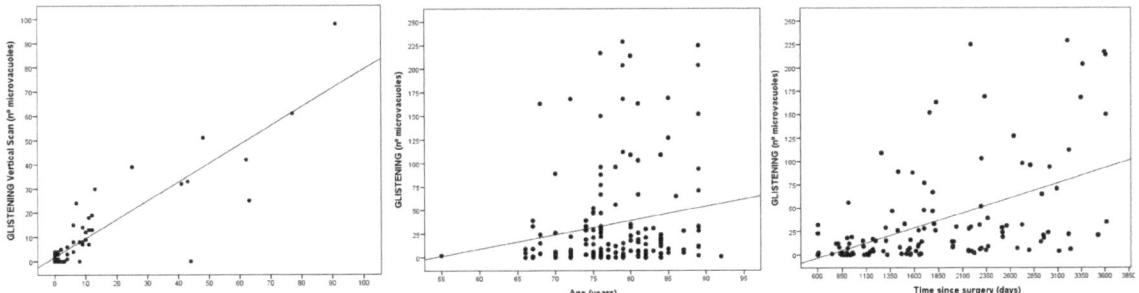

Figure 3. Correlation between horizontal and vertical glistening (**left**), severity of the glistening and age (**center**) and severity of the glistening and time since surgery (**right**).

There was a moderate correlation between the time since surgery and the severity of the glistening (R = 0.497; $p < 0.0001$). In addition, there was a weak correlation between age and the degree of glistening (R = 0.174; $p = 0.034$; Figure 3).

4. Discussion

Optical clarity is an important parameter in the quality assessment of implanted IOLs after cataract surgery [6]. Among different causes of IOL opacifications, glistening is relatively frequent [5]. Glistening or small fluid-filled vacuoles in the IOL material appear in the form of refractive particles that glisten upon slit-lamp examination due to hydration-related phenomena in hydrophobic acrylic lenses when the latter are in aqueous environments.

In the present study, SS-OCT was used to identify, quantify and classify IOL glistening in a simple and objective way. We analyzed the presence of glistening along the entire IOL optic shown on the OCT scans, detecting the absolute number of MVs, seen as HRF, and proposing an OCT-based classification. This classification system presented excellent reproducibility and a very strong correlation between the horizontal and vertical scans. Therefore, the use of only one OCT scan makes it possible to classify the degree of glistening, without the need for a cube or raster scan. Another advantage is that the entire optic in an OCT scan is assessed; it is not limited to a small area of 1 mm^2.

Werner et al. were the first authors to observe glistening through anterior-segment OCT (AS-OCT), by analyzing ex vivo hydrophobic acrylic IOLs explanted because of various complications [21]. They stated that this technique was helpful in analyzing the location and density of the glistening, and AS-OCT scans showed that the glistening was homogeneously distributed within the entire optic, although it was sometimes absent in a small subsurface area. Subsequently, in 2019, Tripathy and Sridhar reported an image describing IOL glistening through OCT in one patient [20]. Glistening takes the form of hyperreflective dots inside the optic of a lens. By contrast, pigment deposits or pseudoexfoliative materials are deposits over the surface of the IOL [21,22].

Currently, one of the most popular glistening-classification systems is the Miyata scale, which is based on slit-lamp images and features the following grades: grade 0, no glistening; grade 1, up to 50/mm^2; grade 2, up to 100/mm^2; and grade 3, 200/mm^2 (considered severe glistening) [19]. Colin et al., who also used slit-lamp images, graded and quantified glistening in a central area measuring 0.75 to 2 mm using Image J, applying different processing techniques. The size limits were set so that the Image J program would recognize

MVs as features with sizes between 0 and 0.001 mm^2. The mean values for the objective grading of the glistening were 26 ± 43 MVs/mm^2 for grade 0, 152 ± 142 MVs/mm^2 for grade 1 and 261 ± 139 MVs/mm^2 for grade 2. Interestingly, in Colin et al.'s study, only four lenses had >400 MVs/mm^2; the maximum observed density was 597 MVs/mm^2 [3]. In the present study, the numbers of MVs were as follows: in grade 0, 1.0 ± 1.4; in grade 1, 9.6 ± 2.5; in grade 2, 20.7 ± 4.6; and in grade 3, 74.5 ± 46.2. The highest number observed was 239.

Similarly, in microscopic images obtained with a digital camera, Yildirim et al. assessed the number of MVs in the central area and four peripheral IOL sections [23]. The software automatically calculated the number of MVs and a modification of the Miyata scale was established: grade 0 (<25 MVs/mm^2); grade 1 (25–100 MVs/mm^2); grade 2 (100–200 MVs/mm^2); and grade 3 (>200 MVs/mm^2). The central section was the region with the highest glistening density.

A similar approach to the quantification of glistening was carried out by Stanojcic et al. [24]. The methodology was based on central vertical slit-lamp images of 10 mm × 2 mm at 40°, on which a 1 × 3 mm grid divided into 1 mm^2 areas was overlayed. The grades of glistening density were assigned according to an 8-point ordinal scale based on increments of 10 glistenings/mm^2 from 0 (grade 0) up to more than 60 (grade 7) [24,25]. Other study groups classified glistening based on MV size (6–25 µm and over 25 µm) [26]. In the present study, based on the OCT resolution, both size groups were detected by using this technology.

In the last few years, a new proposal to classify glistening based on a digital analysis of Scheimpflug images was described by Biwer et al. [8]. They reported a mean glistening count of 2.8 ± 4.8 MV/mm^2. However, the subjective glistening-grading score showed moderate agreement with a counted score based on slit-lamp images. After this study, the authors acknowledged that the Scheimpflug device did not provide images with sufficient resolution to perform a glistening classification.

To date, different proposals have been developed and employed by different authors to assess and classify the glistening on IOLs. However, a direct comparison of the quantification and classification systems using slit-lamp photography (based on a frontal plane of the IOL) with that proposed here, using OCT (based on a transversal plane of the IOL), is difficult. Most authors quantify glistening in IOLs using an optic area of 1 mm^2. By contrast, we analyzed the entire optic IOL OCT-scan visualization, which is approximately 3 mm^2 (6 mm in IOL length and 0.5 mm in IOL thickness). Therefore, this method allows a more comprehensive analysis of IOLs, along with many other advantages.

As Werner et al. recognized, the glistening produced in vitro in their study may result in a morphologic aspect that appears to be stronger on OCT compared with the clinical situation [21]. Therefore, these authors suggested that only clinical studies can confirm whether clinically observed degrees of glistening can be assessed by using AS-OCT. In this regard, the present study demonstrated the ability of this technique to visualize and classify glistening in routine clinical practice.

Interestingly, in the present study, a significant correlation was observed between the time since surgery and the severity of glistening. This was in accordance with the results of a study carried out by Waite et al., who detected an association between the severity index determined by photographs of IOLs and the progression over time [27].

The effect of IOL glistening on visual quality has not yet been thoroughly investigated. The main effect of glistening on vision seems to be an increase in intraocular light scattering and glare, rather than changes in visual acuity [28]. Similarly, Kanclerz et al. found that glistening and subsurface nanoglistening manifest in hydrophobic acrylic IOLs and induce straylight rather than a decrease in visual acuity [1]. A study reported that only MVs greater than 10 µm induce a worsening in the modulation-transfer function [29]. Moreover, Weindler et al. showed that a rather large number of glistenings (>500/ mm^2) is needed to reduce the optical quality [30]. In this line of study, other classification systems have been proposed. Waite et al. suggested employing a severity index, which was defined as the size of the glistenings multiplied by the density of the glistenings (%area) [27], or analyzing the size as a measure of the area (%area/size) [26,31]. Henriksen et al. concluded that glistening %area, at a key size, was correlated with random light scatter [26].

In recent years, IOL manufacturers have tried to improve the fabrication processes and IOL materials to develop glistening-free hydrophobic acrylic polymers. With the introduction of some materials, such as the popular foldable Acrysof IOL (Alcon Laboratories, Inc.), in which this phenomenon often occurs, IOL glistening received clinical and research attention. Using these IOLs, Thomes and Callaghan induced glistening in vitro and compared AcrySof IOLs manufactured in 2003 and 2012 [17], observing a large decrease from 315.7 MV/mm^2 to 39.9 MV/mm^2, respectively [6,32]. Recently, Stanojcic et al. compared two hydrophobic acrylic aspheric monofocal IOLs (Clareon and Tecnis PCB00) in terms of glistening occurrence [25]. At 12 months, the glistening was minimal, with no difference in grade between the groups (p = 0.2). The new Clareon material is promising, with a study reporting no glistening up to 9 years after implantation [30]. The amount of fluid in hydrophobic acrylic materials has been shown to be negatively correlated with the occurrence of glistening, so the relatively high water content of the Clareon CNA0T0 material (1.5%) may explain these findings [32,33].

To the best of our knowledge, this is the first study to propose an OCT-based method to identify and classify IOL glistening. The main advantages are that it is a fast and easy exam, that it is highly reproducible and that the image can be directly assessed in vivo, with no need for image-post-processing techniques. By contrast, slit-lamp photographs with a posterior complex requires the processing of the images, which is a time-consuming method and requires an expert examiner. Even when the repeated images were acquired without any eye-tracking, the repeatability of the quantification and of the classification of the glistening on the IOL was excellent. By providing an objective classification, the method allows prospective evaluation and may serve as a valid tool to study new IOL designs and materials for resistance to glistening formation in clinical trials. As previously stated by Werner et al., AS-OCT may be helpful in assessing the presence, location and density of IOL changes, preventing the misdiagnosis of opacification and the performance of unnecessary procedures, such as posterior capsulotomy or explantation [21].

Our study has several limitations. First, establishing a cut-off point to determine the size in which a MV or HRF is considered as glistening was occasionally challenging. The identification of the smallest MV or HRF was limited by the resolution of the OCT, although we obtained excellent reproducibility. There are no strict criteria to determine how many glistening points are allowed in the determination of glistening-free IOLs [25], although, traditionally, most authors have used 50 MVs/mm^2 as a cutoff [19]. In addition, the density of the MVs or HRF was not considered, so the possible influence of those with a higher density is unknown. In addition, we only studied the central scanning area of the IOLs; although this is the most relevant area, because it includes the visual axis, glistening is usually distributed throughout the entire optic. In the present study, a moderate correlation in the glistening evaluation was observed between both eyes. However, it is well-known that different factors, such as the IOL model and several other factors can affect glistening, and the analysis of inter-eye differences was not the main objective of the present study.

Future studies are warranted to analyze whether glistening progresses over time, as a long follow-up, ideally lasting over 10 years, is needed [24]. Cataract surgery is being performed on increasingly young patients, which, along with the increasing life expectancy, implies that modern IOL needs to maintain optical clarity for several decades [24,25]. The intensity of glistening has been reported to increase for up to 15 years postoperatively, with an increase in surface light scattering on the IOL surface [34]. Studies assessing the possible agreement between OCT-based glistening classification and functional visual tests should be carried out. It would be interesting to establish whether the MV-distribution pattern has clinical relevance. Moreover, future studies should assess the utility of other OCT devices and deep-learning-based algorithms in the provision of automatic descriptions and classifications of glistening; these devices and algorithms may even predict the stability or progression of glistening.

In conclusion, SS-OCT makes it possible to identify, quantify and classify the glistening of IOLs in a simple, objective and reproducible way. This could provide relevant information for the study of the influence of glistening on visual acuity, quality and disability glare.

Author Contributions: Conceptualization, J.I.F.-V., L.D.-P.-G.-d.-L., I.S.-G., V.A.-B., J.Á.F.-V. and A.M.-M.; data curation, J.I.F.-V., V.A.-B. and S.F.-A.; formal analysis, B.B.-B., L.D.-P.-G.-d.-L., I.S.-G., S.F.-A., J.Á.F.-V. and A.M.-M.; investigation, J.I.F.-V., L.D.-P.-G.-d.-L., I.S.-G., V.A.-B. and S.F.-A.; methodology, J.I.F.-V., B.B.-B., V.A.-B. and S.F.-A.; resources, J.Á.F.-V.; software, J.Á.F.-V.; supervision, J.I.F.-V., B.B.-B., L.D.-P.-G.-d.-L., I.S.-G., J.Á.F.-V. and A.M.-M.; validation, L.D.-P.-G.-d.-L.; visualization, A.M.-M.; writing—original draft, J.I.F.-V. and B.B.-B.; writing—review and editing, J.I.F.-V., L.D.-P.-G.-d.-L., I.S.-G., V.A.-B., S.F.-A., J.Á.F.-V. and A.M.-M. All authors have read and agreed to the published version of the manuscript.

Funding: This research received no external funding.

Institutional Review Board Statement: This observational study was conducted in accordance with the Declaration of Helsinki and approved by the Ethics Committee of San Carlos Clinical Hospital.

Informed Consent Statement: Informed consent to use their medical information was obtained from all subjects involved in the study.

Data Availability Statement: Data used to support the findings presented in this study are available on request from the corresponding author.

Conflicts of Interest: The authors declare no conflict of interest.

References

1. Kanclerz, P.; Yildirim, T.M.; Khoramnia, R. A review of late intraocular lens opacifications. *Curr. Opin. Ophthalmol.* **2021**, *32*, 31–44. [CrossRef] [PubMed]
2. Durr, G.M.; Ahmed, I.I.K. Intraocular Lens Complications: Decentration, Uveitis–Glaucoma–Hyphema Syndrome, Opacification, and Refractive Surprises. *Ophthalmology* **2021**, *128*, e186–e194. [CrossRef]
3. Colin, J.; Orignac, I. Glistenings on intraocular lenses in healthy eyes: Effects and associations. *J. Refract. Surg.* **2011**, *27*, 869–875. [CrossRef]
4. Yildirim, T.M.; Schickhardt, S.K.; Wang, Q.; Friedmann, E.; Khoramnia, R.; Auffarth, G.U. Quantitative evaluation of microvacuole formation in five intraocular lens models made of different hydrophobic materials. *PLoS ONE* **2021**, *16*, 1–12. [CrossRef] [PubMed]
5. Grzybowski, A.; Markeviciute, A.; Zemaitiene, R. A narrative review of intraocular lens opacifications: Update 2020. *Ann. Transl. Med.* **2020**, *8*, 1547. [CrossRef] [PubMed]
6. Werner, L. Intraocular Lenses: Overview of Designs, Materials, and Pathophysiologic Features. *Ophthalmology* **2021**, *128*, e74–e93. [CrossRef] [PubMed]
7. Werner, L. Glistenings and surface light scattering in intraocular lenses. *J. Cataract Refract. Surg.* **2010**, *36*, 1398–1420. [CrossRef] [PubMed]
8. Biwer, H.; Schuber, E.; Honig, M.; Spratte, B.; Baumeister, M.; Kohnen, T. Objective classification of glistenings in implanted intraocular lenses using Scheimpflug tomography. *J. Cataract Refract. Surg.* **2015**, *41*, 2644–2651. [CrossRef] [PubMed]
9. Moreno-Montañés, J.; Alvarez, A.; Rodríguez-Conde, R.; Fernández-Hortelano, A. Clinical factors related to the frequency and intensity of glistenings in AcrySof intraocular lenses. *J. Cataract Refract. Surg.* **2003**, *29*, 1980–1984. [CrossRef]
10. Tetz, M.; Jorgensen, M.R. New Hydrophobic IOL Materials and Understanding the Science of Glistenings. *Curr. Eye Res.* **2015**, *40*, 969–981. [CrossRef]
11. Rønbeck, M.; Behndig, A.; Taube, M.; Koivula, A.; Kugelberg, M. Comparison of glistenings in intraocular lenses with three different materials: 12-year follow-up. *Acta Ophthalmol.* **2013**, *91*, 66–70. [CrossRef] [PubMed]
12. Luo, F.; Bao, X.; Qin, Y.; Hou, M.; Wu, M. Subjective Visual Performance and Objective Optical Quality With Intraocular Lens Glistening and Surface Light Scattering. *J. Refract. Surg.* **2018**, *34*, 372–378. [CrossRef] [PubMed]
13. Neuhann, T.; Yildirim, T.M.; Son, H.S.; Merz, P.R.; Khoramnia, R.; Auffarth, G.U. Reasons for explantation, demographics, and material analysis of 200 intraocular lens explants. *J. Cataract Refract. Surg.* **2020**, *46*, 20–26. [CrossRef] [PubMed]
14. Dehoog, E.; Doraiswamy, A. Evaluation of loss in optical quality of multifocal intraocular lenses with glistenings. *J. Cataract Refract. Surg.* **2016**, *42*, 606–612. [CrossRef]
15. Kawahara, S.; Nagai, Y.; Kawakami, E.; Yamanaka, R.; Ida, N.; Takeuchi, M.; Uyama, M.; Miyata, A.; Uchida, N.; Nakajima, K.; et al. Clinical and experimental observation of glistening in acrylic intraocular lenses. Expression of the Varicella Zoster Virus Thymidine Kinase and Cytokines in Patients with Acute Retinal Necrosis Syndrome 2000. Analysis of Proteins During Recovery fr. *J. Jpn. Ophthalmol. Soc.* **2000**, *104*, 349–353.

16. Tognetto, D.; Toto, L.; Sanguinetti, G.; Ravalico, G. Glistenings in foldable intraocular lenses. *J. Cataract Refract. Surg.* **2002**, *28*, 1211–1216. [CrossRef]
17. Thomes, B.E.; Callaghan, T.A. Evaluation of in vitro glistening formation in hydrophobic acrylic intraocular lenses. *Clin. Ophthalmol.* **2013**, *7*, 1529–1534. [CrossRef]
18. Łabuz, G.; Knebel, D.; Auffarth, G.U.; Fang, H.; van den Berg, T.J.; Yildirim, T.M.; Son, H.S.; Khoramnia, R. Glistening Formation and Light Scattering in Six Hydrophobic-Acrylic Intraocular Lenses. *Am. J. Ophthalmol.* **2018**, *196*, 112–120. [CrossRef]
19. Miyata, A.; Uchida, N.; Nakajima, K.; Yaguchi, S. Clinical and experimental observation of glistening in acrylic intraocular lenses. *Jpn. J. Ophthalmol.* **2001**, *45*, 564–569. [CrossRef]
20. Tripathy, K.; Sridhar, U. Optical coherence tomography of intraocular lens glistening. *Indian J. Ophthalmol.* **2019**, *67*, 138–139. [CrossRef]
21. Werner, L.; Michelson, J.; Ollerton, A.; Leishman, L.; Bodnar, Z. Anterior segment optical coherence tomography in the assessment of postoperative intraocular lens optic changes. *J. Cataract Refract. Surg.* **2012**, *38*, 1077–1085. [CrossRef] [PubMed]
22. Fernández-Vigo, J.I.; de-Pablo Gómez de Liaño, L.; Sánchez-Guillen, I.; Macarro-Merino, A.; Fernández-Vigo, C.; García-Feijóo, J.; Fernández-Vigo, J.A. Pseudoexfoliation signs in the anterior segment assessed by optical coherence tomography and Scheimpflug device. *Arch. Soc. Esp. Oftalmol.* **2018**, *93*, 53–59. [CrossRef] [PubMed]
23. Yildirim, T.M.; Fang, H.; Schickhardt, S.K.; Wang, Q.; Merz, P.R.; Auffarth, G.U. Glistening formation in a new hydrophobic acrylic intraocular lens. *BMC Ophthalmol.* **2020**, *20*, 1–7. [CrossRef]
24. Stanojcic, N.; O'Brart, D.P.S.; Maycock, N.; Hull, C.C. Effects of intraocular lens glistenings on visual function: A prospective study and presentation of a new glistenings grading methodology. *BMJ Open Ophthalmol.* **2019**, *4*, e000266. [CrossRef] [PubMed]
25. Stanojcic, N.; O'Brart, D.; Hull, C.; Wagh, V.; Azan, E.; Bhogal, M.; Robbie, S.; Li, J.-P.O. Visual and refractive outcomes and glistenings occurrence after implantation of 2 hydrophobic acrylic aspheric monofocal IOLs. *J. Cataract Refract. Surg.* **2020**, *46*, 986–994. [CrossRef]
26. Henriksen, B.S.; Kinard, K.; Olson, R.J. Effect of intraocular lens glistening size on visual quality. *J. Cataract Refract. Surg.* **2015**, *41*, 1190–1198. [CrossRef] [PubMed]
27. Waite, A.; Faulkner, N.; Olson, R.J. Glistenings in the single-piece, hydrophobic, acrylic intraocular lenses. *Am. J. Ophthalmol.* **2007**, *144*, 143–144. [CrossRef]
28. Hayashi, K.; Hirata, A.; Yoshida, M.; Yoshimura, K.; Hayashi, H. Long-term effect of surface light scattering and glistenings of intraocular lenses on visual function. *Am. J. Ophthalmol.* **2012**, *154*, 240–251.e2. [CrossRef]
29. Geniusz, M.; Zając, M. A technique of experimental and numerical analysis of influence of defects in the intraocular lens on the retinal image quality. *Appl. Digit. Image Process. XXXIX* **2016**, *9971*, 997125. [CrossRef]
30. Weindler, J.N.; Łabuz, G.; Yildirim, T.M.; Tandogan, T.; Khoramnia, R.; Auffarth, G.U. The impact of glistenings on the optical quality of a hydrophobic acrylic intraocular lens. *J. Cataract Refract. Surg.* **2019**, *45*, 1020–1025. [CrossRef]
31. DeHoog, E.; Doraiswamy, A. Evaluation of the impact of light scatter from glistenings in pseudophakic eyes. *J. Cataract Refract. Surg.* **2014**, *40*, 95–103. [CrossRef] [PubMed]
32. Werner, L.; Thatthamla, I.; Ong, M.; Schatz, H.; Garcia-Gonzalez, M.; Gros-Otero, J.; Cañones-Zafra, R.; Teus, M.A. Evaluation of clarity characteristics in a new hydrophobic acrylic IOL in comparison to commercially available IOLs. *J. Cataract Refract. Surg.* **2019**, *45*, 1490–1497. [CrossRef] [PubMed]
33. Packer, M.; Rajan, M.; Ligabue, E.; Heiner, P. Clinical properties of a novel, glistening-free, single-piece, hydrophobic acrylic IOL. *Clin. Ophthalmol.* **2014**, *8*, 421–427. [CrossRef] [PubMed]
34. Miyata, K.; Honbo, M.; Otani, S.; Nejima, R.; Minami, K. Effect on visual acuity of increased surface light scattering in intraocular lenses. *J. Cataract Refract. Surg.* **2012**, *38*, 221–226. [CrossRef] [PubMed]

Disclaimer/Publisher's Note: The statements, opinions and data contained in all publications are solely those of the individual author(s) and contributor(s) and not of MDPI and/or the editor(s). MDPI and/or the editor(s) disclaim responsibility for any injury to people or property resulting from any ideas, methods, instructions or products referred to in the content.

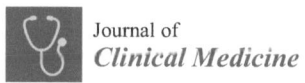

Review

Update on the Utility of Optical Coherence Tomography in the Analysis of the Optic Nerve Head in Highly Myopic Eyes with and without Glaucoma

Bachar Kudsieh [1,2,*], José Ignacio Fernández-Vigo [2,3], Ignacio Flores-Moreno [1], Jorge Ruiz-Medrano [1,4], Maria Garcia-Zamora [1], Muhsen Samaan [5] and Jose Maria Ruiz-Moreno [1,4]

1. Department of Ophthalmology, University Hospital Puerta De Hierro Majadahonda, 28220 Madrid, Spain
2. Centro Internacional de Oftalmologia Avanzada, 28010 Madrid, Spain
3. Department of Ophthalmology, Hospital Clinico San Carlos, Institute of Health Research (IdISSC), 28040 Madrid, Spain
4. Instituto de Microcirugia Ocular (IMO), 28035 Madrid, Spain
5. Barraquer Eye Clinic UAE, Dubai P.O. Box 212619, United Arab Emirates
* Correspondence: bacharkudsieh@gmail.com; Tel.: +34-91-191-60-00

Abstract: Glaucoma diagnosis in highly myopic subjects by optic nerve head (ONH) imaging is challenging as it is difficult to distinguish structural defects related to glaucoma from myopia-related defects in these subjects. Optical coherence tomography (OCT) has evolved to become a routine examination at present, providing key information in the assessment of glaucoma based on the study of the ONH. However, the correct segmentation and interpretation of the ONH data employing OCT is still a challenge in highly myopic patients. High-resolution OCT images can help qualitatively and quantitatively describe the structural characteristics and anatomical changes in highly myopic subjects with and without glaucoma. The ONH and peripapillary area can be analyzed to measure the myopic atrophic-related zone, the existence of intrachoroidal cavitation, staphyloma, and ONH pits by OCT. Similarly, the lamina cribosa observed in the OCT images may reveal anatomical changes that justify visual defects. Several quantitative parameters of the ONH obtained from OCT images were proposed to predict the progression of visual defects in glaucoma subjects. Additionally, OCT images help identify factors that may negatively influence the measurement of the retinal nerve fiber layer (RNFL) and provide better analysis using new parameters, such as Bruch's Membrane Opening-Minimum Rim Width, which serves as an alternative to RNFL measurements in highly myopic subjects due to its superior diagnostic ability.

Keywords: optic nerve head; high myopia; myopic glaucoma; optical coherence tomography; peripapillary atrophy; optic disc tilt; intrachoroidal cavitation; retinal nerve fiber layer

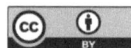

1. Introduction

Population-based studies have shown that myopia is a major risk factor for open-angle glaucoma (OAG) [1,2]. Furthermore, the morbidity rate of glaucoma increases along with the degree of myopia [3]. Hence, the diagnosis of glaucoma in the early stages of the disease in highly myopic eyes is essential for the management and prevention of visual loss.

In highly myopic subjects, the image-based diagnosis of glaucoma is challenging as it is difficult to distinguish structural defects related to glaucoma from myopia-related defects [4]. Optical coherence tomography (OCT) is widely used to measure the optic nerve head (ONH) neuroretinal rim and the peripapillary retinal nerve fiber layer (RNFL), both being the most popular parameters to distinguish glaucoma by clinicians [5].

The anatomical changes caused by the progressive increase in the axial length (AXL) in myopic subjects lead to abnormal positions of the ONH, such as optic disc tilting and torsion [6]. These phenomena result in difficulties in applying the ISNT rule in highly myopic subjects to diagnose the presence of glaucoma [7]. Similarly, in high myopia, the trajectories of the peripapillary nerve fiber layer deviate, hindering the interpretation of OCT measurements [8,9]. Additionally, the visual field (VF) defects in myopic glaucoma subjects are confusing due to their co-occurrence with myopic chorioretinopathy VF defects, making the relation between structural and functional defects in myopic glaucoma weak [10]. The advancement of Swept Source (SS) and Enhanced Depth Imaging (EDI) OCT has enabled clinicians to obtain high-resolution images of the ocular structures, including the deepest layers, which is useful in highly myopic subjects [11]. Through these images, the papillary area can be qualitatively and quantitatively described and these findings can be associated with visual function.

In this review, we summarize and comment on the utility of OCT in identifying and measuring the structural variations and abnormalities of the ONH and peripapillary region in highly myopic subjects with and without glaucoma, including the quantitative and qualitative characteristics of the OCT measurements and the relation of these changes with VF.

In this review, a PubMed search was undertaken in January 2023 using the following search terms: "high myopia", "optic nerve head", "optical coherence tomography", and "glaucoma" and combinations. The abstracts were screened and those relevant to this particular review were retrieved for more detailed analysis.

2. Peripapillary Atrophy

In the peripapillary area of highly myopic subjects, four zones of peripapillary atrophy (PPA) can be differentiated using radial scans of OCT images [12] (Table 1, Figure 1). The alpha PPA (α-PPA) consists of an irregular retinal pigment epithelium (RPE) with the presence of a Bruch's membrane (BM). This area coincides with the clinically observed PPA by retinography. The beta PPA (β-PPA) is characterized by the absence of RPE and the presence of BM. A larger β-PPA area is associated with older age, longer AXL, larger disc area, greater disc ovality, and thinner choroidal thickness [13]. Its presence in glaucoma patients indicates a greater risk of progression and major VF loss [14]. The gamma PPA (γ-PPA) is characterized by the absence of both the RPE and BM, with only the presence of the peripapillary RNFL. This type of PPA is characteristic of myopia and is usually caused by a progressive elongation of the eye regardless of glaucoma. In highly myopic eyes with AXL greater than 26.5 mm, the optic disc area, lamina cribosa (LC) area, and BM opening area increase, leading to a circular γ-PPA and δ-PPA [15]. The delta PPA (δ-PPA) is characterized by the absence of microvessels larger than 50 microns. It is usually within the γ-PPA zone, predisposes to glaucomatous damage, and coincides with the dura mater insertion into the sclera [13,16,17]. The size of the PPA area is usually associated with the AXL, age, and choroidal thickness. Hu et al. described a PPA area of 0.35 mm^2 in subjects with AXL below 24 mm, 0.65 mm^2 when the AXL is between 24 and 27 mm, and 0.78 mm^2 in high myopia (AXL greater than 27 mm^2) [18]. Similarly, in a cross-sectional study including 821 young myopic patients, Chen et al. discovered that every 0.1 mm^2 increase in the PPA area was associated with a 14.93 μm decrease in the macular choroidal thickness (MCT) and a 9.54 μm decrease in the peripapillary choroidal thickness [17]. On the contrary, the PPA area has a negligible or weak correlation with the RNFL thickness [17,18]. Hu et al. found that the PPA area does not usually correlate with the RNFL thickness [18]. In agreement with this, a mild correlation between the PPA and RFNL thickness (R = 0.417, $p < 0.001$) was described by Zhang et al. in a study of 112 patients with a mean AXL of 26.86 ± 0.94 mm [19].

Table 1. ONH characteristics in myopic subjects.

α-PPA	Irregular RPE with the presence of BM
β-PPA	Absence of the RPE and the presence of BM
γ-PPA	Absence of both the RPE and BM with the presence of only the peripapillary RNFL

Table 1. *Cont.*

δ-PPA	Absence of microvessels larger than 50 microns usually within the γ-PPA zone
ONH tilt angle	Angle between two lines: the first line connecting the inner edges of BM on each side of the ONH on the cross-sectional OCT image and a second line connecting the two points of the clinical disc margin along the OCT cross-sectional scan
ONH torsion angle	Angle between the vertical meridian of the line connecting the center of the BMO and fovea and the longest diameter of the BMO-delineated ONH margin defined by OCT
ONH pits	Triangular hyporeflective shape with the apex heading into the interior of the ONH observed in enface images
PICC	Hyporeflective triangular thickening of the choroid with the base at the optic disc border excluding peripapillary large choroidal vessels
PPRS	Cystoid hyporeflective spaces in the peripapillary region around retinal vessels
Peripapillary staphyloma	Arched posterior sclera with less curvature in adjacent regions, the choroid at the edge of the staphyloma is thinned

ONH: optic nerve head; PPA: peripapillary atrophy; RPE: retinal pigment epithelium; BM: Bruch's membrane; RNFL: retinal nerve fibre layer; OCT: optical coherence tomography; BMO: Bruch's membrane opening; PICC: peripapillary intrachoroidal cavitation; PPRS: peripapillary retinoschisis.

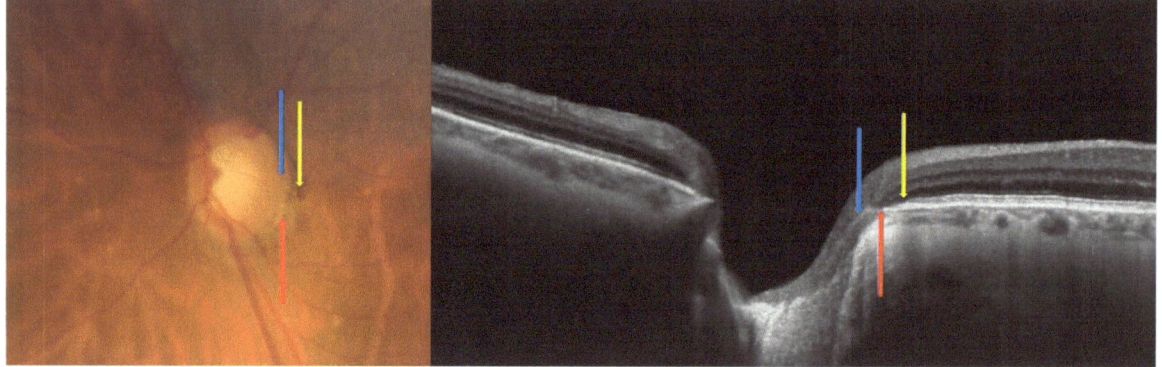

Figure 1. Fundus photography and optical coherence tomography of the peripapillary region of a myopic subject. The blue arrow represents the temporal optic disc margin, the red arrow represents the end of Bruch's membrane (BM), and the yellow arrow represents the end of the retinal pigment epithelium (RPE). The distance from the temporal optic disc margin (blue arrow) to the edge of BM (red arrow) is defined as peripapillary atrophy (PPA) beta and the distance from the edge of BM (red arrow) to the end of RPE is defined as PPA alpha.

3. Tilted Disc in High Myopia

The tilt of the ONH represents an anomalous insertion of the optic nerve in the eyeball in highly myopic subjects. It can be horizontal or vertical, and it has traditionally been evaluated in the images obtained with retinography with the ovality index [20,21]. Recently, the optic nerve tilt angle has been accurately measured in vertical and horizontal scans of OCT images [22]. Hosseini et al. defined the tilt angle as the angle between two lines: the first line connecting the inner edges of the BM on each side of the ONH on the cross-sectional OCT image, and a second line connecting the two points marking the clinical disc margin along the OCT cross-sectional scan (Figure 2). In that study, the median tilt angle was 3.5° (1.2–11.2) [22]. Similarly, Choi et al. found a median temporal and vertical disc tilt using a spectral domain (SD) OCT of 3.60° (1.61° to 6.40°) and 0.00° (−1.03° to 1.62°), respectively, in their study, which included 235 eyes of normal and glaucoma patients with a mean AXL of 24.5 mm. Moreover, they obtained excellent intra- and inter-observer reproducibility for the angle measurements by OCT (ICC = 0.882 and 0.801, respectively) [23]. Tilted optic discs are more frequent in myopic eyes. A study of young myopic subjects revealed that the frequency of tilted optic discs increased with the AXL, being 37.0%, 51.1%, 57.6%, and 70.7% with AXL $\leq$ 24 mm, 24 to 25 mm, 25 to 26 mm, and $\geq$26 mm, respectively [17]. Hosseini et al. demonstrated a positive correlation between the disc tilt angle and AXL (R = 0.399, $p < 0.001$) [22]. A greater tilt in myopic eyes with glaucoma was suggested by Park et al. who observed a significantly greater tilt angle in myopic glaucoma compared to control eyes with similar AXL, being 9.3 ± 6.3° vs. 6.2 ± 4.1°, respectively ($p < 0.05$) [24]. Similarly, Yoon J. Y. et al. found that young myopic glaucomatous eyes showed progressive optic disc tilting during three years of follow-up, increasing from 7.0 ± 3.4 to 8.3 ± 3.8° [25]. The authors attribute these findings in myopic eyes with glaucoma to either continuous AXL enlargement or/and glaucomatous structural change.

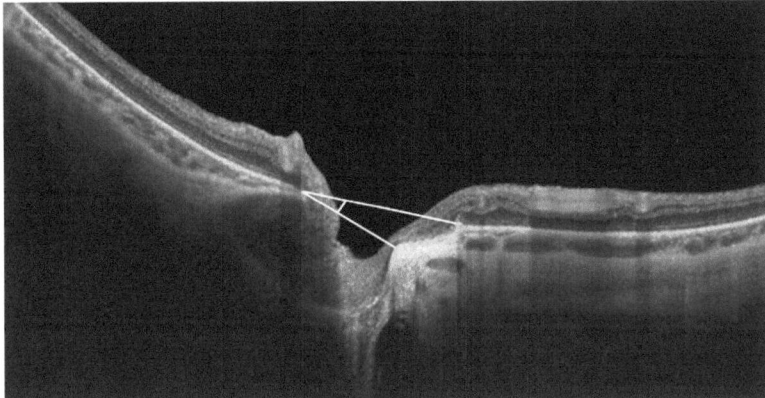

Figure 2. Optic nerve head tilt angle measurement in myopic subject. The tilt angle represents the angle is between the upper white line connecting the inner edges of Bruch's membrane on each side of the optic nerve head on the cross-sectional optical coherence tomography (OCT) image, and the lower white line connecting the two points marking the clinical disc margin along the OCT cross-sectional scan.

The correlation between disc tilt in myopic patients and VF defects has been described by several authors. Hosseini et al. demonstrated a negative correlation with VF defects (R = −0.356, $p < 0.001$). Shoeibi et al. showed arcuate scotoma and generalized depression on the VF in 30% and 30% of myopic eyes with a tilted disc, respectively, observing the lowest average deviation of the VF in the superotemporal quadrant (−4.54 ± 3.16 dB) [26]. In addition, Han et al. described a faster VF progression in myopic OAG with inferiorly tilted discs compared to non-myopic OAG ($p = 0.002$) [27].

Recent studies using OCT have demonstrated that the assessment of the ONH and RNFL are strongly influenced by the optic disc tilt. Refs. [28,29] Shin et al. showed that the disc area, cup volume, and average cup-to-disc-ratio (CDR) obtained by Cirrus HD-OCT were significantly smaller in myopic tilted eyes compared to the non-tilted myopic eyes (1.91 ± 0.81 mm^2 vs. 1.63 ± 0.30 mm^2, 0.53 ± 0.28 mm^2 vs. 0.33 ± 0.19 mm^2 and 0.76 ± 0.09 vs. 0.69 ± 0.11, respectively, all $p < 0.05$). Similarly, they obtained thicker temporal RNFL in the tilted disc group compared with the non-tilted group (62.1 ± 9.0 µm vs. 71.0 ± 12.8 µm, $p < 0.001$). No differences were observed in the macular ganglion cell-inner plexiform layer (GCIPL) thickness between the two groups (72.2 ± 6.5 µm vs. 72.9 ± 5.4 µm, $p = 0.558$) [28]. In agreement with this, Moghadas Sharif et al. found no differences in the central ganglion cell layer (GCL) thickness between tilted and non-tilted high myopic subjects with an AXL > 26 mm (15 µm vs. 15 µm, $p = 0.84$) using Spectralis-OCT (Spectralis; Heidelberg Engineering, Heidelberg, Germany) [29]. Therefore, both groups agreed on the superior glaucoma diagnostic capability of the GCL thickness compared to the RNFL thickness and ONH parameters in the myopic tilted disc patients.

4. Optic Nerve Head Torsion

This represents the rotation of the ONH around the sagittal axis, commonly measured as the angle between the vertical meridian and the longest diameter of the optic disc on fundus photography [30]. More recently, the OCT-based torsion angle was defined as the measurement between the vertical meridian of the line connecting the center of the BMO opening and fovea and the longest diameter of the BMO-delineated ONH margin defined by SD-OCT [31]. Cheng et al. described OCT-based torsion angles of $9.1 \pm 7.4°$, $10.7 \pm 9.1°$, and $11.5 \pm 11.1°$ in healthy subjects with AXL $\leq$ 25 mm, from 25 to 26 mm, and $\geq$26 mm, respectively [32]. Using the Spectralis OCT, Rezapour et al. found a torsion angle of 34.4° (range 29.9 to 39.0) vs. 33.7° (range 27.6 to 39.9) in mild myopia (mean AXL of 24.8 mm, range 24.7 to 25.0) vs. high myopia (mean AXL of 26.8 mm, range 26.6 to 27.0). In addition, they obtained no association between the photograph-based and OCT-based assessment of the torsion angle in high-axial myopic eyes ($p \geq 0.33$ with $R^2 = 0.03$ from 0.0 to 0.21) [33]. It should be highlighted that these different torsion angle values are due to the fact that the OCT-based torsion angle is a BMO-based assessment while the photographed-based torsion angle is measured relative to the clinical disc margin, which does not always correspond with the BMO, especially in myopic eyes.

5. Optic Disc Pits

OCT technology development has helped identify the optic disc pit in normal eyes [34]. In 2007, Shimada et al. first described the optic disc pit in myopic eyes using an OCT ophthalmoscope (C7, NIDEK, Gamagori, Aichi, Japan) [35]. Later, Ohno-Matsui et al. identified the pits using en-face images through vertical and horizontal SS-OCT scans in 16.2% (32/198) of highly myopic eyes (mean AXL: 30 ± 2 mm). Using en-face images, the pits can be observed, such as a triangular hyporeflective shape with the apex heading into the interior of the ONH. In horizontal and vertical OCT images, the optic disc pits were associated with discontinuities of the LC and discontinuous overlying RNFL. The pits were localized in the outer border of the ONH in 34% of cases and the scleral crescent in 64% of cases, being more frequently observed in the temporal conus. Remarkably, in this study, the pits were visible by fundus retinography in only two cases [36].

6. Peripapillary Intrachoroidal Cavitation

Based on OCT manifestations, peripapillary intrachoroidal cavitation (PICC) was first described by Freund et al. as a peripapillary detachment in pathologic myopia [37]. Later, Spaide et al. described the PICC as a suprachoroidal separation using SS-OCT [38]. Recently, Ehongo et al., also based on SS-OCT findings, suggested that the tensile forces of the optic nerve sheaths during adduction cause the collapse of the scleral flange onto the subarachnoid space, leading to PICC [39]. In OCT images, PICC is indeed defined as a hyporeflective triangular thickening of the choroid with the base at the optic disc border (Figure 3A), excluding the peripapillary large choroidal vessels. In their study, which evaluated 884 eyes of highly myopic subjects using SD-OCT (Model Ivue100; Optovue, Fremont, CA, USA), Liu et al. found PICC in 3.6% (32 eyes), frequently affecting the inferior disc (85.7%), followed by multiple locations (9.4%) and superior disc borders (3.1%) [40]. Similarly, Shimada et al. reported PICC in 4.9% of 324 subjects with pathologic myopia [35]. The Beijing Eye Study, however, reported a higher rate (16.9%) [41]. Moreover, Venkatesh et al. found PICC in 55.8% of highly myopic eyes with the presence of a myopic conus and/or the presence of intrascleral vessels near the cavitation [42]. You et al. measured PICC using OCT and showed that the mean width was 4.2 ± 2.3 h of the disc circumference, the mean length being 1363 ± 384 µm [41]. Older age, more myopic spherical equivalent, longer AXL, severe myopic maculopathy, and the presence of posterior staphyloma were associated with the presence of PICC [40,42].

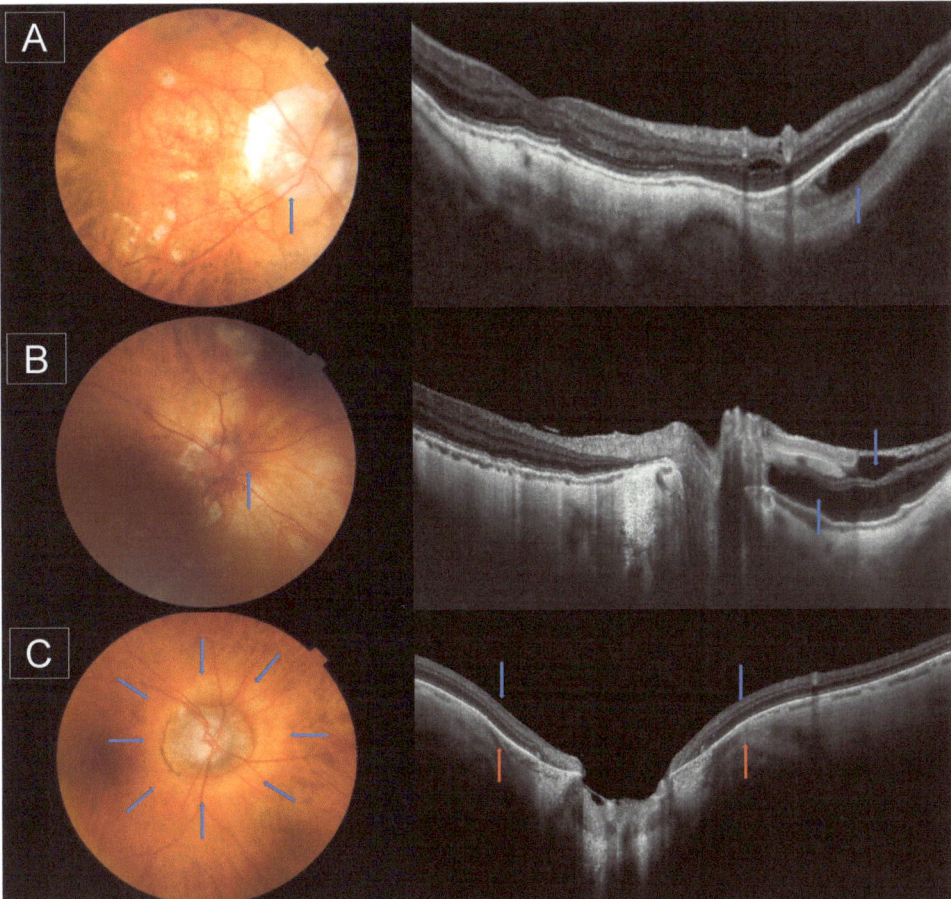

Figure 3. Fundus photography and optical coherence tomography (OCT) of the peripapillary region of a myopic subject. (**A**): Blue arrow represents peripapillary intrachoroidal cavitation observed in the photography as a yellowish peripapillary lesion and in the OCT image as a hyporeflective triangular thickening of the choroid with the base at the optic disc border, (**B**): Blue arrow represents peripapillary retinoschisis observed in the OCT image as cystoid hyporeflective spaces in the peripapillary region around retinal vessels, (**C**): Fundus photography and OCT image of peripapillary staphyloma, blue arrows showing the border of the staphyloma with arched posterior sclera and red arrows showing the thinned choroid at the edge of the staphyloma.

7. Peripapillary Retinoschisis and Holes

Peripapillary retinoschisis (PPRS) is observed in OCT images as cystoid hyporeflective spaces in the peripapillary region around the retinal vessels (Figure 3B) [43]. Shimada et al. demonstrated retinal cysts in 49.5% of 287 highly myopic eyes (AXL > 26.5 mm), only 24.4% of which had been discovered by fundoscopy [44]. In agreement with this, Li et al. found PPRS in 109 eyes (71.7%) with an AXL > 26.5 mm [45]. A higher incidence of PPRS was associated with older age, longer AXL, and the presence of posterior staphyloma [44–46]. Interestingly, Li et al. revealed that the presence of PPRS was negatively associated with the MCT ($\beta = -18.30$, $p < 0.05$) in a recent study that included 645 myopic eyes [47].

The incidence of paravascular lamellar holes in highly myopic eyes ranges between 14% and 31.4%, according to different OCT scan protocols [44,48,49]. Vela et al. described that the holes are mainly distributed in the inferior temporal arcade in 39.9% and are related to staphyloma type V and IX [49]. The pathogenesis of the holes is unknown, although Shimada et al. suggested that the formation of the holes is probably due to the vitreous traction or spontaneous rupture of a cyst [44]. Interestingly, this OCT finding is proposed as an important causative factor for macular retinoschisis as it was noted in 43.1% to 80% of eyes with macular retinoschisis [44].

8. Peripapillary Staphyloma

Peripapillary staphyloma is traditionally evaluated by fundus photography or magnetic resonance imaging (MRI) scans [50]. In 2016, Shinohara et al. described the staphyloma on SS-OCT images in highly myopic eyes (mean AXL 31.1 ± 1 mm), which is characterized by an arched posterior sclera with less curvature in the adjacent regions (Figure 3C). The choroid at the edge of the staphyloma is thinned and is associated with PICC in 52.5% of the cases [51]. Peripapillary staphyloma can also be observed in young myopic subjects. Using ultra-widefield SS-OCT, Tanaka et al. observed the presence of staphyloma in 12.7% of the eyes of subjects younger than 20 years, with a mean AXL of 27.9 mm. Interestingly, they found that the subfoveal choroid and nasal choroid to the ONH were thinner in eyes with a staphyloma than those without [52]. In a recent study of 729 eyes with a mean AXL of 30 ± 2 mm, Shinohara et al. detected posterior staphyloma using ultrawide-field SS-OCT in 482 eyes (66.1%), and it was more frequently detected in eyes with macular retinoschisis (86.0% vs. 61.6%; $p < 0.001$) compared to eyes without macular retinoschisis [53]. It is of clinical relevance that the staphyloma is associated with a greater risk of glaucoma and VF loss [51].

9. Lamina Cribosa in Myopia

A large LC curvature, LC with a reduced thickness, and the presence of focal LC defects have been shown to correlate with highly myopic subjects [54–56] Using SS-OCT, Miki et al. observed LC defects in eight eyes with high myopia but without glaucoma (22.9%) vs. 28 eyes (41.8%) in high myopia with glaucoma ($p = 0.0009$). In this study, 79.5% of patients with LC defects had corresponding damage in the VF. Interestingly, other factors, such as visual acuity, intraocular pressure, disc ovality, or a PPA area, did not differ significantly between eyes with and without LC defects [54]. Sawada et al. used EDI SD-OCT B-scans to classify the defects into LC defects (with a diameter > 100 µm) and large pores with a diameter of 60 to 100 µm. They demonstrated that highly myopic eyes with glaucoma had more LC defects and larger pores than myopic eyes without glaucoma (3.8 vs. 0.8 and 1.9 vs. 1.6, respectively), both being more commonly located on the temporal side of the ONH. Interestingly, in this study, the number of temporal LC defects was associated with paracentral VF scotoma, whereas the number of inferior and superior LC defects was associated with the presence of superior and inferior VF defects [55].

Similarly, Han et al. used EDI SD-OCT to classify LC defects in myopic eyes into LC holes that were defined as a localized discontinuity of the LC, or LC disinsertion type defects defined as a posteriorly displaced laminar insertion with a downward slope at the far periphery of the LC toward the neural canal wall. Moreover, they noted more LC defects in myopic eyes with glaucoma than without glaucoma (65.7% vs. 27.8%, $p < 0.001$). These disinsertion-type LC defects were associated with the presence of glaucoma, AXL, and disc tilt angle, and they were found at the γ- PPA zone ($R = 0.71$, $p < 0.001$), while the location of hole-type LC defects did not correlate with the location of the γ-zone PPA ($R = 0.07$, $p = 0.73$) [56]. Table 2 summarizes the qualitative and quantitative measurable ONH characteristics in myopic subjects.

Table 2. Measurable ONH characteristics in myopic subjects.

PPA area	- 0.35 mm^2 in AXL < 24 mm [18] - 0.65 mm^2 in AXL 24 to 27 mm [18] - 0.78 mm^2 in AXL > 27 mm [18] - 0.1 mm^2 increase in PPA area for every 14.93-μm decrease in MCT [18] - 0.1 mm^2 increase in PPA area for every 9.54-μm decrease in peripapillary CT [18] - Week correlation with RNFL (R = 0.417, p < 0.001) [19]

ONH Tilt	- Tilt angle 3.5° (1.2–11.2) [22]
	- Temporal tilt angle 3.60° (1.61–6.40°) [23]
	- Vertical tilt angle 0.00° (−1.03° to 1.62°) [23]
	- Tilt in myopic glaucoma vs. myopic 9.3 ± 6.3° vs. 6.2 ± 4.1° (p < 0.05) [24]
	- Tilt angle in myopic glaucoma during 3 years of follow-up 8.3 ± 3.8° vs. 7.0 ± 3.4 [25]
	- Tilt angle correlation with VF (r = −0.356, p < 0.001) [22]
	- Lower deviation of the VF in the superotemporal quadrant (−4.54 ± 3.16 dB) in myopic with tilted ONH [26]
	- Myopic tilted vs. non-tilted myopic [28]
	   ○ Disc area 1.91 ± 0.81 mm^2 vs. 1.63 ± 0.30 mm^2 (p < 0.05)
	   ○ Cup volume 0.53 ± 0.28 mm^2 vs. 0.33 ± 0.19 mm^2, (p < 0.05)
	   ○ CDR 0.76 ± 0.09 vs. 0.69 ± 0.11, (p < 0.05)
	   ○ Temporal RNFL 62.1 ± 9.0 μm vs. 71.0 ± 12.8 μm, (p < 0.001)
	   ○ GCIPL 72.2 ± 6.5 μm vs. 72.9 ± 5.4 μm, (p = 0.558)

ONH torsion	- Torsion angle 9.1 ± 7.4° AXL ≤ 25 mm [32] - Torsion angle 10.7 ± 9.1° AXL from 25 to 26 mm [32] - Torsion angle 11.5 ± 11.1° AXL ≥ 26 mm [32] - Torsion angle 34.4° (range 29.9 to 39.0) vs. 33.7° (range 27.6 to 39.9) in mild 24.8 mm (range 24.7 to 25.0) vs. high 26.8 mm (range 26.6 to 27.0) myopic eyes [33]

ONH pits	- 16.2% of high myopic eyes (AXL 30 ± 2 mm) [36]
	   ○ 34% localized in the outer border of the ONH
	   ○ 64% localized in the scleral crescent

PICC	- PICC in 3.6% of myopic eyes [40]
	   ○ Inferior disc border (85.7%)
	   ○ Multiple locations (9.4%)
	   ○ Superior disc borders (3.1%).
	- PICC in 4.9% of pathologic myopia eyes [35]
	- PICC in 16.9% of myopic eyes [41]
	- PICC mean width = 4.2 ± 2.3 h of the disc circumference [41]
	- PICC mean length = 1363 ± 384 μm [41]

PPRS	- PPRS 49.5% of high myopic eyes (AXL > 26.5) [44] - PPRS (71.7%) high myopic eyes with AXL > 26.5 mm [45] - PPRS presence was negatively associated with MCT (β = −18.30, p < 0.05) [47]
PP hols	- The incidence ranges between 14% and 31.4% [44,47–49] - 39.9% distributed in the inferior temporal arcade [49] - Related to staphyloma V and IX [49] - Found in 43.1% of eyes with macular retinoschisis [49] - Found in 80.0% of eyes with macular retinoschisis [44].
PP staphyloma	- 12.7% of eyes of subjects younger than 20 years with mean AXL of 27.9 mm [52] - 66.1% of eyes with mean AXL of 30 ± 2 mm [53] - 86.0% vs. 61.6% (p < 0.001) in eyes with macular retinoschisis vs. without macular retinoschisis [53] - Associated with PICC in 52.5% of the cases [51]

Table 2. *Cont.*

LC	• Present in 22.9% vs. 41.8% (*p* < 0.05) in high myopic vs. high myopic with glaucoma [54] • Present in 27.8% vs. 65.7% (*p* < 0.001) in high myopic vs. high myopic with glaucoma [56] • 79.5% of patients with LC defects had corresponding damage in VF [54] • The number of LC defects with a diameter > 100 μm: 3.8 vs. 0.8 in myopic eyes with vs. without glaucoma [55] • The number of large pores with a diameter of 60 to 100 μm: 1.9 vs. 1.6 in myopic eyes with vs. without glaucoma [55] • Disinsertion-type LC defects were associated with glaucoma, AXL, and disc tilt angle (R = 0.71, *p* < 0.001) [56]

ONH: optic nerve head; PPA: peripapillary atrophy; AXL: Axial length; MCT: macular choroidal thickness; CT: choroidal thickness; RNFL: retinal nerve fiber layer; VF: visual field; CDR: cup to disc ratio; GCIPL: macular ganglion cell-inner plexiform layer; PP: peripapillary; PPIC: peripapillary intrachoroidal cavitation; PPRS: peripapillary retinoschisis; LC: lamina cribrosa.

10. RNFL Measurement in Myopic Eyes: Anatomy

As the AXL increases, the retina is shifted temporally, resulting in the thickening of the RNFL in the temporal quadrant and its thinning in the other quadrants, especially the nasal [57]. In the superior-temporal region, the RNFL trajectories are associated with the course of the retinal vessels, while in the inferior-temporal region, they are associated with the course of the retinal vessels and disc torsion. This implies that, in 7.5% of the myopes, the RNFL raphe rotated enough to produce a false nasal step in the VF and is, generally, in poor agreement with the ISNT rule (67% in high myopes vs. 8% in emmetropes) [8]. In a population-based study of 5387 participants, Wagner et al. described that the angle between the peaks of the peripapillary RNFL in the upper and lower hemispheres decreased by, $-5.86°$ with a 1 mm increase in AXL [58].

11. Factors Affecting RNFL Measurement

The peripapillary RNFL thickness measurement is one the most useful parameters to distinguish abnormal eyes in multiple ocular diseases. Measuring the RNFL thickness in myopic eyes is challenging as many factors may affect the measurements. Segmentation errors may occur due to incorrect delineation of the retinal layers, reaching up to 46.3% of the OCT scans [59]. Such artifacts are especially likely to occur in high myopia due to the anatomical features of the myopic ONH, such as extensive PPA, that makes RNFL recognition difficult, or due to the presence of intraretinal cyst-like anomalies that generate a false thickening of the RNFL [60]. Suwan et al. observed that manual correction was necessary for 32% vs. 56% of RNFL OCT scans of myopic eyes and myopic eyes with glaucoma, respectively ($p < 0.001$). Additionally, they showed that the glaucoma diagnostic capability of the global RNFL increased significantly after this correction, increasing the areas under the curve (AORUC) from 0.827 to 0.886 ($p = 0.017$) [61].

In addition, most commercial OCT devices do not include a database of highly myopic patients, which leads to false out-of-normal limit results when compared with healthy subject databases. In a study conducted on 193 healthy myopic eyes, 52 (26.9%) of the subjects showed at least one false positive red sign ($p > 0.001$) on the RNFL thickness map when comparing the measurements with the non-myopic data. This percentage increased to 62.8% in the case of high myopia (AXL > 26 mm) [60]. Seol et al., in a comparative validity study, implemented a myopic database to improve the Cirrus SD-OCT (Cirrus SD-OCT Carl Zeiss Meditec Inc) diagnostic ability in myopic glaucoma. The myopic normative database showed a higher specificity than the built-in normative database according to the quadrant RNFL thickness, clock-hour RNFL thickness, and GCIPL thickness (71% vs. 91%, 53% vs. 81%, and 66% vs. 91%, respectively; all $p < 0.001$) [62].

Similarly, the mean RNFL thickness may be affected by the magnification due to an increased AXL. This is because OCT devices have been configured to measure the RNFL thickness at a fixed angular distance, centered on the ONH, leading to a larger measuring circle when the AXL increases [63].

A large myopic optic disc may overestimate the RNFL thickness due to a shorter distance from the OCT scanning circle to the disc margin as the RNFL thickness becomes thinner with the increasing distance from the disc margin. Seo et al., using a Cirrus HD-OCT in 168 young myopic subjects, found that the average OCT RNFL thickness increased significantly with the optic disc area (5.35 µm/mm^2, $p < 0.001$), while there was no significant correlation between the average GCIPL thickness and the ONH area [64].

A high optic disc tilt angle in myopic subjects may cause errors in the examination of the peripapillary area due to the difficulty in delaminating the center of the optic disc and the center of the opening of the BM, both being centers usually used to perform the RNFL thickness calculation. Additionally, eyes with optic tilt tend to have a thicker temporal RNFL thickness due to retina convergence towards the macular region [65]. Moghadas Sharif et al. found a significantly thicker temporal RNFL thickness in highly myopic subjects (AXL > 26 mm) with tilted ONH vs. no tilted ONH (29 µm vs. 25 µm $p = 0.004$) [29], while no significant differences were demonstrated in the average RNFL thickness between the tilted and non-tilted ONH [29,66] Finally, the presence of peripapillary detachment in pathologic myopia may lead to a misidentification of the outer profile of the RNFL. Kamal Salah et al. observed a thicker global RNFL thickness in myopic subjects with and without peripapillary detachment (88.2 ± 25 µm vs. 72.7 ± 16 µm, $p = 0.001$) [67].

12. RNFL Thickness Measurement by OCT

The mean RNFL thickness is usually reduced in highly myopic patients compared to emmetropic patients (89.8 ± 9 µm vs. 110.9 ± 10 µm, respectively, $p > 0.001$) [68]. Therefore, the RNFL thickness is negatively correlated with the AXL. Singh et al. and Kang et al. found that the mean RNFL thickness decreased by 3.74 µm and 2.2 µm, respectively, for each mm increase in the AXL [69,70] Additionally, this thinning of the RNFL in highly myopic eyes is not uniformly distributed, being greater in the lower quadrant (134.8 ± 17 µm vs. 109.9 ± 15 µm, $p > 0.001$) in emmetropes vs. high myopes, respectively. It has also been observed that myopic eyes have a significantly greater rate of decline in RNFL during follow-up than controls. In subjects between 30 and 39 years old, Lee et al. observed that the RNFL loss was 0.95 µm/year vs. 0.57 µm/year in myopic vs. healthy subjects; 1.69 µm/year vs. 0.48 µm/year in myopic vs. healthy subjects aged 40 to 49, and the loss rate was 1.70 µm/year vs. 0.63 µm/year in myopic vs. healthy subjects in the group from 50 to 59 years [71]. Similarly, myopic subjects with glaucoma have a higher rate of RNFL loss than non-myopic glaucoma subjects. Biswas et al. found that, during follow-up (>60 months), myopic eyes with AXL ≥ 26.0 and ≥26.5 mm had an average rate loss in RNFL thickness of 0.15 and 0.16 µm/year, faster than eyes with AXL < 26 and 26.5 mm, respectively [72].

Taking into account all of the aforementioned factors, the peripapillary RNFL thickness should be used with caution to distinguish healthy from glaucoma highly myopic subjects. Seo et al. showed that the best RNFL sectors for diagnosing glaucoma in patients with high myopia were the temporal-inferior sector and the inferior quadrant (AUROC were 0.974 and 0.951, respectively) [64]. Similarly, Rolle et al., using Fourier-Domain-OCT (FD-OCT RTVue-100; Optovue, Fremont, CA, USA), found that the average RNFL yielded the best diagnostic ability for the diagnosis of glaucoma in patients with AXL > 25 mm, followed by the superior and inferior RNFL, reaching AUROC of 0.883, 0.858, and 0.872, respectively [73]. As the macular parameters are not significantly affected by high myopia, recent studies have established that the macular ganglion cells' layer thickness has higher diagnostic power and progression analysis than the peripapillary RNFL thickness in high myopia [74–76], the inferotemporal macular GCIPL thickness being the best parameter for myopic glaucoma discrimination [74].

13. Bruch's Membrane Opening-Minimum Rim Width

The Bruch's membrane opening-minimum rim width (BMO-MRW) represents the minimum distance between the BM opening and the internal limiting membrane (Figure 4). BMO-

MRW measurements may have higher accuracy in detecting glaucoma than RNFL [77,78]. Sastre-Ibañez et al. reported no correlation between the AXL and BMO-MRW in moderate myopic subjects. In this study, which used Spectralis SD-OCT and Glaucoma Premium Module Edition (GPME) software version 6.0c, they showed that the number of sectors classified as being outside of the normal limits was significantly lower compared to the RNFL analysis 0.2 ± 0.6 vs. 0.7 ± 1.1, respectively ($p = 0.023$) [79]. Wang et al. found that the BMO-MRW classified a significantly lower percentage of eyes as being outside the normal limits in at least one quadrant than the RNFL thickness (4% vs. 34.67%; $p < 0.01$) [80]. Similarly, Uzair et al. noted that the specificity was better with the OCT BMO-MRW (85.7%) than with the RNFL (66.7%). Moreover, they observed a higher agreement between the glaucoma expert classification and BMO-MRW based classification ($\kappa = 0.800$, $p < 0.001$), rather than the RNFL-based classification ($\kappa = 0.480$, $p < 0.001$), to identify subjects outside of the normal limits [81]. This indicated that BMO-MRW measurement reduced the false-positive rate caused by myopia. Table 3 summarizes the characteristics of the RNFL measurement in highly myopic subjects.

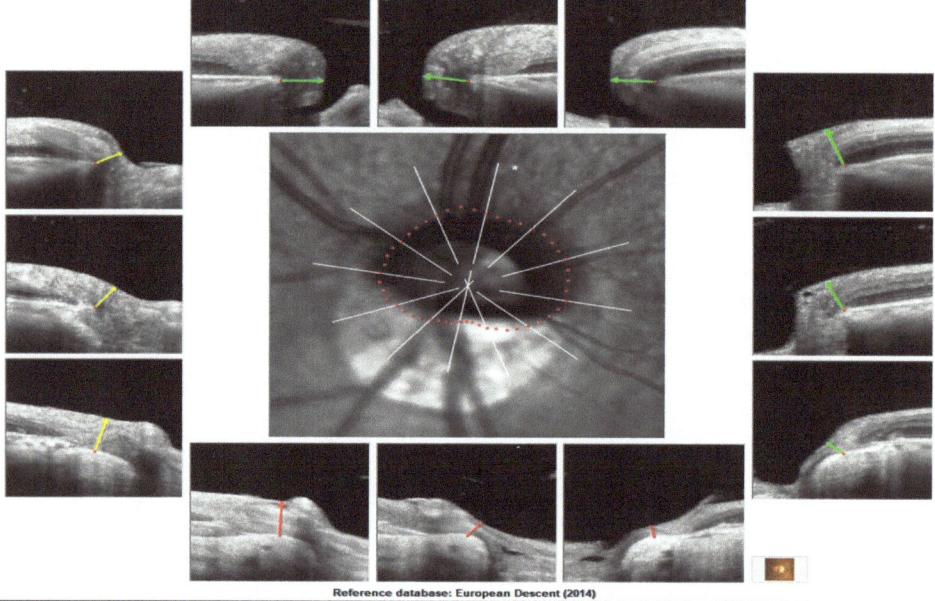

Figure 4. Bruch's membrane opening-minimum rim width (BMO-MRW) measurement in a high myopic patient. Green, yellow, and red lines represent the least distance between Bruch's membrane opening and the internal limiting membrane. Green, yellow, and red color of the lines represent the classification of BMO-MRW measurement within normal limits, borderline and out of normal limits, respectively.

Table 3. Characteristics of RNFL measurement in highly myopic subjects.

- Segmentations errors up to 46.3% of the OCT scans [59].
- The manual correction was necessary for myopic eyes and myopic eyes with glaucoma in 32% vs. 56% ($p < 0.001$) of the RNFL scan [61].
- 26.9% of the subjects showed at least one false positive red sign on the RNFL thickness map based on non-myopic data [82].
- 62.8% of subjects with AXL > 26 mm showed at least one false positive red sign on the RNFL thickness map based on non-myopic data [82].
- RNFL specificity of glaucoma diagnosis: 71% vs. 91% ($p < 0.001$) myopic normative database vs. built-in normative database [62].

Table 3. *Cont.*

- RNFL thickness: 88.2 ± 25 µm vs. 72.7 ± 16 µm, ($p = 0.001$) in myopic subjects with and without peripapillary detachment [67].
- The mean RNFL thickness: 110.9 ± 10 µm vs. 89.8 ± 9 µm in highly myopic patients compared to emmetropic patients ($p < 0.001$) [69].
- RNFL thickness decreased by 3.74 µm for each mm of increase in AXL [69].
- RNFL thickness decreased by 2.2 µm for each mm of increase in AXL [70].
- Progressive thinning of RNFL in myopic vs. non-myopic subjects [71]
    - Aged 30 to 39 years old: 0.95 µm/year vs. 0.57 µm/year
    - Aged 40 to 49 years old: 1.69 µm/year vs. 0.48 µm/year
    - Aged 50 to 59 years old: 1.70 µm/year vs. 0.63 µm/year
- Best diagnostic ability of glaucoma in patients with high myopia [64]
    - Temporal-inferior sector: AUROC of 0.974
    - Inferior quadrant: AUROC of 0.951 [64]
- Best diagnostic ability of glaucoma in patients with AXL > 25 mm [73]
    - Average RNFL: AUROC of 0.883
    - Superior RNFL: AUROC of 0.858
    - Inferior RNFL: AUROC 0.872
- The number of sectors classified as outside of normal limits in BMO-MRW classification vs. RNFL classification 0.2 ± 0.6 vs. 0.7 ± 1.1 ($p = 0.023$) [79].
- Percentage of eyes as outside normal limits in BMO-MRW classification vs. RNFL classification: 4% vs. 34.67% ($p < 0.01$) [80].
- Specificity for glaucoma diagnosis in BMO-MRW classification vs. RNFL classification: 85.7% vs. 66.7% [81].
- No correlation between AXL and BMO-MRW in moderate myopic subjects [79].

RNFL: retinal nerve fibre layer; OCT: ocular coherence tomography; AXL; axial length; AUROC: area under the receiver operating characteristic; BMO-MRW: Bruch's membrane opening-minimum rim width.

14. Conclusions

The diagnosis of glaucoma and its severity by ONH imaging in highly myopic subjects is still a key challenge in clinical practice. In recent years, OCT has become the mainstay for ONH study, offering high-resolution images of the papillary and peripapillary region in highly myopic eyes. This imaging technique allows clinicians to describe the qualitative typical characteristics of the myopic ONH and quantify them with measurable parameters. A larger β-PPA area is associated with older age, a longer AXL, and thinner choroidal thickness. ONH tilt is more frequent in myopic eyes and is usually greater in myopic eyes with glaucoma, with a negative correlation with VF defects. Peripapillary intrachoroidal cavitation is associated with severe myopic maculopathy and the presence of posterior staphyloma. Myopic eyes with glaucoma have larger and more LC defects than eyes without glaucoma.

A correction of segmentations errors and the use of a myopic database should be considered to increase the ability of RNFL measurement to distinguish eyes outside of the normal range. Both the macular GCL and BMO-MRW may reduce the false-positive results caused by myopia and are promising parameters for the diagnosis of glaucoma. The OCT results were obtained from transversal or retrospective studies with no comparative study samples. Therefore, future prospective studies with large samples are needed to confirm the aforementioned findings. It will be interesting to have a standard scanning protocol in the future to explore ONH in myopic eyes.

Author Contributions: Conceptualization, B.K. and J.I.F.-V.; Methodology, B.K., J.I.F.-V., M.G.-Z. and J.R.-M.; Writing—Original Draft Preparation, B.K., J.I.F.-V, M.S. and I.F.-M.; Writing—Review & Editing, B.K., J.I.F.-V and M.G.-Z.; Visualization, M.G.-Z., I.F.-M. and J.R.-M.; Supervision, B.K., M.S. and J.M.R.-M. All authors have read and agreed to the published version of the manuscript.

Funding: This research received no external funding.

Institutional Review Board Statement: Not applicable.

Informed Consent Statement: Not applicable.

Data Availability Statement: Not applicable.

Conflicts of Interest: The authors declare no conflict of interest.

References

1. Mitchell, P.; Hourihan, F.; Sandbach, J.; Wang, J.J. The relationship between glaucoma and myopia. *Ophthalmology* **1999**, *106*, 2010–2015. [CrossRef] [PubMed]
2. Xu, L.; Wang, Y.; Wang, S.; Wang, Y.; Jonas, J.B. High Myopia and Glaucoma Susceptibility. *Ophthalmology* **2007**, *114*, 216–220. [CrossRef] [PubMed]
3. Ha, A.; Kim, C.Y.; Shim, S.R.; Chang, I.B.; Kim, Y.K. Degree of Myopia and Glaucoma Risk: A Dose-Response Meta-analysis. *Am. J. Ophthalmol.* **2022**, *236*, 107–119. [CrossRef]
4. Tan, N.Y.Q.; Sng, C.C.A.; Jonas, J.B.; Wong, T.Y.; Jansonius, N.M.; Ang, M. Glaucoma in myopia: Diagnostic dilemmas. *Br. J. Ophthalmol.* **2019**, *103*, 1347–1355. [CrossRef] [PubMed]
5. Hood, D.C.; La Bruna, S.; Tsamis, E.; Thakoor, K.A.; Rai, A.; Leshno, A.; de Moraes, C.G.; Cioffi, G.A.; Liebmann, J.M. Detecting glaucoma with only OCT: Implications for the clinic, research, screening, and AI development. *Prog. Retin. Eye Res.* **2022**, *90*, 101052. [CrossRef] [PubMed]
6. Jonas, J.B.; Panda-Jonas, S. The Optic Nerve Head in High Myopia/Abnormalities of the Intrapapillary and Parapapillary Region. In *Pathologic Myopia*; Springer International Publishing: Cham, Switzerland, 2021; pp. 167–176. [CrossRef]
7. Qiu, K.; Wang, G.; Lu, X.; Zhang, R.; Sun, L.; Zhang, M. Application of the ISNT rules on retinal nerve fibre layer thickness and neuroretinal rim area in healthy myopic eyes. *Acta Ophthalmol.* **2018**, *96*, 161–167. [CrossRef] [PubMed]
8. Bedggood, P.; Mukherjee, S.; Nguyen, B.N.; Turpin, A.; McKendrick, A.M. Geometry of the Retinal Nerve Fibers From Emmetropia Through to High Myopia at Both the Temporal Raphe and Optic Nerve. *Investig. Opthalmol. Vis. Sci.* **2019**, *60*, 4896. [CrossRef]
9. Qiu, K.; Zhang, M.; Wu, Z.; Nevalainen, J.; Schiefer, U.; Huang, Y.; Jansonius, N.M. Retinal nerve fiber bundle trajectories in Chinese myopic eyes: Comparison with a Caucasian based mathematical model. *Exp. Eye Res.* **2018**, *176*, 103–109. [CrossRef]
10. Chang, R.T.; Singh, K. Myopia and glaucoma. *Curr. Opin. Ophthalmol.* **2013**, *24*, 96–101. [CrossRef]
11. Akagi, T.; Hangai, M.; Kimura, Y.; Ikeda, H.O.; Nonaka, A.; Matsumoto, A.; Akiba, M.; Yoshimura, N. Peripapillary Scleral Deformation and Retinal Nerve Fiber Damage in High Myopia Assessed With Swept-Source Optical Coherence Tomography. *Am. J. Ophthalmol.* **2013**, *155*, 927–936.e1. [CrossRef]
12. Jonas, J.B.; Jonas, S.B.; Jonas, R.A.; Holbach, L.; Panda-Jonas, S. Histology of the Parapapillary Region in High Myopia. *Am. J. Ophthalmol.* **2011**, *152*, 1021–1029. [CrossRef] [PubMed]
13. Vianna, J.R.; Malik, R.; Danthurebandara, V.M.; Sharpe, G.P.; Belliveau, A.C.; Shuba, L.M.; Chauhan, B.C.; Nicolela, M.T. Beta and Gamma Peripapillary Atrophy in Myopic Eyes With and Without Glaucoma. *Investig. Opthalmol. Vis. Sci.* **2016**, *57*, 3103. [CrossRef]
14. Ha, A.; Kim, Y.W.; Lee, J.; Bak, E.; Han, Y.S.; Kim, Y.K.; Park, K.H.; Jeoung, J.W. Morphological characteristics of parapapillary atrophy and subsequent visual field progression in primary open-angle glaucoma. *Br. J. Ophthalmol.* **2021**, *105*, 361–366. [CrossRef] [PubMed]
15. Wang, Y.X.; Panda-Jonas, S.; Jonas, J.B. Optic nerve head anatomy in myopia and glaucoma, including parapapillary zones alpha, beta, gamma and delta: Histology and clinical features. *Prog. Retin. Eye Res.* **2021**, *83*, 100933. [CrossRef]
16. Sung, M.S.; Heo, H.; Piao, H.; Guo, Y.; Park, S.W. Parapapillary atrophy and changes in the optic nerve head and posterior pole in high myopia. *Sci. Rep.* **2020**, *10*, 4607. [CrossRef] [PubMed]
17. Chen, Q.; He, J.; Yin, Y.; Zhou, H.; Jiang, H.; Zhu, J.; Ohno-Matsui, K.; Zou, H.; Fan, Y.; Xu, X. Impact of the Morphologic Characteristics of Optic Disc on Choroidal Thickness in Young Myopic Patients. *Investig. Opthalmol. Vis. Sci.* **2019**, *60*, 2958. [CrossRef]
18. Hu, G.; Chen, Q.; Xu, X.; Lv, H.; Du, Y.; Wang, L.; Yin, Y.; Fan, Y.; Zou, H.; He, J.; et al. Morphological Characteristics of the Optic Nerve Head and Choroidal Thickness in High Myopia. *Investig. Opthalmol. Vis. Sci.* **2020**, *61*, 46. [CrossRef]
19. Zhang, F.; Liu, X.; Wang, Y.; Wang, Q.; Zheng, M.; Chang, F.; Mao, X. Characteristics of the optic disc in young people with high myopia. *BMC Ophthalmol.* **2022**, *22*, 477. [CrossRef]
20. Giuffrè, G. Chorioretinal degenerative changes in the tilted disc syndrome. *Int. Ophthalmol.* **1991**, *15*, 1–7. [CrossRef]
21. Vongphanit, J.; Mitchell, P.; Wang, J.J. Population prevalence of tilted optic disks and the relationship of this sign to refractive error. *Am. J. Ophthalmol.* **2002**, *133*, 679–685. [CrossRef]
22. Hosseini, H.; Nassiri, N.; Azarbod, P.; Giaconi, J.; Chou, T.; Caprioli, J.; Nouri-Mahdavi, K. Measurement of the Optic Disc Vertical Tilt Angle With Spectral-Domain Optical Coherence Tomography and Influencing Factors. *Am. J. Ophthalmol.* **2013**, *156*, 737–744.e1. [CrossRef]
23. Choi, J.A.; Park, H.-Y.L.; Shin, H.-Y.; Park, C.K. Optic Disc Tilt Direction Determines the Location of Initial Glaucomatous Damage. *Investig. Opthalmol. Vis. Sci.* **2014**, *55*, 4991. [CrossRef]
24. Park, H.-Y.L.; Choi, S.I.; Choi, J.-A.; Park, C.K. Disc Torsion and Vertical Disc Tilt Are Related to Subfoveal Scleral Thickness in Open-Angle Glaucoma Patients With Myopia. *Investig. Opthalmol. Vis. Sci.* **2015**, *56*, 4927. [CrossRef] [PubMed]
25. Yoon, J.Y.; Sung, K.R.; Yun, S.-C.; Shin, J.W. Progressive Optic Disc Tilt in Young Myopic Glaucomatous Eyes. *Korean J. Ophthalmol.* **2019**, *33*, 520. [CrossRef] [PubMed]
26. Shoeibi, N.; Moghadas Sharif, N.; Daneshvar, R.; Ehsaei, A. Visual field assessment in high myopia with and without tilted optic disc. *Clin. Exp. Optom.* **2017**, *100*, 690–694. [CrossRef]

27. Han, J.C.; Lee, E.J.; Kim, S.H.; Kee, C. Visual Field Progression Pattern Associated with Optic Disc Tilt Morphology in Myopic Open-Angle Glaucoma. *Am. J. Ophthalmol.* **2016**, *169*, 33–45. [CrossRef]
28. Shin, H.-Y.; Park, H.-Y.L.; Park, C.K. The effect of myopic optic disc tilt on measurement of spectral-domain optical coherence tomography parameters. *Br. J. Ophthalmol.* **2015**, *99*, 69–74. [CrossRef] [PubMed]
29. Moghadas Sharif, N.; Shoeibi, N.; Ehsaei, A.; Mallen, E.A.H. Optical Coherence Tomography and Biometry in High Myopia with Tilted Disc. *Optom. Vis. Sci.* **2016**, *93*, 1380–1386. [CrossRef]
30. How, A.C.S. Population Prevalence of Tilted and Torted Optic Discs Among an Adult Chinese Population in Singapore. *Arch. Ophthalmol.* **2009**, *127*, 894. [CrossRef] [PubMed]
31. Park, H.-Y.L.; Lee, K.-I.; Lee, K.; Shin, H.Y.; Park, C.K. Torsion of the Optic Nerve Head Is a Prominent Feature of Normal-Tension Glaucoma. *Investig. Ophthalmol. Vis. Sci.* **2015**, *56*, 156–163. [CrossRef]
32. Cheng, D.; Ruan, K.; Wu, M.; Qiao, Y.; Gao, W.; Lian, H.; Shen, M.; Bao, F.; Yang, Y.; Zhu, J.; et al. Characteristics of the Optic Nerve Head in Myopic Eyes Using Swept-Source Optical Coherence Tomography. *Investig. Opthalmol. Vis. Sci.* **2022**, *63*, 20. [CrossRef] [PubMed]
33. Rezapour, J.; Tran, A.Q.; Bowd, C.; El-Nimri, N.W.; Belghith, A.; Christopher, M.; Brye, N.; Proudfoot, J.A.; Dohleman, J.; Fazio, M.A.; et al. Comparison of Optic Disc Ovality Index and Rotation Angle Measurements in Myopic Eyes Using Photography and OCT Based Techniques. *Front. Med.* **2022**, *9*, 872658. [CrossRef] [PubMed]
34. Uzel, M.M.; Karacorlu, M. Optic disk pits and optic disk pit maculopathy: A review. *Surv. Ophthalmol.* **2019**, *64*, 595–607. [CrossRef] [PubMed]
35. Shimada, N.; Ohno-Matsui, K.; Nishimuta, A.; Tokoro, T.; Mochizuki, M. Peripapillary Changes Detected by Optical Coherence Tomography in Eyes with High Myopia. *Ophthalmology* **2007**, *114*, 2070–2076. [CrossRef]
36. Ohno-Matsui, K.; Akiba, M.; Moriyama, M.; Shimada, N.; Ishibashi, T.; Tokoro, T.; Spaide, R.F. Acquired Optic Nerve and Peripapillary Pits in Pathologic Myopia. *Ophthalmology* **2012**, *119*, 1685–1692. [CrossRef]
37. Freund, K.B. Peripapillary Detachment in Pathologic Myopia. *Arch. Ophthalmol.* **2003**, *121*, 197. [CrossRef] [PubMed]
38. Spaide, R.F.; Akiba, M.; Ohno-Matsui, K. Evaluation Of Peripapillary Intrachoroidal Cavitation With Swept Source and Enhanced Depth Imaging Optical Coherence Tomography. *Retina* **2012**, *32*, 1037–1044. [CrossRef]
39. Ehongo, A.; Bacq, N.; Kisma, N.; Dugauquier, A.; Alaoui Mhammedi, Y.; Coppens, K.; Bremer, F.; Leroy, K. Analysis of Peripapillary Intrachoroidal Cavitation and Myopic Peripapillary Distortions in Polar Regions by Optical Coherence Tomography. *Clin. Ophthalmol.* **2022**, *16*, 2617–2629. [CrossRef] [PubMed]
40. Liu, R.; Li, Z.; Xiao, O.; Zhang, J.; Guo, X.; Loong Lee, J.T.; Wang, D.; Lee, P.; Jong, M.; Sankaridurg, P.; et al. Characteristics of Peripapillary Intrachoroidal Cavitation in Highly Myopic Eyes. *Retina* **2021**, *41*, 1057–1062. [CrossRef] [PubMed]
41. You, Q.S.; Peng, X.Y.; Chen, C.X.; Xu, L.; Jonas, J.B. Peripapillary Intrachoroidal Cavitations. The Beijing Eye Study. *PLoS ONE* **2013**, *8*, e78743. [CrossRef]
42. Venkatesh, R.; Jain, K.; Aseem, A.; Kumar, S.; Yadav, N.K. Intrachoroidal cavitation in myopic eyes. *Int. Ophthalmol.* **2020**, *40*, 31–41. [CrossRef] [PubMed]
43. Ohno-Matsui, K.; Hayashi, K.; Tokoro, T.; Mochizuki, M. Detection of paravascular retinal cysts before using OCT in a highly myopic patient. *Graefe's Arch. Clin. Exp. Ophthalmol.* **2006**, *244*, 642–644. [CrossRef]
44. Shimada, N.; Ohno-Matsui, K.; Nishimuta, A.; Moriyama, M.; Yoshida, T.; Tokoro, T.; Mochizuki, M. Detection of Paravascular Lamellar Holes and Other Paravascular Abnormalities by Optical Coherence Tomography in Eyes with High Myopia. *Ophthalmology* **2008**, *115*, 708–717. [CrossRef]
45. Li, T.; Wang, X.; Zhou, Y.; Feng, T.; Xiao, M.; Wang, F.; Sun, X. Paravascular abnormalities observed by spectral domain optical coherence tomography are risk factors for retinoschisis in eyes with high myopia. *Acta Ophthalmol.* **2018**, *96*, e515–e523. [CrossRef] [PubMed]
46. Chebil, A.; Ben Achour, B.; Maamouri, R.; Ben Abdallah, M.; El Matri, L. Étude des anomalies péripapillaires en SD OCT dans la myopie forte. *J. Fr. Ophtalmol.* **2014**, *37*, 635–639. [CrossRef]
47. Li, M.; Ye, L.; Hu, G.; Chen, Q.; Sun, D.; Zou, H.; He, J.; Zhu, J.; Fan, Y.; Xu, X. Relationship Between Paravascular Abnormalities and Choroidal Thickness in Young Highly Myopic Adults. *Transl. Vis. Sci. Technol.* **2022**, *11*, 18. [CrossRef]
48. Kamal-Salah, R.; Morillo-Sanchez, M.J.; Rius-Diaz, F.; Garcia-Campos, J.M. Relationship between paravascular abnormalities and foveoschisis in highly myopic patients. *Eye* **2015**, *29*, 280–285. [CrossRef] [PubMed]
49. Vela, J.I.; Sánchez, F.; Díaz-Cascajosa, J.; Mingorance, E.; Andreu, D.; Buil, J.A. Incidence and distribution of paravascular lamellar holes and their relationship with macular retinoschisis in highly myopic eyes using spectral-domain oct. *Int. Ophthalmol.* **2016**, *36*, 247–252. [CrossRef]
50. Ohno-Matsui, K. Proposed Classification of Posterior Staphylomas Based on Analyses of Eye Shape by Three-Dimensional Magnetic Resonance Imaging and Wide-Field Fundus Imaging. *Ophthalmology* **2014**, *121*, 1798–1809. [CrossRef] [PubMed]
51. Shinohara, K.; Moriyama, M.; Shimada, N.; Yoshida, T.; Ohno-Matsui, K. Characteristics of Peripapillary Staphylomas Associated With High Myopia Determined by Swept-Source Optical Coherence Tomography. *Am. J. Ophthalmol.* **2016**, *169*, 138–144. [CrossRef] [PubMed]
52. Tanaka, N.; Shinohara, K.; Yokoi, T.; Uramoto, K.; Takahashi, H.; Onishi, Y.; Horie, S.; Yoshida, T.; Ohno-Matsui, K. Posterior staphylomas and scleral curvature in highly myopic children and adolescents investigated by ultra-widefield optical coherence tomography. *PLoS ONE* **2019**, *14*, e0218107. [CrossRef] [PubMed]

53. Shinohara, K.; Tanaka, N.; Jonas, J.B.; Shimada, N.; Moriyama, M.; Yoshida, T.; Ohno-Matsui, K. Ultrawide-Field OCT to Investigate Relationships between Myopic Macular Retinoschisis and Posterior Staphyloma. *Ophthalmology* **2018**, *125*, 1575–1586. [CrossRef]
54. Miki, A.; Ikuno, Y.; Asai, T.; Usui, S.; Nishida, K. Defects of the Lamina Cribrosa in High Myopia and Glaucoma. *PLoS ONE* **2015**, *10*, e0137909. [CrossRef] [PubMed]
55. Sawada, Y.; Araie, M.; Ishikawa, M.; Yoshitomi, T. Multiple Temporal Lamina Cribrosa Defects in Myopic Eyes with Glaucoma and Their Association with Visual Field Defects. *Ophthalmology* **2017**, *124*, 1600–1611. [CrossRef] [PubMed]
56. Han, J.C.; Cho, S.H.; Sohn, D.Y.; Kee, C. The Characteristics of Lamina Cribrosa Defects in Myopic Eyes With and Without Open-Angle Glaucoma. *Investig. Opthalmol. Vis. Sci.* **2016**, *57*, 486. [CrossRef] [PubMed]
57. Fan, Y.Y.; Jonas, J.B.; Wang, Y.X.; Chen, C.X.; Wei, W. Bin Horizontal and vertical optic disc rotation. The Beijing Eye Study. *PLoS ONE* **2017**, *12*, e0175749. [CrossRef] [PubMed]
58. Wagner, F.M.; Hoffmann, E.M.; Nickels, S.; Fiess, A.; Münzel, T.; Wild, P.S.; Beutel, M.E.; Schmidtmann, I.; Lackner, K.J.; Pfeiffer, N.; et al. Peripapillary Retinal Nerve Fiber Layer Profile in Relation to Refractive Error and Axial Length: Results From the Gutenberg Health Study. *Transl. Vis. Sci. Technol.* **2020**, *9*, 35. [CrossRef]
59. Liu, Y.; Simavli, H.; Que, C.J.; Rizzo, J.L.; Tsikata, E.; Maurer, R.; Chen, T.C. Patient Characteristics Associated With Artifacts in Spectralis Optical Coherence Tomography Imaging of the Retinal Nerve Fiber Layer in Glaucoma. *Am. J. Ophthalmol.* **2015**, *159*, 565–576.e2. [CrossRef]
60. Kim, Y.W.; Park, K.H. Diagnostic Accuracy of Three-Dimensional Neuroretinal Rim Thickness for Differentiation of Myopic Glaucoma From Myopia. *Investig. Opthalmol. Vis. Sci.* **2018**, *59*, 3655. [CrossRef]
61. Suwan, Y.; Rettig, S.; Park, S.C.; Tantraworasin, A.; Geyman, L.S.; Effert, K.; Silva, L.; Jarukasetphorn, R.; Ritch, R. Effects of Circumpapillary Retinal Nerve Fiber Layer Segmentation Error Correction on Glaucoma Diagnosis in Myopic Eyes. *J. Glaucoma* **2018**, *27*, 971–975. [CrossRef]
62. Seol, B.R.; Kim, D.M.; Park, K.H.; Jeoung, J.W. Assessment of Optical Coherence Tomography Color Probability Codes in Myopic Glaucoma Eyes After Applying a Myopic Normative Database. *Am. J. Ophthalmol.* **2017**, *183*, 147–155. [CrossRef]
63. Budenz, D.L.; Anderson, D.R.; Varma, R.; Schuman, J.; Cantor, L.; Savell, J.; Greenfield, D.S.; Patella, V.M.; Quigley, H.A.; Tielsch, J. Determinants of Normal Retinal Nerve Fiber Layer Thickness Measured by Stratus OCT. *Ophthalmology* **2007**, *114*, 1046–1052. [CrossRef]
64. Seo, S.; Lee, C.E.; Jeong, J.H.; Park, K.H.; Kim, D.M.; Jeoung, J.W. Ganglion cell-inner plexiform layer and retinal nerve fiber layer thickness according to myopia and optic disc area: A quantitative and three-dimensional analysis. *BMC Ophthalmol.* **2017**, *17*, 22. [CrossRef] [PubMed]
65. Hwang, Y.H.; Yoo, C.; Kim, Y.Y. Myopic Optic Disc Tilt and the Characteristics of Peripapillary Retinal Nerve Fiber Layer Thickness Measured by Spectral-domain Optical Coherence Tomography. *J. Glaucoma* **2012**, *21*, 260–265. [CrossRef]
66. Lee, J.E.; Sung, K.R.; Park, J.M.; Yoon, J.Y.; Kang, S.Y.; Park, S.B.; Koo, H.J. Optic disc and peripapillary retinal nerve fiber layer characteristics associated with glaucomatous optic disc in young myopia. *Graefe's Arch. Clin. Exp. Ophthalmol.* **2017**, *255*, 591–598. [CrossRef] [PubMed]
67. Kamal Salah, R.; Morillo-Sánchez, M.J.; García-Ben, A.; Rius-Diaz, F.; Cilveti-Puche, Á.; Figueroa-Ortiz, L.; García-Campos, J.M. The Effect of Peripapillary Detachment on Retinal Nerve Fiber Layer Measurement by Spectral Domain Optical Coherence Tomography in High Myopia. *Ophthalmologica* **2015**, *233*, 209–215. [CrossRef] [PubMed]
68. Tai, E.L.M.; Ling, J.L.; Gan, E.H.; Adil, H.; Wan-Hazabbah, W.H. Comparison of peripapillary retinal nerve fiber layer thickness between myopia severity groups and controls. *Int. J. Ophthalmol.* **2018**, *11*, 274–278. [CrossRef] [PubMed]
69. Sharma, R.; Singh, D.; Agarwal, E.; Mishra, S.K.; Dada, T. Assessment of Retinal Nerve Fiber Layer Changes by Cirrus High-definition Optical Coherence Tomography in Myopia. *J. Curr. Glaucoma Pract.* **2017**, *11*, 52–57. [CrossRef] [PubMed]
70. Kang, S.H.; Hong, S.W.; Im, S.K.; Lee, S.H.; Ahn, M.D. Effect of Myopia on the Thickness of the Retinal Nerve Fiber Layer Measured by Cirrus HD Optical Coherence Tomography. *Investig. Opthalmol. Vis. Sci.* **2010**, *51*, 4075. [CrossRef]
71. Lee, M.-W.; Kim, J.; Shin, Y.-I.; Jo, Y.-J.; Kim, J.-Y. Longitudinal Changes in Peripapillary Retinal Nerve Fiber Layer Thickness in High Myopia. *Ophthalmology* **2019**, *126*, 522–528. [CrossRef]
72. Biswas, S.; Biswas, P. Longitudinal Evaluation of the Structural and Functional Changes Associated with Glaucoma in Myopia. *Optom. Vis. Sci.* **2020**, *97*, 448–456. [CrossRef]
73. Rolle, T.; Bonetti, B.; Mazzucco, A.; Dallorto, L. Diagnostic ability of OCT parameters and retinal ganglion cells count in identification of glaucoma in myopic preperimetric eyes. *BMC Ophthalmol.* **2020**, *20*, 373. [CrossRef] [PubMed]
74. Seol, B.R.; Jeoung, J.W.; Park, K.H. Glaucoma Detection Ability of Macular Ganglion Cell-Inner Plexiform Layer Thickness in Myopic Preperimetric Glaucoma. *Investig. Opthalmol. Vis. Sci.* **2015**, *56*, 8306. [CrossRef]
75. Shoji, T.; Sato, H.; Ishida, M.; Takeuchi, M.; Chihara, E. Assessment of Glaucomatous Changes in Subjects with High Myopia Using Spectral Domain Optical Coherence Tomography. *Investig. Opthalmol. Vis. Sci.* **2011**, *52*, 1098. [CrossRef] [PubMed]
76. Scuderi, G.; Fragiotta, S.; Scuderi, L.; Iodice, C.M.; Perdicchi, A. Ganglion Cell Complex Analysis in Glaucoma Patients: What Can It Tell Us? *Eye Brain* **2020**, *12*, 33–44. [CrossRef] [PubMed]
77. Reis, A.S.C.; O'Leary, N.; Yang, H.; Sharpe, G.P.; Nicolela, M.T.; Burgoyne, C.F.; Chauhan, B.C. Influence of Clinically Invisible, but Optical Coherence Tomography Detected, Optic Disc Margin Anatomy on Neuroretinal Rim Evaluation. *Investig. Opthalmol. Vis. Sci.* **2012**, *53*, 1852. [CrossRef] [PubMed]

78. Malik, R.; Belliveau, A.C.; Sharpe, G.P.; Shuba, L.M.; Chauhan, B.C.; Nicolela, M.T. Diagnostic Accuracy of Optical Coherence Tomography and Scanning Laser Tomography for Identifying Glaucoma in Myopic Eyes. *Ophthalmology* **2016**, *123*, 1181–1189. [CrossRef]
79. Sastre-Ibañez, M.; Martinez-de-la-Casa, J.M.; Rebolleda, G.; Cifuentes-Canorea, P.; Nieves-Moreno, M.; Morales-Fernandez, L.; Saenz-Frances, F.; Garcia-Feijoo, J. Utility of Bruch membrane opening-based optic nerve head parameters in myopic subjects. *Eur. J. Ophthalmol.* **2018**, *28*, 42–46. [CrossRef] [PubMed]
80. Wang, G.; Zhen, M.; Liu, S.; Qiu, K.; Liu, C.; Wang, J.; Zhang, M. Diagnostic Classification of Bruch's Membrane Opening-Minimum Rim Width and Retinal Nerve Fiber Layer Thickness in Myopic Eyes by Optical Coherence Tomography. *Front. Med.* **2021**, *8*, 729523. [CrossRef]
81. Uzair, N.; Shamim, M.; Mamoon, S.A.; Naz, S.; Feroz, L.; Kumari, K. Comparison of retinal nerve fibre layer versus bruch membrane opening-minimum rim width as an optical coherence tomography-based marker for glaucoma in myopia. *J. Coll. Physicians Surg. Pak.* **2021**, *31*, 162–165. [CrossRef]
82. Bak, E.; Lee, K.M.; Kim, M.; Oh, S.; Kim, S.H. Angular Location of Retinal Nerve Fiber Layer Defect: Association with Myopia and Open-Angle Glaucoma. *Investig. Opthalmol. Vis. Sci.* **2020**, *61*, 13. [CrossRef] [PubMed]

Disclaimer/Publisher's Note: The statements, opinions and data contained in all publications are solely those of the individual author(s) and contributor(s) and not of MDPI and/or the editor(s). MDPI and/or the editor(s) disclaim responsibility for any injury to people or property resulting from any ideas, methods, instructions or products referred to in the content.

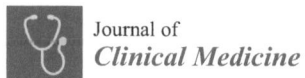

Article

Assessment by Optical Coherence Tomography of Short-Term Changes in IOP-Related Structures Caused by Wearing Scleral Lenses

Juan Queiruga-Piñeiro [1,2,*], Alberto Barros [1,2], Javier Lozano-Sanroma [1,2], Andrés Fernández-Vega Cueto [1,2,3], Ignacio Rodríguez-Uña [1,2,3,*] and Jesús Merayo-LLoves [1,2,3]

1. Instituto Universitario Fernández-Vega, Fundación de Investigación Oftalmológica, Universidad de Oviedo, 33012 Oviedo, Spain; alberto.barros@fernandez-vega.com (A.B.); javilo@fernandez-vega.com (J.L.-S.); afvc@fernandez-vega.com (A.F.-V.C.); merayo@fio.as (J.M.-L.)
2. Instituto de Investigación Sanitaria del Principado de Asturias (ISPA), 33011 Oviedo, Spain
3. Department of Surgery and Medical-Surgical Specialities, Universidad de Oviedo, 33006 Oviedo, Spain
* Correspondence: juan.queiruga@fernandez-vega.com (J.Q.-P.); irodriguezu@fernandez-vega.com (I.R.-U.); Tel.: +34-985240-141 (J.Q.-P. & I.R.-U.)

Abstract: Background: The mechanism that could increase intraocular pressure (IOP) during scleral lens (SL) wear is not fully understood, although it may be related to compression of the landing zone on structures involved in aqueous humor drainage. Methods: Thirty healthy subjects were fitted with two SLs of different sizes (L1 = 15.8 mm, L2 = 16.8 mm) for 2 h in the right eye and left eye as a control. Central corneal thickness (CCT), parameters of iridocorneal angle (ICA), Schlemm's canal (SC), and optic nerve head were measured before and after wearing both SLs. IOP was measured with a Perkins applanation tonometer before and after lens removal and with a transpalpebral tonometer before, during (0 h, 1 h, and 2 h), and after lens wear. Results: CCT increased after wearing L1 (8.10 ± 4.21 µm; $p < 0.01$) and L2 (9.17 ± 4.41 µm; $p < 0.01$). After L1 removal, the ICA parameters decreased significantly ($p < 0.05$). With L2 removal, nasal and temporal SC area and length were reduced ($p < 0.05$). An increased IOP with transpalpebral tonometry was observed at 2 h of wearing L1 (2.55 ± 2.04 mmHg; $p < 0.01$) and L2 (2.53 ± 2.22 mmHg; $p < 0.01$), as well as an increased IOP with Perkins applanation tonometry after wearing L1 (0.43 ± 1.07 mmHg; $p = 0.02$). Conclusions: In the short term, SL resulted in a slight increase in IOP in addition to small changes in ICA and SC parameters, although it did not seem to be clinically relevant in healthy subjects.

Keywords: scleral lenses; intraocular pressure; iridocorneal angle; Schlemm's canal; optic nerve head; optical coherence tomography; transpalpebral tonometry; Perkins applanation tonometry

Citation: Queiruga-Piñeiro, J.; Barros, A.; Lozano-Sanroma, J.; Fernández-Vega Cueto, A.; Rodríguez-Uña, I.; Merayo-LLoves, J. Assessment by Optical Coherence Tomography of Short-Term Changes in IOP-Related Structures Caused by Wearing Scleral Lenses. *J. Clin. Med.* **2023**, *12*, 4792. https://doi.org/10.3390/jcm12144792

Academic Editor: José Ignacio Fernández-Vigo

Received: 21 June 2023
Revised: 12 July 2023
Accepted: 18 July 2023
Published: 20 July 2023

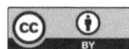

Copyright: © 2023 by the authors. Licensee MDPI, Basel, Switzerland. This article is an open access article distributed under the terms and conditions of the Creative Commons Attribution (CC BY) license (https://creativecommons.org/licenses/by/4.0/).

1. Introduction

Multiple studies demonstrated an increase in intraocular pressure (IOP) with scleral lens (SL) wear [1–6]. This increase varies according to the tonometer used [2,3,6] and the wearing time [1,2,6,7]. The transpalpebral tonometer (TT) is one of the few tonometers designed to perform IOP measurements with SLs in situ [1,2,4,8]. The largest increases in IOP, between 4.4 and 5.5 mmHg, have been obtained with this instrument during the wearing of SLs [1,2], but it has shown poor agreement with Goldmann applanation tonometry (GAT), considered the gold standard [9–11]. The GAT has also observed a slight increase in IOP after lens removal, around 1 mmHg, because measurements cannot be made during SL wear [4,6]. The pneumotonometer presents a good correlation between corneal and scleral IOP measurements in healthy subjects [12,13], so it has also been used to measure IOP during SL wear [2,14]. Nau et al. [14] reported that scleral IOP measurements made while wearing SLs were not accurate and, similar to Fogt et al. [2], observed that scleral IOP was approximately 6 mmHg higher than corneal IOP. Similarly, scleral IOP measurement with the rebound tonometer during SL wearing showed a poor correlation with corneal IOP [15]. These studies do not observe an increase in IOP during the wearing of SLs; however, they measure IOP at the sclera with tonometers that are calibrated to obtain corneal measurements [2,14,15].

Suction forces have been mentioned as one of the possible reasons for the increase in IOP [3,16,17]. This elevation would be caused by the loss of FR during the settling of the SL, which would increase the subatmospheric pressure under the lens; however, this is unlikely to occur [18]. Furthermore, studies evaluating suction forces during lens wear rule out their presence [5,19]. Another possibility is that the compression produced by the support SL area on the episcleral veins and adjacent structures, such as the iridocorneal angle (ICA) or Schlemm's canal (SC), increases resistance to aqueous humor outflow [18,20]. The use of a SL with a larger diameter could decrease compression by distributing the weight over a wider bearing surface [14,21], compared to a smaller diameter lens, in which a greater displacement of intraocular fluid due to tangential flattening could increase IOP [14]. Larger diameter SLs [16,22] and lens fittings with a lower initial fluid reservoir (FR) in the central zone [16] were found to produce less settling. However, the validity of this hypothesis remains questionable, as several studies have not found a relationship between IOP and compression produced by SLs of different diameters [1,2].

SLs overlie several structures on which they can produce morphologic changes, including the cornea; lens wear longer than eight hours induced an incidence of oedema of about two percent [16,23–25], due to the central lens thickness and FR that make oxygen flow difficult [26]. However, this oedema is lower in incidence than the physiological oedema by around four percent, which occurs during sleep [24]. Studies that have analyzed the changes produced by SLs in the trabecular iris angle (TIA) have found no changes over four hours of wear [27] or after lens removal [1,27]. In the landing zone, the greatest compression occurs in the adjacent conjunctival/episcleral tissue, while in the scleral tissue, this compression is less than two percent [28]. Despite the fact that the changes in this tissue are small, the impact that SLs have on the SC has not been studied.

The optic nerve head has also been analyzed, searching for possible changes resulting from IOP increases after the use of SLs [8,29]. The Bruch's membrane opening relative to the minimum ring amplitude (BMO-MRW), measured by OCT, is a parameter able to detect these changes with a robustness and sensitivity similar to the retinal nerve fiber layer (RNFL) analysis [30]. However, the results obtained are controversial; while some studies found a reduction in this parameter during six hours of SL wear [29], others did not find changes in the same time frame or after SL removal, as well as no relationship between BMO-MRW and IOP [8].

Previous studies have separately assessed the changes produced by SLs either in the different anterior segment structures or in IOP. The aim of this work was to evaluate, in a comprehensive and combined way, the short-term changes produced by SLs in the cornea, ICA, and SC structures and measurements with AS-OCT, as well as in IOP, including the structural parameters of the optic nerve head with OCT.

2. Materials and Methods

This longitudinal, prospective study was conducted in accordance with the Declaration of Helsinki and was approved by the Research Ethics Committee of the Principado de Asturias (protocol number 2020.490). All participants signed the informed consent form explaining the nature and objectives of the study. Thirty healthy subjects were recruited for this study. They underwent a complete ophthalmologic examination, including a detailed anamnesis, visual acuity, retinoscopy, noncycloplejic automated refraction, biomicroscopic examination of the anterior segment, fundus examination with a 90 D lens, Posner lens gonioscopy, Perkins applanation tonometry (PAT), and corneal topography. Exclusion criteria were previous refractive surgery, family history of glaucoma, medication that produces an increase in IOP (corticosteroids, anxiolytics, antidepressants, etc., cup/disc ratio > 0.5 or with eye-to-eye asymmetry > 0.2, refractive errors < -6 D, visible horizontal iris diameter

(HVID) > 12.30 mm, ICA $\leq$ grade 3 (Shaffer scale) [31], synechiae or pigmentation grade 3+ or greater (Spaeth scale) [32] measured by gonioscopy, IOP $\geq$ 21 mmHg, and SL users. All study subjects were advised to avoid drinking coffee or caffeinated beverages for at least 24 h before the assessment.

In the study protocol, prior to the screening process, it was determined that the right eye would be fitted with the SL (the study eye), while the left eye remained without a lens (the control eye). The order of measurements was also established. First, the optic nerve head and SC parameters were measured with the Optovue. Next, ICA and CCT parameters were measured with the CASIA2. Finally, IOP was measured first with the TT, which was the least invasive tonometer, and then with the PAT. A period of time was left between the measurements of both tonometers to avoid bias in the measurements.

2.1. Scleral Contact Lenses

A 15.8 mm diameter lens (L1) and a 16.8 mm diameter lens (L2) (Paflufocon B) (ICD Flexfit, Lenticon, Spain) were adapted from a trial box of 5 lenses of each diameter and 200 μm steps in sagittal height with a landing zone (steep +5). Lens fitting was performed according to the fitting guide provided by the manufacturer, starting from an initial fluid reservoir (FR) thickness between 250 and 400 μm (Figure 1). It was verified that the landing zone was aligned with the sclera in all patients and that there were no whitening and/or compression areas. All participants had the L1 inserted first. The investigator was instructed to exert minimal pressure during lens insertion and removal. Physiological saline 0.9% (Braun Medical S.A., Barcelona, Spain) was instilled into all lenses for application. The patient was instructed to avoid physical exertion and forced and prolonged palpebral closure during the 2 h of lens wear. A period of one week was left between the insertion of both SLs.

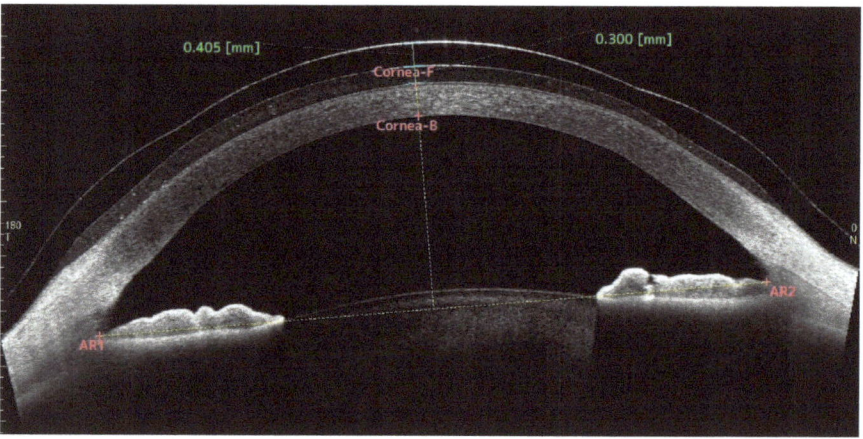

Figure 1. Lens thickness and fluid reservoir thickness measured with CASIA2 at the time of SL insertion (0 h).

2.2. Measurement of IOP

IOP measurements were performed with two tonometers. The Perkins MK2 (PAT) (Haag-Streig Holding, Harlow, UK) is a portable Goldmann applanation tonometer. It was used to test diurnal variations in IOP by taking 3 measurements in each eye between 08:00 and 10:00 a.m., as well as to measure IOP before insertion and after removal of the SL in the study eye and control eye. A drop of fluorescein sodium (2.5 mg) and oxybuprocaine hydrochloride (4 mg) (Colircusí Fluotest, Alcon Healthcare S.A., Barcelona, Spain) was instilled for measurements. The tonometer was calibrated every week, following the device's manual.

The Diaton transpalpebral tonometer (TT, Ryazan State Instrument-Making Enterprise, Ryazan, Russia) is based on a ballistic principle to determine IOP. It was used to measure IOP before insertion, during wear (0 h, 1 h, and 2 h), and after removal of the lens in the study eye and in the control eye. With the patients seated, they were asked to tilt their heads back and look straight ahead, forming a 45° angle with their line of gaze. Subsequently, the upper eyelid was slightly lifted, leaving the sclerocorneal limbus visible, and the tonometer was placed vertically to the eyelid, 1 mm behind the tarsus. When the device stops emitting sound, it means that it is ready to perform the measurement, which occurs automatically when the rod touches the eyelid. The tonometer takes several measurements and averages them.

2.3. Measurement of Iridocorneal Angle (ICA) and Schlemm Channel (SC) Parameters

The CASIA2 (Tomey, Nagoya, Japan) is a swept source OCT (SS-OCT) designed for anterior segment study (AS-OCT) that allows quantitative analysis of ICA and other anterior segment parameters. The ICA parameters measured were trabecular iris angle (TIA500), trabecular iris area (TISA500), angle opening distance (AOD500), and angle recess area (ARA500) at 500 µm from the scleral spur (SS) in the horizontal (0–180°) and vertical (90–270°) axes (Figure 2), in addition to the trabecular iris contact index (ITC index). Another parameter that was also measured was the central corneal thickness (CCT).

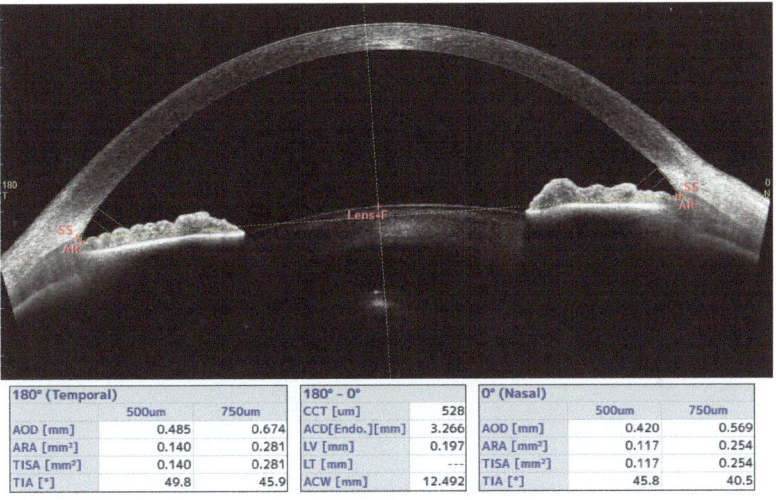

Figure 2. ICA parameters measured with CASIA2 in the horizontal axis (0–180°) before insertion of the SL.

All these measurements were performed before lens insertion and after lens removal in the study eye, except for CCT, which was also performed in the control eye. This device was also used to measure parameters related to SLs, such as sagittal ocular height (SAG-OC) in the horizontal (0–180°) and vertical (90–270°) axes before lens insertion, lens thickness in these axes at the time of insertion (0 h), and central FR thickness during wear (0 h, 1 h, and 2 h) in these same axes (Figure 1). Finally, the mean value of the central FR thickness and lens thickness obtained in both axes was calculated.

The Optovue RTVue 100 (Optovue, Fremont, CA, USA) is a spectral domain OCT (SD-OCT) incorporating CAM-L and CAM-S modules for anterior segment scanning. The CAM-S module, with a scan size of 2 mm × 2 mm, has higher resolution, so it was used to measure the length and area of the SC in the nasal and temporal regions. To perform the measurements in the same area, the patient was asked to maintain fixation on the central point shown by the device. At that time, the arrow shown by the device on the screen and indicating the location of the scan was placed above the limbus, leaving the same distance on both sides of the limbus, while the perpendicular straight line cutting the arrow was placed tangent to the limbus. The quality of the images was checked with the indicator provided by the device, and measurements were taken before insertion and after removal of the lens.

2.4. Measurement of Optic Nerve Head Parameters

The Optovue RTVue (Optovue, Fremont, CA, USA) was also used to analyze the optic nerve head by removing the CAM-S module. In addition, RNFL thickness, neuroretinal ring area (NRA), and neuroretinal ring volume (NRV) were measured in the study eye and control eye before and after removal of the SL.

2.5. Statistical Analysis

A sample size calculation was performed with statistical software Granmo version 7.12 (Institut Municipal d'investigacio' Mèdica; Barcelona, Spain), considering mean IOP as the main variable. A risk of $\alpha = 0.05$ and $\beta = 0.20$ was accepted in a bilateral test. Twenty-four subjects were necessary to detect a statistically significant difference greater than or equal to 3 mmHg with a standard deviation of 5 mmHg. A total of thirty-two subjects were recruited, and thirty finally completed all the tests. Statistical analysis was performed with SPSS® for Windows (version 22.0; SPSS Inc.; Chicago, IL, USA). Three measurements of all parameters were performed, and the mean was calculated.

The normality of the sample was assessed with the Saphiro–Wilk test. For the comparison of the mean values of the parameters studied before and after removing the lens and the correlation between the measurements, the repeated measures t-test and Pearson's correlation test were used, respectively. The Wilcoxon test and Spearman's correlation were applied when the sample did not have a normal distribution. Changes in all parameters analyzed were calculated as Δ equaling the mean value after lens removal minus the mean value before lens insertion. A multivariate linear regression model was employed to study the relationship between several variables. Intrasession repeatability of TT and PAT was calculated by within-subject standard deviation (Sw), which was used for within-subject precision (Sw $\times$ 1.96), repeatability (2.77 $\times$ Sw), and coefficient of variation (CV), defined as CV = Sw/mean $\times$ 100 [%]. The agreement in IOP measurements between the two tonometers was studied using Bland and Altman plots, where 95% of the difference or limits of agreement (LoA) were between 1.96 and the standard deviation (SD) of the mean difference. The degree of statistical significance was $p < 0.05$.

3. Results

Thirty-two subjects who visited the Instituto Oftalmológico Fernández-Vega between June 2021 and May 2022 participated in this study. Two of them did not complete the protocol because, at the end of the period wearing the first lens, they decided to drop out voluntarily. The descriptive characteristics of the sample are shown in Table 1.

Table 1. Sample descriptive characteristics.

Characteristics	Value
Participants (n)	30
Sex (male/female)	14/16
CL wearers (yes/no)	11/19
Age (years)	28.97 ± 5.62
SAG-OC (0–180°) (µm)	3751.80 ± 194.09
SAG-OC (90–270°) (µm)	3758.47 ± 189.50
HVID (mm)	12.09 ± 0.16
SE (D)	−1.18 ± 1.39

CL = contact lenses; SAG-OC = sagittal ocular height; HVID = horizontal visible iris diameter; SE = spherical equivalent. Data are expressed as mean ± SD.

3.1. Scleral Contact Lenses

The mean sagittal depth was 3940.00 ± 167.33 µm with L1 and 3980.00 ± 198.96 µm with L2 ($p = 0.01$). The mean thicknesses of L1 (399.62 ± 45.21 µm) and L2 (399.85 ± 50.35 µm) were similar ($p = 0.89$).

3.2. Central Fluid Reservoir

The initial central FR with L1 was 355.08 ± 85.81 µm, and with L2 it was 352.50 ± 74.56 µm ($p = 0.89$). After 2 h of wearing the SL, the central FR with L1 was reduced by 137.50 ± 40.97 µm, and with L2 by 117.50 ± 41.81 µm ($p = 0.04$).

3.3. Central Corneal Thickness

The initial CCT was 537.53 ± 34.10 µm with L1 and 545.63 ± 33.70 µm with L2 ($p = 0.37$). After 2 h of wearing the SL, there was an increase in CCT with L1 with respect to the initial value of 8.10 ± 4.21 µm ($p < 0.01$), representing an increase of 1.50%. After L2 wearing, the CCT increased by 9.17 ± 4.41 µm ($p < 0.01$), which is equivalent to an increase in CCT of 1.71%.

In the control eye, no difference in initial CCT was observed with L1 (539.03 ± 28.04 µm) and with L2 (539.27 ± 23.61 µm) ($p = 0.42$). After 2 h, matching the removal of the SL in the study eye, the CCT did not undergo significant changes with L1 (−0.87 ± 6.53 µm) ($p = 0.46$) and L2 (0.70 ± 6.31 µm) ($p = 0.55$), representing a reduction of 0.16% and an increase of 0.13%, respectively. In the study eye and control eye, no differences were observed in the initial CCT with L1 ($p = 0.46$) and L2 ($p = 0.53$).

Using a multivariate linear regression model, it was tested whether the change in CCT in the study eye was related to lens thickness (LT) and initial FR (0 h), finding no relationship with the variables studied in L1 (constant = 2.32, LT = 0.02, FR = 0.00, $R^2 = 0.03$, $p = 0.66$) and L2 (constant = 2.96, LT = 0.02, FR = 0.00, $R^2 = 0.07$, $p = 0.38$).

3.4. Iridocorneal Angle and Schlemm's Canal Parameters

The ICA parameters (TIA500, TISA500, AOD500, and ARA500) in the axes 0–180° and 90–270° and the ITC analysis, as well as the SC (length and area of the SC in the nasal and temporal areas), showed no significant differences when comparing the values obtained before L1 and L2 insertion ($p > 0.05$). A decrease in ICA parameters was observed with L1 except in TISA500 and ARA500 (90–270°) (Figure 3) and in the ITC index. Similar to this parameter, no changes were observed with L2 (Table 2).

Table 2. Changes in ICA and SC parameters after wearing SLs.

		Before Lens (Mean ± SD)	After Lens (Mean ± SD)	Δ (Mean ± SD)	p
ICA parameters					
TIA500	L1	47.55 ± 14.19	44.80 ± 12.14	−2.72 ± 5.33	0.01 *
0–180° (°)	L2	47.90 ± 13.74	46.43 ± 14.17	−1.54 ± 4.86	0.09
TIA500	L1	46.71 ± 12.76	44.10 ± 12.50	−2.30 ± 5.26	0.02 *
90–270° (°)	L2	46.46 ± 12.75	44.86 ± 12.59	−1.60 ± 5.24	0.11
TISA500	L1	0.21 ± 0.08	0.20 ± 0.08	−0.02 ± 0.04	0.01 *
0–180° (mm²)	L2	0.21 ± 0.08	0.20 ± 0.08	−0.01 ± 0.03	0.38
TISA500	L1	0.20 ± 0.08	0.19 ± 0.07	−0.01 ± 0.03	0.06
90–270° (mm²)	L2	0.20 ± 0.07	0.19 ± 0.07	0.00 ± 0.04	0.43
AOD500	L1	0.61 ± 0.24	0.53 ± 0.24	−0.08 ± 0.12	<0.01 *
0–180° (mm)	L2	0.59 ± 0.24	0.56 ± 0.24	−0.03 ± 0.11	0.14
AOD500	L1	0.56 ± 0.23	0.49 ± 0.22	−0.07 ± 0.12	0.00 *
90–270° (mm)	L2	0.53 ± 0.18	0.52 ± 0.19	−0.01 ± 0.10	0.72
ARA500	L1	0.23 ± 0.09	0.22 ± 0.09	−0.02 ± 0.05	0.04 *
0–180° (mm²)	L2	0.22 ± 0.09	0.22 ± 0.08	−0.01 ± 0.04	0.47

Table 2. Cont.

		Before Lens (Mean ± SD)	After Lens (Mean ± SD)	Δ (Mean ± SD)	p
ARA500 90–270° (mm^2)	L1	0.21 ± 0.08	0.20 ± 0.08	−0.01 ± 0.04	0.09
	L2	0.21 ± 0.07	0.21 ± 0.07	−0.01 ± 0.04	0.61
ITC index (%)	L1	3.26 ± 9.00	4.53 ± 12.08	1.28 ± 4.53	0.19
	L2	2.62 ± 7.92	4.03 ± 9.83	1.52 ± 7.99	0.15
SC parameters					
SC Nasal Lenght (μm)	L1	260.56 ± 51.87	252.91 ± 43.05	−8.66 ± 50.57	0.36
	L2	261.51 ± 47.22	235.56 ± 37.96	−25.96 ± 46.60	0.01 *
SC Temp Lenght (μm)	L1	269.51 ± 54.99	261.56 ± 57.87	−7.96 ± 42.96	0.32
	L2	275.71 ± 54.22	249.21 ± 55.76	−26.50 ± 45.36	<0.01 *
SC Nasal Area (μm^2)	L1	5411.11 ± 1603.84	4977.78 ± 1637.52	−433.33 ± 1411.91	0.10
	L2	5777.78 ± 1967.81	4733.34 ± 1450.06	−1044.44 ± 1852.27	<0.01 *
SC Temp. Area (μm^2)	L1	6022.22 ± 1909.71	5111.11 ± 1749.29	−911.11 ± 1324.49	<0.01 *
	L2	5944.45 ± 1830.11	5088.89 ± 1623.42	−855.56 ± 1601.45	0.01 *

ICA = iridocorneal angle; TIA500 = trabecular iris angle; AOD500 = angle opening distance; ARA500 = angle recess area; TISA500 = iris-trabecular area; ITC = iris-trabecular contact; SC = Schlemm's channel; Δ = the difference between the values after and before lens wear (Negative values show a decrease and positive values an increase). The asterisk (*) in the table indicates significant differences ($p < 0.05$).

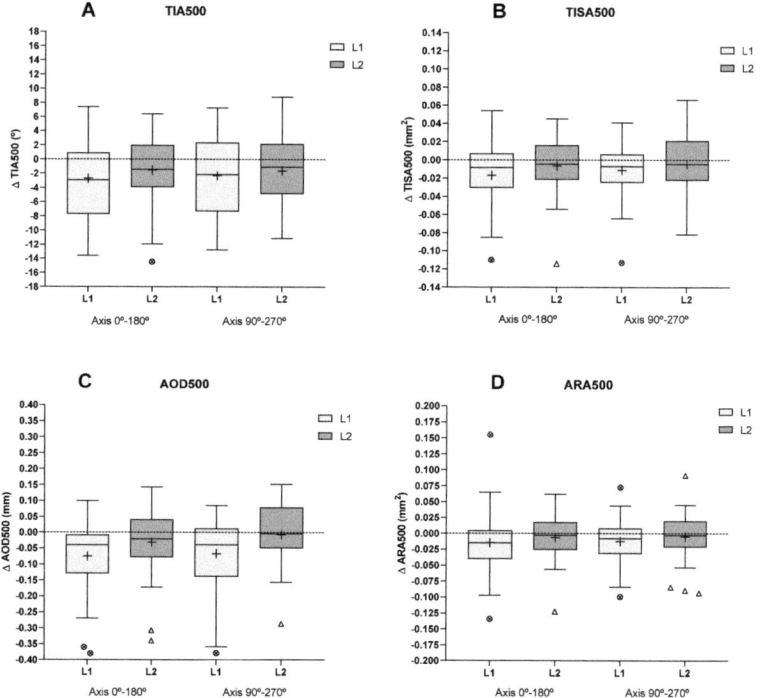

Figure 3. The box plot shows the change (Δ) in ICA parameters after L1 and L2 removals relative to pre-insertion values. (**A**) trabecular iris angle (TIA500); (**B**) trabecular iris area (TISA500); (**C**) angle opening distance (AOD500); (**D**) angle recess area (ARA500). The line inside the box represents the median, and the cross represents the mean. The lower and upper borders of the boxes represent the 25th and 75th percentiles, the lower and upper bars show the 10th and 90th percentiles, and the dots and triangles show the outliers for each lens. The dashed horizontal line indicates no change. Δ represents the difference between the values after and before lens wear (Negative values show a decrease and positive values an increase).

In contrast, SC area and length decreased in the nasal and temporal sectors after wearing L2. With L1, a decrease in SC area was only observed in the temporal sector (Table 2).

The relationship between changes in the ICA and SC parameters and changes in IOP with L1 and L2 in the study eye was studied. A positive correlation was observed between the Δ IOP PAT and the Δ ITC with L1 ($\rho = 0.44$, $p = 0.02$) and L2 ($\rho = 0.45$, $p = 0.01$). The rest of the results can be seen in Appendix A.

3.5. Intraocular Pressure (IOP)

In the study eye, no differences in IOP PAT were observed before L1 and L2 insertion ($p = 0.85$). Before L1 insertion, IOP PAT in the study eye and control eye were not different ($p = 0.75$). However, with L2, significant differences in IOP PAT were obtained ($p = 0.01$). In the study eye, after both lenses were removed, IOP increased, while in the control eye it decreased (Table 3).

Table 3. Measurement of IOP with the PAT before and after wearing SLs in the study eye and the control eye.

	Time	Study Eye (Right Eye)			Control Eye (Left Eye)		
		IOP (Mean ± SD)	Δ IOP (Mean ± SD)	p	IOP (Mean ± SD)	Δ IOP (Mean ± SD)	p
L1	BL	11.09 ± 1.66	-	-	11.14 ± 1.75	-	-
	AL	11.54 ± 2.82	0.46 ± 1.07	0.02 *	11.09 ± 1.66	−0.06 ± 0.77	0.87
L2	BL	11.02 ± 1.63	-	-	11.61 ± 1.79	-	-
	AL	11.25 ± 1.86	0.23 ± 1.16	0.44	11.29 ± 1.86	−0.32 ± 1.16	0.04 *

BL = before the lens; AL = after removing the lens. Δ = the difference between the values after and before lens wear (Negative values show a decrease and positive values an increase). The asterisk (*) in the table indicates significant differences ($p < 0.05$).

Before L1 insertion, IOP TT was different in the study eye and control eye ($p = 0.08$), while with L2, it was not different ($p = 0.44$). In the study eye, IOP TT was not different before L1 and L2 insertion ($p = 0.90$). In this eye, IOP TT increased significantly during L1 and L2 wearing, while in the control eye, no changes were observed during the same time (Table 4 and Figure 4).

Table 4. Measurement of IOP with the TT before, during, and after wearing SLs in the study eye and the control eye.

	Time	Study Eye (Right Eye)			Control Eye (Left Eye)		
		IOP (Mean ± SD)	ΔIOP (Mean ± SD)	p	IOP (Mean ± SD)	Δ IOP (Mean ± SD)	p
L1	BL	10.70 ± 2.80	-	-	9.90 ± 2.92	-	-
	0 h	11.63 ± 2.82	0.93 ± 2.34	0.04	10.08 ± 3.00	0.18 ± 1.32	1.00
	1 h	12.73 ± 2.87	2.03 ± 1.79	<0.01 *	10.19 ± 2.93	0.29 ± 1.19	1.00
	2 h	13.25 ± 3.26	2.55 ± 2.04	<0.01 *	10.07 ± 3.13	0.17 ± 1.68	1.00
	AL	10.95 ± 3.15	0.24 ± 1.69	1.00	9.90 ± 2.76	0.00 ± 1.31	1.00
L2	BL	10.79 ± 2.66	-	-	10.56 ± 2.38	-	-
	0 h	12.02 ± 2.73	1.23 ± 1.49	<0.01 *	9.96 ± 2.40	−0.30 ± 1.35	1.00
	1 h	12.91 ± 2.49	2.12 ± 1.99	<0.01 *	10.03 ± 2.85	−0.22 ± 1.86	1.00
	2 h	13.32 ± 3.22	2.53 ± 2.22	<0.01 *	10.39 ± 3.20	0.13 ± 1.89	1.00
	AL	11.37 ± 2.84	0.58 ± 1.38	0.29	10.57 ± 2.85	0.31 ± 1.32	1.00

BL = before lens fitting; 0 h = immediately after lens fitting; 1 h = one hour after fitting; 2 h = two hours after fitting; AL = after lens removal. Δ = the difference between the several time intervals with respect to BL (Negative values show a decrease and positive values an increase). The asterisk (*) in the table indicates significant differences ($p < 0.05$).

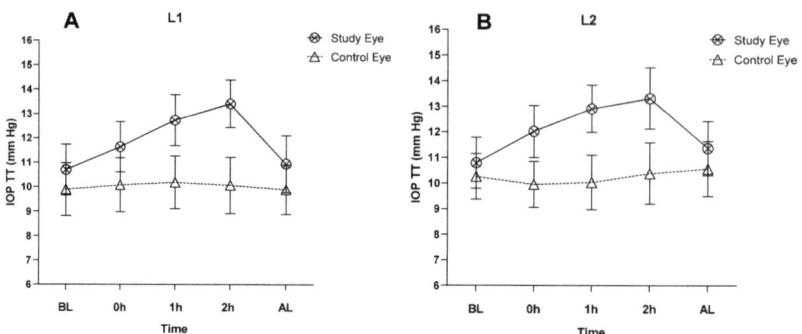

Figure 4. IOP with TT before, during, and after wearing the SL in the study eye and the control eye. (**A**) L1 (15.8 mm lens); (**B**) L2 (16.8 mm lens).

In the study eye, ΔCCT was not related to ΔIOP PAT (r = 0.01; p = 0.96) nor to ΔIOP TT (r = −0.15; p = 0.44) after wearing L1. The ΔCCT observed with L2 was also unrelated to ΔIOP PAT (r = −0.26; p = 0.17) and ΔIOP TT (r = 0.31; p = 0.09).

In the control eye, there was also no relationship between ΔCCT and ΔIOP PAT (ρ = −0.12; p = 0.54) and ΔIOP TT (ρ = 0.23; p = 0.22) with L1 wear, nor with ΔIOP PAT (ρ = −0.11; p = 0.56) and ΔIOP TT (ρ = −0.18; p = 0.34) with L2 wear.

These results showed individual variability in IOP values. IOP TT in the study eye after wearing L1 decreased in 11 patients (36.67%), showed no change in 5 patients (16.67%), and increased in 15 patients (50.00%), with one of them increasing by 4 mmHg. After wearing L2, IOP TT decreased in 7 patients (23.33%), showed no change in 5 patients (16.67%), and increased in 18 patients (60.00%), with one of them increasing up to 3.33 mmHg.

However, while wearing the lens, IOP TT with L1 increased in 28 patients (93.33%). Of these 28 patients, 18 (60.00%) had an increase ≥ 2 mmHg, and 4 (13.33%) had an increase ≥ 5 mmHg. With L2, IOP TT increased in 26 patients (86.67%), with an increase ≥ 2 mmHg in 19 patients (63.33%) and ≥5 mmHg in 3 patients (10.00%).

The comparison between the mean IOP values between TT and PAT was performed with the 60 measurements obtained before the insertion of both lenses in the study eye (30 measurements from L1 and 30 from L2). The IOP PAT (11.05 ± 1.63 mmHg) was slightly higher than the IOP TT (10.74 ± 2.71 mmHg), but this difference was not significant (p = 0.44). The correlation between the measurements of both instruments was moderate (ρ = 0.50, p = 0.01). The repeatability of PAT and TT was 4.56 and 7.57, respectively. The CV was higher with the TT (25.43%) than with the PAT (14.90%). The agreement between PAT and TT was 0.31 ± 2.11 mmHg (LoA from −4.48 to 5.08) (Figure 5).

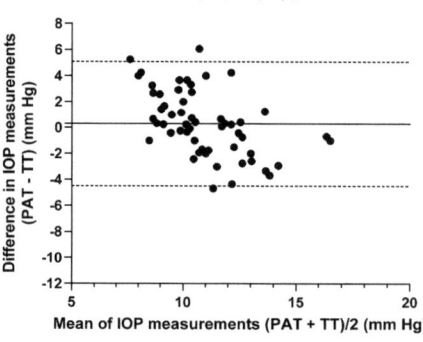

Figure 5. Bland and Altman plot of IOP agreement between TT and PAT. Mean difference of 0.31 ± 2.11 mmHg; limits of agreement (LoA) from −4.48 to 5.08.

3.6. Optic Nerve Head Parameters

No significant differences were observed when comparing RNFL thickness ($p = 0.38$), NRA ($p = 0.50$), and NRV ($p = 0.19$) values with OCT before L1 and L2 insertion in the study eye. We also compared the values before L1 insertion in the study eye and control eye without finding differences in RNFL thickness ($p = 0.16$), NRA ($p = 0.52$), or NRV ($p = 0.27$) values. Similar results were found when comparing RNFL thickness ($p = 0.12$), NRA ($p = 0.85$), and NRV ($p = 0.51$) values in the study eye and the control eye with L2.

RNFL thickness, NRA, and NRV values also did not experience significant changes after removal of L1 and L2 in the study eye and control eye (Table 5).

Table 5. Changes in the retinal nerve fiber layer (RFNL) and optic nerve head parameters while wearing L1 and L2 in the study and control eyes.

		Study Eye (Right Eye)				Control Eye (Left Eye)			
		Before (Mean ± SD)	After (Mean ± SD)	Δ (Mean ± SD)	*p*	Before (Mean ± SD)	After (Mean ± SD)	Δ (Mean ± SD)	*p*
L1	RNFLt (μm)	107.76 ± 10.60	108.04 ± 10.25	0.28 ± 2.32	0.51	109.02 ± 9.90	109.04 ± 9.80	0.20 ± 2.06	0.96
	NRA (mm^2)	1.67 ± 0.39	1.63 ± 0.42	−0.04 ± 0.12	0.09	1.64 ± 0.34	1.65 ± 0.35	0.01 ± 0.15	0.65
	NRV (mm^3)	0.24 ± 0.08	0.23 ± 0.09	−0.01 ± 0.03	0.34	0.24 ± 0.11	0.24 ± 0.11	0.00 ± 0.03	0.66
L2	RNFL (μm)	106.95 ± 9.50	106.70 ± 10.64	−0.26 ± 2.82	0.62	108.23 ± 10.35	107.93 ± 9.93	−0.30 ± 3.48	0.64
	NRA (mm^2)	1.65 ± 0.41	1.64 ± 0.42	−0.01 ± 0.12	0.71	1.65 ± 0.34	1.66 ± 0.34	0.01 ± 0.11	0.93
	NRV (mm^3)	0.23 ± 0.09	0.23 ± 0.09	0.00 ± 0.02	0.45	0.23 ± 0.10	0.24 ± 0.11	0.01 ± 0.02	0.15

RNFLt = retinal nerve fiber layer thickness; NRA = neuroretinal rim area; NRV = neuroretinal rim volume. Δ = the difference between the values after and before lens wearing (Negative values show a decrease and positive values an increase).

The relationship between changes produced in optic nerve head parameters and IOP was also evaluated. In the study eye, an inverse correlation was observed between ΔIOP TT and ΔNRA ($\rho = -0.37$, $p = 0.04$) with L1, while in the control eye, ΔIOP TT and ΔRNFL ($\rho = -0.41$, $p = 0.02$) with L1 and ΔIOP PAT and ΔNRV ($\rho = -0.46$, $p = 0.01$) with L2 were also related (Appendix B).

4. Discussion

In the present study, a reduction in FR of 137.50 μm with L1 and 117.50 μm with L2 was found after two hours of wear. Other studies have reported reductions in FR between 76 and 133 μm after six and eight hours of wear [22,33,34]. The greatest decrease occurs mainly in the first two to four hours after insertion [22]. Moreover, this decrease in FR varies with lens design and diameter [16,22], being lower in larger SLs. This is probably because the larger SL rests further away from the limbus, where the episclera is thicker [35]. Additionally, due to the changes in FR during the two hours of L1 and L2 wear, there was an increase of 8.10 and 9.17 μm, respectively, in CCT. This increase was greater than the ratio established by Munford et al. [36] of 1 μm per hour with a high-permeability SL (DK 120) and is consistent with the increase observed in some studies that evaluated SLs during eight hours of wearing [16,23]. However, the oedema observed in this study (<2%) is lower than the physiological oedema that occurs during sleep (4%) [24]. The cause of this oedema is insufficient oxygen supply to the cornea, known as hypoxia, due to the thickness of the lens [37]. In the case of SLs, in addition to the thickness of the lens itself, the thickness of the FR also plays a role. However, the multivariate model showed that the increase in CCT with lens wear was not related to lens thickness or initial FR. This may be due to the DK of the lens, which, in preventing hypoxia, is more important than the thickness of the FR [24].

The studies that evaluated the influence of the SLs on the AIC did not observe any changes [1,27]. However, these studies measure AIC globally [1] or in the temporal area [27], so changes in a specific meridian may go undetected. In addition, AIC analysis is performed with a Scheimpflug camera system, which provides limited resolution of the AIC [38]. In this study, TIA500, TISA500, AOD500, and ARA500 were analyzed in the principal axes, 0–180° and 90–270°, with CASIA 2, an AS-OCT that allows visualization of the AIC at a higher resolution [39]. A decrease in all parameters was found in the horizontal meridian after the smallest lens diameter (L1). In this meridian, the sclera becomes flatter, and thus the SL produces a higher mechanical pressure in this area [40], which may cause changes in adjacent structures such as the ICA and subsequently in its parameters. In the vertical meridian, the decrease in TIA500 and AOD500 may be related to greater compression of the SL on the conjunctiva in the upper zone due to the mechanical pressure exerted by the eyelids [28]. Furthermore, unlike the horizontal meridian, no changes in parameters such as TISA500 and ARA500, which represent areas, were observed in this meridian. This may be because these parameters need more compression to observe significant changes compared to TIA500 and AOD500, which do not represent an area. The ITC was the only ICA parameter studied globally for which no change was observed. It has been seen that TIA is less than 23.2° if there is an iridotrabecular contact [41]. However, the highest reduction in TIA after SL wear, regardless of axis, was −2.72° with L1 and −1.60° with L2, resulting in a final value of 44.80° and 44.86°, respectively. These values are considerably higher than the limit established by Fernandez-Vigo et al. [41], so the relevance of the observed changes is limited. A similar situation occurred with AOD, which is a standardized parameter in the assessment of angular opening. In patients with angular closure, the value of this parameter was 0.2 mm [42]. However, this value is again considerably lower compared with that obtained in this study after wearing both SCLs (L1 = 0.49 mm and L2 = 0.52 mm).

In the SC, the area and length were reduced in the horizontal meridian after wearing the largest diameter lens (L2). The SC is located deeply in the corneoscleral tissue, covering more than two-thirds of its thickness [43]. The compression produced by the SL landing zone in this tissue is small (2% of its thickness) compared to 30% in the conjunctival/episcleral tissue [28]. However, the SC is not a rigid structure; it collapses (invisible) with increasing IOP [44]. It has been observed that the CS area decreased by 30% with an IOP increase of 23.2 mmHg [45]. In this study, although the CS area decreased by 18.07% in the nasal zone and 15.02% in the temporal zone after wearing L2, the 0.58 mmHg increase in IOP with the TT and 0.23 mmHg with the PAT was considerably less than that observed by Kageman et al. [45]. Furthermore, IOP with both tonometers was not related to CS area or CS length, which also decreased in both areas after L2 use and is a more reproducible parameter [46]. Therefore, an increase in IOP due to CS compression with L2 in healthy patients seems improbable. However, this compression may have different implications for IOP in patients with glaucoma, in whom the CS area is smaller [46,47].

Changes in the CS with L2 (larger diameter) are possibly related to a slightly posterior location of this structure with respect to the AIC, where changes are observed with L1 (smaller diameter), as the size of the supporting area is the same for both LSs (1.5 mm).

During the two hours of wearing both SLs, a similar increase in IOP measured with the TT was observed in the study eye, while the control eye showed little change. A slightly higher increase (between 4.4 and 5.5 mmHg) was also observed by several authors who measured IOP with TT during one and four hours of wearing SLs of different sizes [1,2]. However, Fogt et al. [2] observed a rapid increase in IOP of 4.4 mmHg with the 15.2 mm lens and 5.0 mmHg with the 18.2 mm lens at the time of insertion, which persisted during lens wear. The decrease in the elasticity of the tissue adjacent to the lens landing zone in the superior sector, where the compression is greatest and the TT measurements are made, was attributed as a possible cause of the increase in IOP with this tonometer during lens wear [2]. Possibly, this fact occurs in this study because, despite being lower, a rapid increase was observed at the time of insertion (L1 = 0.93 mmHg, L2 = 1.23 mmHg). However, this different IOP behavior at the time of insertion in both studies may be due to the different tonicity of the eyelids of the sample tested as well as the characteristics of the scleral tissue. In this study, IOP was also measured with the PAT, with a slight increase in the study eye and a decrease in the control eye, although changes in IOP were not related to changes in CCT. The PAT measurements are comparable to the GAT [48] that was used in several studies to measure IOP after removal of SLs in patients with keratoconus and ocular surface disease [4,6,49]. In one of them, Shanhazi et al. [49] did not find an association between changes in IOP and CCT caused by wearing SLs. In this study, the relationship between changes in IOP and ICA was also studied as one of the possible hypotheses leading to an increase in IOP. A positive correlation was only observed between the ΔIOP PAT and the ΔITC index after wearing both SLs, although this finding is of limited clinical importance. According to some reports with the previous version of the AS-OCT platform used in the present study (CASIA SS-1000, Tomey, Nagoya, Japan), results greater than 35% for the ITC index provide good diagnostic ability for angle closure [50], which can also be associated with high IOP [51]. However, in this study, the ITC index before insertion of both SLs was <3.5%, and it increased by 1.28% with L1 and 1.52% with L2. As there was hardly any relationship between changes in IOP, ICA, and SC with SL wearing in this study with healthy subjects, it seems unlikely that an IOP increase could be due to changes in these structures. By contrast, authors think that IOP changes might be related to the degree of scleral applanation (or indentation) associated with the greater volume of displaced intraocular fluid [18]. However, Xu et al. [52] established cut-off points that, except for TIA500 (15.16°), TISA500 (0.046 mm^2), AOD500 (0.104 mm), and ARA500 (0.047 mm^2), were related to IOP. Although the study was conducted in the Asian population, it cannot be excluded that the changes produced by SL wear in subjects with AIC parameters close to these values may lead to an increase in IOP.

Before insertion of both SLs, IOP PAT was slightly higher than IOP TT (0.31 mmHg), with moderate correlation and agreement between tonometers. By contrast, Formisano et al. [4] observed a consistent difference in IOP values (around 5 mmHg) between these tonometers before and after removal of SLs in patients with keratoconus. However, most studies in healthy and keratoconus patients have shown a poor/moderate correlation and agreement [9–11,53]. PAT showed lower CV and repeatability, similar to other studies [54,55]. However, TT is accurate when IOP measurements with GAT are between 11 and 21 mmHg [56]. In this range, according to the instructions provided by the manufacturer, the error of TT is 2 mmHg. However, the increase in IOP at two hours of wear with both lenses (L1 = 2.55 mmHg and L2 = 2.53 mmHg) was greater than the tonometer error, which would indicate that there is an increase in IOP during this time. Furthermore, the percentage of subjects who had an increase in IOP $\geq$ 2 mmHg during both SL wear was at least 60%, but similar to other studies, the intersubject variability was high [1,5].

RFNL thickness and optic nerve head parameters were also studied to indirectly determine the possible consequences of the potential IOP increase during SL wear. Other works studied changes in BMO-MRW under the same conditions, with different results [8,29]. This parameter is associated with an increase in IOP [30], and its position is susceptible to changes in IOP [57]. Therefore, it is possible that the difference in the IOP value and/or the position of the BMO-MRW between the two studies is the reason for the discrepancy in the results. However, no relationship between BMO-MRW and IOP has been observed with SLs [8]. In this study, changes found in RNFL thickness, NRA, and NRV values with the wearing of SLs were minimal or not clinically significant. Furthermore, most of the changes in these parameters are not related to changes in IOP with TT and PAT in the study eye. Only a positive relationship is observed between changes in NRA and IOP with TT after wearing L1. However, RFNL thickness, which is a parameter sensitive to IOP fluctuations [58], has also been related to changes in IOP TT in the L1 control eye. Similarly, the observed changes in NRV, which were also related to IOP changes with PAT in the L2 control eye, were of the same magnitude as those observed in the study eye after wearing L2. In addition, the changes observed in RFNL thickness and NRV after wearing both SLs are similar to the fluctuations shown by these parameters during the day [59,60].

Therefore, it is most likely that these observed changes in optic nerve head parameters after wearing both SLs are related to fluctuations in the eye itself and not to changes in IOP. However, these changes could be relevant in patients with glaucomatous damage, where small fluctuations in IOP produce changes in RFNL thickness that are predictive of glaucoma [58].

One of the limitations of this study was that, when examining the AIC and SC with different AS-OCT, the distance of these structures to the center of the eye and the centration of the lens were not taken into account. This may result in the decentration of the smaller lens resting in the area where the larger diameter lens does, and conversely, this is one of the possible reasons for the reduction in the SC area with L1. Therefore, it cannot be categorically said that the changes in the different structures are due to a specific lens size.

In the future, it would be important to establish a standard method for measuring IOP with SLs. In addition, it would be interesting to assess the changes produced by these types of contact lenses in ICA and SC in subjects with different angle widths, higher IOPs, and/or susceptibility to developing glaucomatous disease, as well as optic nerve head monitoring.

5. Conclusions

In the short term, SLs resulted in a slight increase in IOP as well as small changes in CCT, ICA, and SC, although they do not seem to be clinically relevant in healthy subjects. TT showed a moderate concordance with PAT; however, their measurements are not interchangeable in SL wearers.

Author Contributions: Conceptualization, J.Q.-P. and A.B.; methodology, J.Q.-P. and I.R.-U.; software, J.Q.-P. and J.L.-S.; validation, J.Q.-P. and A.B.; formal analysis, J.Q.-P. and J.L.-S.; investigation, J.Q.-P.; resources, A.F.-V.C.; data curation, J.Q.-P., A.B. and J.L.-S.; writing—original draft preparation, J.Q.-P.; writing—review and editing, J.Q.-P. and I.R.-U.; visualization, I.R.-U.; supervision, I.R.-U and J.M.-L.; project administration, A.F.-V.C.; funding acquisition, A.F.-V.C and J.M.-L. All authors have read and agreed to the published version of the manuscript.

Funding: This research was funded by a grant RD21/0002/0041 (Instituto de Salud Carlos III).

Institutional Review Board Statement: The study was conducted in accordance with the Declaration of Helsinki, and approved by Committee on Ethics of the Principality of Asturias with the code number 2020.490 of 28 November 2020.

Informed Consent Statement: Informed consent was obtained from all subjects involved in the study.

Data Availability Statement: All the obtained data used to support the findings of this study are available from the corresponding author upon reasonable request.

Acknowledgments: The authors want to especially acknowledge the devoted work and support of medical, optometrist and technical staff at the Instituto Oftalmológico Fernández-Vega.

Conflicts of Interest: The authors declare no conflict of interest.

Appendix A

Table A1. Correlation between the changes in IOP and ICA parameters after SL wearing.

	Lens	ΔIOP TT		ΔIOP PAT	
		Correlation	p	Correlation	p
ICA parameters					
ΔTIA500	L1	0.19	0.31	−0.23	0.22
0–180° axis (°)	L2	−0.27	0.21	0.03	0.89
ΔTIA500	L1	0.24	0.21	−0.26	0.17
90–270° axis (°)	L2	0.02	0.94	0.19	0.32
ΔTISA500	L1	0.21	0.24	−0.21	0.27
0–180° axis (mm^2)	L2	−0.04	0.82	0.05	0.81

Table A1. Cont.

	Lens	ΔIOP TT Correlation	p	ΔIOP PAT Correlation	p
ΔTISA500	L1	0.22	0.25	0.05	0.79
90–270° axis (mm^2)	L2	−0.11	0.57	0.22	0.25
ΔAOD500	L1	0.32	0.09	0.08	0.69
0–180° axis (mm)	L2	0.13	0.50	0.05	0.81
ΔAOD500	L1	0.29	0.12	0.15	0.42
90–270° axis (mm)	L2	−0.04	0.83	0.15	0.43
ΔARA500	L1	0.14	0.46	−0.12	0.52
0–180° axis (mm^2)	L2	0.10	0.59	0.08	0.66
ΔARA500	L1	0.10	0.59	−0.09	0.64
90–270° axis (mm^2)	L2	−0.10	0.59	0.04	0.85
ΔITC index	L1	0.08	0.67	0.44	0.02 *
(%)	L2	0.09	0.64	0.45	0.01 *
SC parameters					
SC Nasal Lenght	L1	0.07	0.71	0.05	0.78
(μm)	L2	0.26	0.16	0.16	0.42
SC Temp. Lenght	L1	0.29	0.12	0.19	0.32
(μm)	L2	−0.11	0.58	0.05	0.81
SC Nasal Área	L1	−0.19	0.31	0.24	0.21
(μm^2)	L2	0.26	0.17	0.14	0.45
SC Temp. Área	L1	0.00	1.00	−0.03	0.87
(μm^2)	L2	−0.07	0.71	0.03	0.88

IOP TT = Intraocular pressure with transpalpebral tonometry. IOP PAT = Intraocular pressure with perkins tonometry applanation; TIA500 = Trabecular iris angle; TISA500 = Trabecular iris area; AOD500 = Angle opening distance; ARA500 = Angle recess area; SC = Schlemm's channel; Δ = represents the change obtained from the difference of the value when removing the SL minus the value before inserting the lenses. The asterisk (*) in the table indicates significant differences ($p < 0.05$).

Appendix B

Table A2. Correlation between changes in IOP and optic nerve head parameters after wearing SL.

	Parameters	Lens	Study Eye (Right Eye) Correlation	p	Control Eye (Left Eye) Correlation	p
Δ IOP TT (mmHg)	ΔRNFL (μm)	L1	−0.10	0.60	−0.41	0.02 *
		L2	0.04	0.85	0.15	0.42
	ΔNRA (μm^2)	L1	−0.37	0.04 *	0.15	0.44
		L2	0.00	0.99	0.25	0.19
	ΔNRV (μm^3)	L1	−0.34	0.07	0.07	0.73
		L2	0.00	0.99	0.25	0.18
Δ IOP PAT (mmHg)	ΔRNFL (μm)	L1	0.33	0.07	−0.34	0.06
		L2	0.05	0.81	−0.10	0.58
	ΔNRA (μm^2)	L1	0.11	0.56	0.19	0.30
		L2	0.13	0.50	−0.35	0.06
	ΔNRV (μm^3)	L1	0.12	0.52	0.25	0.19
		L2	−0.12	0.52	−0.46	0.01 *

IOP TT = Intraocular pressure with transpalpebral tonometry. IOP PAT = Intraocular pressure with perkins tonometry applanation; RNFL = Retinal nerve fibre layer; NRA = Neuroretinal rim area; NRV = Neuroretinal rim volume. Δ = represents the change obtained from the difference of the value when removing the SL minus the value before inserting the lenses. The asterisk (*) in the table indicates significant differences ($p < 0.05$).

References

1. Michaud, L.; Samaha, D.; Giasson, C.J. Intra-Ocular Pressure Variation Associated with the Wear of Scleral Lenses of Different Diameters. *Contact Lens Anterior Eye* **2019**, *42*, 104–110. [CrossRef] [PubMed]
2. Fogt, J.S.; Nau, C.B.; Schornack, M.; Shorter, E.; Nau, A.; Harthan, J.S. Comparison of Pneumatonometry and Transpalpebral Tonometry Measurements of Intraocular Pressure during Scleral Lens Wear. *Optom. Vis. Sci.* **2020**, *97*, 711–719. [CrossRef] [PubMed]

3. Aitsebaomo, A.P.; Wong-Powell, J.; Miller, W.; Amir, F. Influence of Scleral Lens on Intraocular Pressure. *J. Contact Lens Res. Sci.* **2019**, *3*, e1–e9. [CrossRef]
4. Formisano, M.; Franzone, F.; Alisi, L.; Pistella, S.; Spadea, L. Effects of Scleral Contact Lenses for Keratoconus Management on Visual Quality and Intraocular Pressure. *Ther. Clin. Risk Manag.* **2021**, *17*, 79–85. [CrossRef]
5. Cheung, S.Y.; Collins, M.J.; Vincent, S.J. The Impact of Short-Term Fenestrated Scleral Lens Wear on Intraocular Pressure. *Contact Lens Anterior Eye* **2020**, *43*, 585–588. [CrossRef]
6. Kramer, E.G.; Vincent, S.J. Intraocular Pressure Changes in Neophyte Scleral Lens Wearers: A Prospective Study. *Contact Lens Anterior Eye* **2020**, *43*, 609–612. [CrossRef]
7. Porcar, E.; Montalt, J.C.; España-Gregori, E.; Peris-Martínez, C. Impact of Corneoscleral Contact Lens Usage on Corneal Biomechanical Parameters in Keratoconic Eyes. *Eye Contact Lens* **2019**, *45*, 318–323. [CrossRef]
8. Walker, M.K.; Pardon, L.P.; Redfern, R.; Patel, N. IOP and Optic Nerve Head Morphology during Scleral Lens Wear. *Optom. Vis. Sci.* **2020**, *97*, 661–668. [CrossRef]
9. Lam, A.K.C.; Lam, C.H.; Chan, R. The Validity of a Digital Eyelid Tonometer (TGDc-01) and Its Comparison with Goldmann Applanation Tonometry—A Pilot Study. *Ophthalmic Physiol. Opt.* **2005**, *25*, 205–210. [CrossRef]
10. Doherty, M.D.; Carrim, Z.I.; O'Neill, D.P. Diaton Tonometry: An Assessment of Validity and Preference against Goldmann Tonometry. *Clin. Exp. Ophthalmol.* **2012**, *40*, e171–e175. [CrossRef]
11. Wisse, R.P.L.; Peeters, N.; Imhof, S.M.; van der Lelij, A. Comparison of Diaton Transpalpebral Tonometer with Applanation Tonometry in Keratoconus. *Int. J. Ophthalmol.* **2016**, *18*, 395–398. [CrossRef]
12. Lee, J.H.; Sanchez, L.R.; Porco, T.; Han, Y.; Campomanes, A.G.D.A. Correlation of Corneal and Scleral Pneumatonometry in Pediatric Patients. *Ophthalmology* **2018**, *125*, 1209–1214. [CrossRef]
13. Kapamajian, M.A.; De Cruz, J.; Hallak, J.A.; Vajaranant, T.S. Correlation Between Corneal and Scleral Pneumatonometry: An Alternative Method for Intraocular Pressure Measurement. *Am. J. Ophthalmol.* **2013**, *156*, 902–906.e1. [CrossRef]
14. Nau, C.B.; Schornack, M.M.; Mclaren, J.W.; Sit, A.J. Intraocular Pressure after 2 Hours of Small-Diameter Scleral Lens Wear. *Eye Contact Lens* **2016**, *42*, 350–353. [CrossRef]
15. Fedotova, K.; Zhu, W.; Astakhov, S.Y.; Novikov, S.A.; Grabovetskiy, V.R.; Nikolaenko, V.P. Intraocular Pressure with Miniscleral Contact Lenses. *Vestn. Oftalmol.* **2021**, *137*, 52–58. [CrossRef]
16. Esen, F.; Toker, E. Influence of Apical Clearance on Mini-Scleral Lens Settling, Clinical Performance, and Corneal Thickness Changes. *Eye Contact Lens Sci. Clin. Pract.* **2017**, *43*, 230–235. [CrossRef]
17. Vincent, S.J.; Alonso-Caneiro, D.; Collins, M.J. Evidence on Scleral Contact Lenses and Intraocular Pressure. *Clin. Exp. Optom.* **2017**, *100*, 87–88. [CrossRef]
18. McMonnies, C.W. A Hypothesis That Scleral Contact Lenses Could Elevate Intraocular Pressure. *Clin. Exp. Optom.* **2016**, *99*, 594–596. [CrossRef]
19. Lotocky, J.; Cosgrove, J.; Slate, F. Do Scleral Lenses Suck? An Analysis of What Really Happens as Scleral Lenses "Settle". In Proceedings of the Global Specialty Lens Symposium, Las Vegas, NV, USA, 25–27 January 2018.
20. Fadel, D.; Kramer, E. Potential Contraindications to Scleral Lens Wear. *Contact Lens Anterior Eye* **2019**, *42*, 92–103. [CrossRef]
21. Bergmanson, J.P.G.; Martinez, J.G. Size Does Matter: What Is the Corneo-Limbal Diameter? *Clin. Exp. Optom.* **2017**, *100*, 522–528. [CrossRef]
22. Kauffman, M.J.; Gilmartin, C.A.; Bennett, E.S.; Bassi, C.J. A Comparison of the Short-Term Settling of Three Scleral Lens Designs. *Optom. Vis. Sci.* **2014**, *91*, 1462–1466. [CrossRef] [PubMed]
23. Vincent, S.J.; Alonso-caneiro, D.; Collins, M.J.; Beanland, A.; Lam, L. Hypoxic Corneal Changes Following Eight Hours. *Optom. Vis. Sci.* **2016**, *93*, 293–299. [CrossRef] [PubMed]
24. Hyun, Y.; Meng, C.; Kim, Y.H.; Tan, B.; Lin, M.C.; Radke, C.J. Central Corneal Edema with Scleral-Lens Wear. *Curr. Eye Res.* **2018**, *43*, 1305–1315. [CrossRef]
25. Vincent, S.J.; Alonso-Caneiro, D.; Collins, M.J. Corneal Changes Following Short-Term Miniscleral Contact Lens Wear. *Contact Lens Anterior Eye* **2014**, *37*, 461–468. [CrossRef]
26. Michaud, L.; van der Worp, E.; Brazeau, D.; Warde, R.; Giasson, C.J. Predicting Estimates of Oxygen Transmissibility for Scleral Lenses. *Contact Lens Anterior Eye* **2012**, *35*, 266–271. [CrossRef] [PubMed]
27. Obinwanne, C.J.; Echendu, D.C.; Agbonlahor, O.; Dike, S. Changes in Scleral Tonometry and Anterior Chamber Angle after Short-Term Scleral Lens Wear. *Optom. Vis. Sci.* **2020**, *97*, 720–725. [CrossRef]
28. Alonso-Caneiro, D.; Vincent, S.J.; Collins, M.J. Morphological Changes in the Conjunctiva, Episclera and Sclera Following Short-Term Miniscleral Contact Lens Wear in Rigid Lens Neophytes. *Contact Lens Anterior Eye* **2016**, *39*, 53–61. [CrossRef]
29. Samaha, D.; Michaud, L. Bruch Membrane Opening Minimum Rim Width Changes during Scleral Lens Wear. *Eye Contact Lens* **2021**, *47*, 295–300. [CrossRef]
30. Pardon, L.P.; Harwerth, R.S.; Patel, N.B. Neuroretinal Rim Response to Transient Changes in Intraocular Pressure in Healthy Non-Human Primate Eyes. *Exp. Eye Res.* **2020**, *193*, 107978. [CrossRef]
31. Shaffer, R.N. A New Classification of the Glaucomas. *Trans. Am. Ophthalmol. Soc.* **1960**, *58*, 219–225.
32. Spaeth, G.L. The Normal Development of the Human Anterior Chamber Angle: A New System of Descriptive Grading. *Trans. Ophthalmol. Soc. UK* **1971**, *91*, 709–739.
33. Caroline, J.P.; Andre, P.A. Scleral lens Settling. *Contact Lens Spectr.* **2012**, *27*, 1.

34. Michaud, L. Variation of Clearance with Mini-Scleral Lenses. In Proceedings of the Global Specialty Lens Symposium, Las Vegas, NV, USA, 23–26 January 2014.
35. Bergmanson, J.P. *Clinical Ocular Anatomy and Physiology*; Texas Eye Research and Technology Center: Houston, TX, USA, 2011.
36. Mountford, J.; Carkeet, N.; Carney, L. Corneal Thickness Changes during Scleral Lens Wear: Effect of Gas Permeability. *Int. Contact Lens Clin.* **1994**, *21*, 19–22. [CrossRef]
37. Bruce, A.S.; Brennan, N.A. Corneal Pathophysiology with Contact Lens Wear. *Surv. Ophthalmol.* **1990**, *35*, 25–58. [CrossRef]
38. De Leon, J.M.S.; Tun, T.A.; Perera, S.A.; Aung, T. Angle Closure Imaging: A Review. *Curr. Ophthalmol. Rep.* **2013**, *1*, 80–88. [CrossRef]
39. Cumba, R.J.; Radhakrishnan, S.; Bell, N.P.; Nagi, K.S.; Chuang, A.Z.; Lin, S.C.; Mankiewicz, K.A.; Feldman, R.M. Reproducibility of Scleral Spur Identification and Angle Measurements Using Fourier Domain Anterior Segment Optical Coherence Tomography. *J. Ophthalmol.* **2012**, *2012*, 487309. [CrossRef]
40. Macedo-de-Araújo, R.J.; van der Worp, E.; González-Méijome, J.M. In Vivo Assessment of the Anterior Scleral Contour Assisted by Automatic Profilometry and Changes in Conjunctival Shape after Miniscleral Contact Lens Fitting. *J. Optom.* **2019**, *12*, 131–140. [CrossRef]
41. Fernández-Vigo, J.I.; De-Pablo-Gómez-De-Liaño, L.; Fernández-Vigo, C.; Sánchez-Guillén, I.; Santos-Bueso, E.; Martínez-de-la-Casa, J.M.; García-Feijóo, J.; Fernández-Vigo, J.Á. Quantification of Trabecular-Iris Contact and Its Prevalence by Optical Coherence Tomography in a Healthy Caucasian Population. *Eur. J. Ophthalmol.* **2017**, *27*, 417–422. [CrossRef]
42. Mansouri, K.; Sommerhalder, J.; Shaarawy, T. Prospective Comparison of Ultrasound Biomicroscopy and Anterior Segment Optical Coherence Tomography for Evaluation of Anterior Chamber Dimensions in European Eyes with Primary Angle Closure. *Eye* **2010**, *24*, 233–239. [CrossRef]
43. Usui, T.; Tomidokoro, A.; Mishima, K.; Mataki, N.; Mayama, C.; Honda, N.; Amano, S.; Araie, M. Identification of Schlemm's Canal and Its Surrounding Tissues by Anterior Segment Fourier Domain Optical Coherence Tomography. *Investig. Ophthalmol. Vis. Sci.* **2011**, *52*, 6934–6939. [CrossRef]
44. Steglitz, K. Schlemm's Canal under the Scanning Electron Microscope. *Ophthalmic Res.* **1971**, *45*, 37–45.
45. Kagemann, L.; Wang, B.; Wollstein, G.; Ishikawa, H.; Nevins, J.E.; Nadler, Z.; Sigal, I.A.; Bilonick, R.A.; Schuman, J.S. IOP Elevation Reduces Schlemm's Canal Cross-Sectional Area. *Investig. Ophthalmol. Vis. Sci.* **2014**, *55*, 1805–1809. [CrossRef] [PubMed]
46. Hong, J.; Xu, J.; Wei, A.; Wen, W.; Chen, J.; Yu, X.; Sun, X. Spectral-Domain Optical Coherence Tomographic Assessment of Schlemm's Canal in Chinese Subjects with Primary Open-Angle Glaucoma. *Ophthalmology* **2013**, *120*, 709–715. [CrossRef] [PubMed]
47. Kagemann, L.; Wollstein, G.; Ishikawa, H.; Bilonick, R.A.; Brennen, P.M.; Folio, L.S.; Gabriele, M.L.; Schuman, J.S. Identification and Assessment of Schlemm's Canal by Spectral-Domain Optical Coherence Tomography. *Investig. Ophthalmol. Vis. Sci.* **2010**, *51*, 4054–4059. [CrossRef]
48. Arora, R.; Bellamy, H.; Austin, M.W. Applanation Tonometry: A Comparison of the Perkins Handheld and Goldmann Slit Lamp-Mounted Methods. *Clin. Ophthalmol.* **2014**, *8*, 605–610. [CrossRef]
49. Shahnazi, K.C.; Isozaki, V.L.; Chiu, G.B. Effect of Scleral Lens Wear on Central Corneal Thickness and Intraocular Pressure in Patients With Ocular Surface Disease. *Eye Contact Lens Sci. Clin. Pract.* **2019**, *46*, 341–347. [CrossRef]
50. Baskaran, M.; Ho, S.W.; Tun, T.A.; How, A.C.; Perera, S.A.; Friedman, D.S.; Aung, T. Assessment of Circumferential Angle-Closure by the Iris-Trabecular Contact Index with Swept-Source Optical Coherence Tomography. *Ophthalmology* **2013**, *120*, 2226–2231. [CrossRef]
51. Chong, R.S.; Sakata, L.M.; Narayanaswamy, A.K.; Ho, S.; He, M.; Baskaran, M.; Wong, T.Y.; Perera, S.A.; Aung, T. Relationship between Intraocular Pressure and Angle Configuration: An Anterior Segment OCT Study. *Investig. Ophthalmol. Vis. Sci.* **2013**, *54*, 1650–1655. [CrossRef]
52. Xu, B.Y.; Burkemper, B.; Lewinger, J.P.; Jiang, X.; Pardeshi, A.A.; Richter, G.; Torres, M.; McKean-Cowdin, R.; Varma, R. Correlation between Intraocular Pressure and Angle Configuration Measured by OCT: The Chinese American Eye Study. *Ophthalmol. Glaucoma* **2018**, *1*, 158–166. [CrossRef]
53. Bali, S.J.; Bhartiya, S.; Sobti, A.; Dada, T.; Panda, A. Comparative Evaluation of Diaton and Goldmann Applanation Tonometers. *Ophthalmologica* **2012**, *228*, 42–46. [CrossRef]
54. Sánchez Pavón, I.; Cañadas, P.; Martin, R. Repeatability and Agreement of Intraocular Pressure Measurement among Three Tonometers. *Clin. Exp. Optom.* **2020**, *103*, 808–812. [CrossRef] [PubMed]
55. Molero-Senosiaín, M.; Morales-Fernández, L.; Saenz-Francés, F.; García-Feijoo, J.; Martínez-de-la-Casa, J.M. Analysis of Reproducibility, Evaluation, and Preference of the New IC100 Rebound Tonometer versus ICare PRO and Perkins Portable Applanation Tonometry. *Eur. J. Ophthalmol.* **2020**, *30*, 1349–1355. [CrossRef] [PubMed]
56. Li, Y.; Shi, J.; Duan, X.; Fan, F. Transpalpebral Measurement of Intraocular Pressure Using the Diaton Tonometer versus Standard Goldmann Applanation Tonometry. *Graefes Arch. Clin. Exp. Ophthalmol.* **2010**, *248*, 1765–1770. [CrossRef]
57. Patel, N.; McAllister, F.; Pardon, L.; Harwerth, R. The Effects of Graded Intraocular Pressure Challenge on the Optic Nerve Head. *Exp. Eye Res.* **2018**, *169*, 79–90. [CrossRef] [PubMed]
58. Fortune, B.; Yang, H.; Strouthidis, N.G.; Cull, G.A.; Grimm, J.L.; Downs, J.C.; Burgoyne, C.F. The Effect of Acute Intraocular Pressure Elevation on Peripapillary Retinal Thickness, Retinal Nerve Fiber Layer Thickness, and Retardance. *Investig. Ophthalmol. Vis. Sci.* **2009**, *50*, 4719–4726. [CrossRef]

59. Kamppeter, B.A.; Jonas, J.B. Fluctuations Depending on Time of Day in Measurements of the Optic Disc Using Confocal Laser Canning Tomography. *Ophthalmologe* **2006**, *103*, 40–42. [CrossRef]
60. Ashraf, H.; Nowroozzadeh, M.H. Diurnal Variation of Retinal Thickness. *Optom. Vis. Sci.* **2014**, *91*, 615–623. [CrossRef]

Disclaimer/Publisher's Note: The statements, opinions and data contained in all publications are solely those of the individual author(s) and contributor(s) and not of MDPI and/or the editor(s). MDPI and/or the editor(s) disclaim responsibility for any injury to people or property resulting from any ideas, methods, instructions or products referred to in the content.

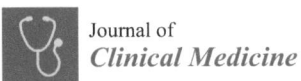 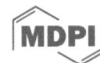

Article

Evaluation of Retinal Blood Flow in Patients with Monoclonal Gammopathy Using OCT Angiography

Cecilia Czakó [1,*], Dóra Gerencsér [1], Kitti Kormányos [1], Klaudia Kéki-Kovács [1], Orsolya Németh [2], Gábor Tóth [1], Gábor László Sándor [1], Anita Csorba [1], Achim Langenbucher [3], Zoltán Zsolt Nagy [1], Gergely Varga [4], László Gopcsa [5], Gábor Mikala [5], Illés Kovács [1,6,†] and Nóra Szentmáry [1,7,†]

1. Department of Ophthalmology, Semmelweis University, 1085 Budapest, Hungary
2. Department of Ophthalmology, Markusovszky University Teaching Hospital, 9700 Szombathely, Hungary
3. Experimental Ophthalmology, Saarland University, 66424 Homburg, Germany
4. 3rd Department of Internal Medicine and Haematology, Semmelweis University, 1085 Budapest, Hungary
5. Department of Haematology and Stem Cell-Transplantation, South-Pest Central Hospital-National Institute for Hematology and Infectious Diseases, 1097 Budapest, Hungary
6. Department of Ophthalmology, Weill Cornell Medical College, New York City, NY 10065, USA
7. Dr. Rolf M. Schwiete Center for Limbal Stem Cell and Congenital Aniridia Research, Saarland University, 66424 Homburg, Germany
* Correspondence: cecilia.czako@gmail.com
† These authors contributed equally to this work.

Abstract: Background: Monoclonal gammopathy (MG) is characterized by monoclonal protein overproduction, potentially leading to the development of hyperviscosity syndrome. Objective: To assess retinal circulation using optical coherence tomography angiography (OCTA) parameters in patients with monoclonal gammopathy. Methods: OCTA measurements were performed using the Optovue AngioVue system by examining 44 eyes of 27 patients with MG and 62 eyes of 36 control subjects. Superficial and deep retinal capillary vessel density (VD SVP and DVP) in the whole 3 × 3 mm macular and parafoveal area, foveal avascular zone (FAZ) area, and central retinal thickness (CRT) were measured using the AngioAnalytics software. The OCTA parameters were evaluated in both groups using a multivariate regression model, after controlling for the effect of imaging quality (SQ). Results: There was no significant difference in age between the subjects with monoclonal gammopathy and the controls (63.59 ± 9.33 vs. 58.01 ± 11.46 years; $p > 0.05$). Taking into account the effect of image quality, the VD SVP was significantly lower in the MG group compared to the control group (44.54 ± 3.22% vs. 46.62 ± 2.84%; $p < 0.05$). No significant differences were found between the two groups regarding the other OCTA parameters ($p > 0.05$). Conclusions: A decreased superficial retinal capillary vessel density measured using OCTA in patients with MG suggests a slow blood flow, reduced capillary circulation, and consequent tissue hypoperfusion. An evaluation of retinal circulation using OCTA in cases of monoclonal gammopathy may be a sensitive method for the non-invasive detection and follow-up of early microcirculatory dysfunction caused by increased viscosity.

Keywords: monoclonal gammopathy; multiple myeloma; hyperviscosity syndrome; optical coherence tomography angiography

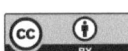

1. Introduction

Monoclonal gammopathies are characterized by the proliferation of clonal plasma cells, resulting in the presence of serum M-protein, also known as paraproteinemia [1]. The most common form of the disease is monoclonal gammopathy of undetermined significance (MGUS). MGUS occurs in 3% of individuals aged 50 or older and 5% of those 70 years of age or older [2]. According to the International Myeloma Working Group (IMWG), MGUS is characterized by the presence of serum M-protein less than 3 g/dL, monoclonal plasma cells less than 10% in the bone marrow, and the absence of end-organ damage associated with plasma cell proliferative disorder—such as bone lesions, anemia, hypercalcemia, and renal insufficiency [3]. The most common type of M-protein is IgG (69%), followed by IgM (17%), IgA (11%), or biclonal (3%). Patients with IgG and IgA monoclonal gammopathy tend to progress to multiple myeloma (MM) and rarely, to light chain (AL) amyloidosis. Nevertheless, those with IgM monoclonal immunoglobulin overproduction may progress to Non-Hodgkin's lymphoma, Waldenström's macroglobulinemia (WM), chronic lymphocytic leukemia, and AL amyloidosis. MGUS is considered to be a premalignant condition, as the risk of progression to MM is 1% per year for patients with IgG MGUS and the risk of progression to WM is 1.5% for those with IgM MGUS. The cumulative risk of progression is 10% at 10 years, 18% at 20 years, and 36% at 40 years. Associations between MGUS and other conditions such as renal disease, polyneuropathy, and also ocular conditions were recently described, where the presence of the M-protein may contribute to the development of organ dysfunctions [4].

Ocular manifestations of monoclonal gammopathy are not common and mainly affect the anterior segment. Ophthalmic disorders are due to the deposition of monoclonal kappa light chain immunoglobulins in the ocular tissues or hyperviscosity syndrome from increased circulating serum immunoglobulins. Proptosis, conjunctival and corneal crystalline deposits, copper deposition in Descemet's membrane, maculopathy with serous macular detachment, autoimmune retinopathy, central retinal vein occlusion, and hyperviscosity-related retinopathy have been described in the literature [5–10]. Crystalline keratopathy may be present as corneal deposits of immunoglobulin light chains in less than 1% of patients with monoclonal gammopathy [11]. Retinal vascular manifestations include venous dilatation, retinal hemorrhages, cotton wool spots, and microaneurysms. These findings have been attributed to hyperviscosity due to elevated levels of circulating immunoglobulins, which is most frequently observed in Waldenström's macroglobulinemia, where the large molecular weight serum IgM pentamer leads to aggregation and a significant increase in serum viscosity [12]. Ocular symptoms may be the initial presentation of monoclonal gammopathy; as a result, earlier detection may allow closer monitoring for its progression to multiple myeloma or Waldenström's macroglobulinemia.

Optical coherence tomography angiography (OCTA) is increasingly becoming a promising and important imaging technique in ophthalmology due to its ability to non-invasively visualize the different retinal and choroidal vascular layers. Instead of intravenous dye injection, OCTA uses motion contrast technology to image the blood flow by detecting the movement of red blood cells. OCTA is a useful imaging modality for evaluating ophthalmological diseases such as diabetic retinopathy, age-related macular degeneration, retinal artery and vein occlusions, and glaucoma. Moreover, besides a visualization of the retinal and choroidal vasculature, OCTA provides numerous data on retinal blood flow; thus, it is highly suitable for objective follow-ups on different diseases [13].

Due to the less frequent involvement of the posterior segment in monoclonal gammopathy, only a few papers have been published assessing retinal circulation using OCT angiography [14–16]. As retinal blood flow may reflect the systemic blood circulation, an easy method for recognizing even mild circulatory changes can have many benefits, such as early diagnosis and the detection of progression, the possibility of a closer follow-up of these patients, and monitoring the effect of systemic therapies, as well as the prevention of complications affecting other organs. Given the possible increase in blood viscosity and decrease in circulation in paraproteinemia, our purpose in this study was to evaluate retinal blood flow using OCT angiography in patients with monoclonal gammopathy.

2. Materials and Methods

In this cross-sectional study, 44 eyes of 27 patients with monoclonal gammopathy (11 male and 16 female, mean age: 63.59 ± 9.33 years) were recruited from the Department of Hematology and Stem Cell-Transplantation of the South-Pest Central Hospital, National Institute for Hematology and Infectious Diseases (Budapest, Hungary) and the 3rd Department of Internal Medicine, Semmelweis University (Budapest, Hungary). The patients were diagnosed and treated between 1997 and 2020. The study was conducted according to the Declaration of Helsinki, concerning the relevant national and local requirements, and was approved by the National Drug Agency's Ethical Review Board for Human Research (OGYÉI/50115/2018). All subjects gave their written informed consent. Regarding the hematological diagnosis, MGUS was diagnosed in 3 (11.11%), multiple myeloma in 21 (77.77%), smoldering myeloma in 1 (3.7%), and amyloidosis in 2 (7.4%) patients. As a control group, 62 eyes of 36 age-matched healthy individuals (11 male and 25 female, mean age: 58.01 ± 11.46 years) were involved in the study.

Patients with diabetes and those with any history of intraocular surgery, previous intravitreal anti-VEGF injection or laser treatment, or other ophthalmological diseases—such as glaucoma, age-related macular degeneration, vitreomacular disease, or refractive errors > 6 diopters—were excluded from the study. All the patients underwent OCT angiography imaging using the Optovue AngioVue OCT angiography system (2017.1 software version, phase 7.0 update) with an SSADA (split-spectrum amplitude-decorrelation angiography) software algorithm, by which 3 × 3 mm OCT angiograms were performed, centered at the macula. The superficial retinal vessel density (SVD) and deep retinal vessel density (DVD) were evaluated in the central 3 × 3 mm and parafoveal area, and the size of the foveal avascular zone (FAZ) at the level of the superficial capillary plexus and central retinal thickness (CRT) were measured using the built-in automated AngioAnalytics software of the OptoVue system. The parafoveal area was defined as a ring-shaped region with an inner radius of 1.5 mm from the center of the fovea, excluding a central foveal 0.5 mm radius area. Scans with segmentation errors at the superficial or deep vascular plexus level and images with artifacts (double vessel pattern, dark areas from blink, white line artifacts, and vessel discontinuities induced by microsaccades) were excluded from the study. Only OCT angiograms with a scan quality (SQ) index of 6 or above were accepted for further analysis—as recommended by OptoVue as a threshold for acceptable image quality.

Statistical Analysis

The statistical analysis was performed with SPSS software (version 27.0, IBM, Armonk, NY, USA). The effect of the image quality on the OCTA parameters was assessed with a multivariable regression analysis using generalized estimating equation (GEE) models. This test enabled adjustments to be made for the within-subject correlation of the parameters (right vs. left eye) by taking into account the between-eye correlations. Moreover, the inclusion of scan quality as a covariate in GEE models permits one to simultaneously control for its effect on the dependent variables, providing valid p values for group comparisons.

3. Results

There were no significant differences in terms of age and gender between the monoclonal gammopathy and healthy control groups ($p > 0.05$).

The values of the SQ ranged from 6 to 9, with an overall mean of 7.05 ± 1.12 in the eyes with monoclonal gammopathy and 7.83 ± 1.03 in the normal subjects ($p = 0.001$). The superficial retinal vessel density values showed a significant positive correlation with the SQ values in both groups (beta: 0.9, 95%CI: 0.19–1.61; $p = 0.01$), but there was no significant correlation between the SQ and other OCTA parameters ($p > 0.05$ for all the parameters). The superficial retinal vessel density was significantly decreased in the central 3 × 3 mm macular area in the patients with monoclonal gammopathy compared to the healthy individuals, after controlling for the effect of signal quality in a multivariable regression model (Figure 1). However, no significant difference was found regarding the superficial retinal vessel density in the parafoveal zone, the deep retinal vessel density both in the 3 × 3 mm macular and parafoveal zone, the foveal avascular zone (FAZ) area, and the central retinal thickness (CRT) values between the two groups (Table 1).

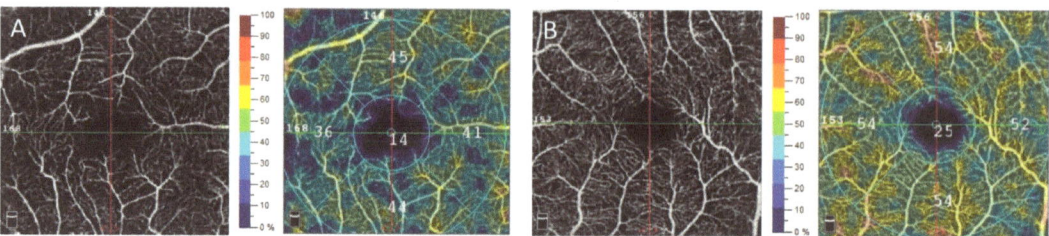

Figure 1. En-face OCT angiogram and retinal vessel density map of the superficial retinal vascular plexus measured in the 3 × 3 mm macular using by OptoVue AngioVue OCT angiography in a patient with monoclonal gammopathy (**A**), and a healthy subject (**B**). OCT: optical coherence tomography.

Table 1. OCTA parameters in patients with monoclonal gammopathy and healthy individuals.

	Monoclonal Gammopathy ($n = 44$)	Healthy Controls ($n = 62$)	p
VD SVP—3 × 3 mm central macular area (%)	44.54 ± 3.22	46.62 ± 2.84	0.04
VD DVP—3 × 3 mm central macular area (%)	48.59 ± 3.23	49.76 ± 3.99	0.77
VD SVP—parafoveal area (%)	47.54 ± 3.60	49.57 ± 2.95	0.08
VD DVP—parafoveal area (%)	51.13 ± 3.24	52.00 ± 3.99	0.93
FAZ (mm^2)	0.293	0.289	0.91
CRT (μm)	263.73	254.95	0.22

OCTA: optical coherence tomography angiography, VD: vessel density, SVP: superficial vascular plexus, DVP: deep vascular plexus, FAZ: foveal avascular zone, CRT: central retinal thickness, and p: the difference between the two groups after controlling for scan quality in multivariable models.

4. Discussion

Monoclonal gammopathy may have several ocular manifestations, affecting most ocular tissues, and these are not uncommonly the first symptom of the disease. In a previous paper, our study group evaluated the ocular signs and ocular comorbidities in 80 patients with monoclonal gammopathy. According to our results, ocular surface disease and cataracts are more common in subjects with monoclonal gammopathy than in age-matched controls [7]. We also demonstrated that increased corneal light scattering in the central 10 mm annular zone and increased keratocyte hyperreflectivity, evaluated using Pentacam and in vivo confocal microscopy, respectively, may give rise to a suspicion of monoclonal gammopathy [8]. Nevertheless, in contrast to the anterior segment involvement in this population, we have much less knowledge about the involvement of the posterior segment. Due to the alterations in the systemic circulation in monoclonal gammopathy, quantitative measurements of retinal blood flow using OCT angiography could offer an easy and fast method for detecting even subtle circulatory changes.

In monoclonal gammopathy, owing to the high level of paraproteins, major hemorheological changes occur in the circulation that may be as serious as hyperviscosity syndrome. Hypergammaglobulinemia—especially Waldenström macroglobulinemia—is the most frequent cause of hyperviscosity syndrome. An increase in blood viscosity can result from either erythrocyte aggregation or an increased plasma viscosity. These changes depend on the plasma concentration, as well as the molecular size of the paraprotein, with a threshold for the onset of hyperviscosity for IgG of >15 g/dL, for IgA of >1 g/dL, and for IgM of >3 g/dL. Accordingly, symptomatic hyperviscosity in Waldenström macroglobulinemia is more common, affecting 10–30% of patients, than IgG myeloma (2–6%) is [17]. Nevertheless, after taking into account the above exclusion criteria, patients with Waldenström macroglobulinemia were not included in our present study; only MGUS, multiple myeloma, smoldering myeloma, and amyloidosis subjects could be analyzed. In monoclonal gammopathy, an increased blood viscosity causes sluggish blood flow and decreased microvascular circulation, leading to the hypoperfusion of tissues. The classic triad of hyperviscosity syndrome consists of mucosal or skin bleeding, neurological deficits, and visual disturbances [18]. Ophthalmic findings include venous dilation, flame hemorrhages, papilledema, exudates, and microaneurysm formation. The most severe ophthalmic manifestation of hyperviscosity syndrome is central retinal vein or artery occlusion, which can result in irreversible vision loss [5].

Physiologically, blood flow is influenced by blood velocity, vessel diameter, and whole-blood viscosity, which is determined by hematocrit, plasma viscosity, red cell aggregation, and deformability [19]. A previous study conducted by Uggla et al. examined the hemorheological patterns of 87 patients with monoclonal gammopathy, including MM (n = 52), MGUS (n = 30), and WM (n = 5). Of the MG patients, 71% had a plasma viscosity above the reference limit and 40% were above the whole-blood viscosity limit [20]. Another study group observed significant increases in whole-blood viscosity and plasma viscosity, as well as a marked decrease in erythrocyte deformability in MGUS patients compared to controls [19].

OCT angiography is a new imaging technique based on optical coherence tomography that can visualize the functional blood vessels in the eye by detecting the variation in the OCT signal caused by moving particles. During image acquisition, repeated OCT scans are performed at the same location of the retina, and the backscattered OCT signals from the moving red blood cells in the vessels are differentiated from the backscattered OCT signals from static structural tissue [21]. Commercially available OCTA devices are typically used to create en-face images with red blood cell movement occurring within a range from 0.3 to 3 mm/s. As human retinal capillary flow speeds have been estimated to be in the range of 0.4–3.0 mm/s, this suggests that SSADA is well suited for detailed angiography down to the capillary level [22].

After performing OCT angiography studies examining various ophthalmological diseases, different systemic disorders are also increasingly becoming the focus of the research into this novel imaging technique. The major advantage offered by OCT angiography is that it is an excellent non-invasive tool for screening and monitoring vascular diseases, allowing for closer follow-ups of these patients. Several studies have been published using OCT angiography in systemic diseases, such as hypertension, diabetes mellitus, coronary artery disease, carotid artery stenosis, preeclampsia, kidney disease, and hematological disorders. Previous reports have illustrated that OCT angiography can detect retinal microvascular alterations in systemic hypertension and high cardiovascular risks. Therefore, monitoring these changes before irreversible end-organ damage occurs could prevent life-threatening hypertensive-related complications [23,24]. Since OCTA has become available, numerous studies have reported changes in the retinal microvasculature of patients with diabetes. Our study group demonstrated that, regardless of the duration of diabetes, a reduced retinal vessel density was linked to a significantly increased rate of diabetic retinopathy, and as a consequence, OCTA metrics may serve as prognostic biomarkers for the prediction of early-onset diabetic retinopathy [25]. We also analyzed the retinal circulation of patients with severe carotid artery stenosis using OCT angiography and found that carotid surgery resulted in a significant improvement in retinal blood flow, both ipsi- and contralaterally, independent of systemic factors. This finding corroborates those of Lee et al. [26,27]. Accordingly, OCT angiography could also help in the assessment of cerebral circulation changes related to carotid artery stenosis. Another recent study described that subjects with end-stage renal disease receiving hemodyalisis showed a decreased flow density in the superficial capillary and choriocapillary plexus in OCTA imaging, and that flow density was negatively correlated with hemodyalisis treatment. In contrast, the deep capillary plexus appeared to be more resilient towards hemodynamic changes caused by hemodyalisis treatment [28]. Additionally, OCT angiography may also be beneficial for neurological research to advance our understanding of the pathophysiology of multiple sclerosis, Alzheimer's disease, and several optic neuropathies [29]. According to the results published in the literature, OCT angiography provides extremely useful information concerning the blood flow both in the retina and in the whole body. There is an increasing number of studies that are devoted to expanding the usability of OCT angiography in the management of systemic diseases, which previously did not include assessments of the retinal vasculature [30].

Currently, there have only been a few reported studies on OCT angiographic evaluations of the retinal circulation in patients with monoclonal gammopathy. A previous report described a case of hyperviscosity retinopathy due to Waldenström macroglobulinemia, with no abnormalities on OCT angiography [14]. However, in a study conducted by Li et al., OCT angiography showed characteristic changes in both the retinal and choroidal vasculatures in a patient with Waldenström macroglobulinemia retinopathy, as macula edema presented as petaloid cysts in the outer plexiform layer, the capillary network of the macula was blurred and irregular, and there were augmented choroidal large blood vessels [15]. Considering the exclusion criteria, OCTA measurements of patients with Waldenström macroglobulinemia were not included in our study for further statistical analysis.

In the present study, the superficial retinal vessel density measured using OCT angiography was significantly decreased in the eyes of the patients with monoclonal gammopathy compared to the controls. Nevertheless, we found no significant differences regarding the other OCTA parameters—the deep retinal vessel density, foveal avascular zone area, and central retinal thickness—between the two groups. In line with our findings, Dursun et al. detected a decreased vessel density in the superficial and deep macular retinal areas and papillary and peripapillary regions measured with OCT angiography, suggesting a decreased blood flow and possible ischemia in patients with multiple myeloma. However, they did not take into account the effect of image quality on the OCTA parameters, which is inevitable for the appropriate assessment of the values, as well as for longitudinal patient follow-up [16,31,32].

Consistent with our prior findings, in the current study, the image quality (SQ index) was positively correlated with the superficial retinal vessel density values in both groups, demonstrating that the OCTA parameters are significantly different in scans with a lower image quality compared to those with better quality [31,32].

Furthermore, we classified the patients with monoclonal gammopathy according to the International Staging System (ISS) and Revised ISS, based on their serum levels of albumin, β2 microglobulin, and lactate dehydrogenase (LDH), and the presence of high-risk chromosomal abnormalities (CA) [33,34]. In our study, 16 patients were assigned to ISS stage I (59%), 3 patients to ISS stage II (11%), and 8 patients to ISS stage III (30%), whereas 15 patients were assigned to R-ISS stage I (56%), 10 patients to R-ISS stage II (37%), and 2 patients to R-ISS stage III (7%). According to the ISS and Revised ISS, we found no significant difference regarding the OCTA parameters between the different-stage groups. Nevertheless, given that the blood tests of the patients with monoclonal gammopathy and the OCT angiographic examinations were not performed simultaneously, in our study, these data were not included in the manuscript for further statistical analysis, owing to a possible change in blood flow occurring between the two visits.

Monoclonal gammopathy is associated with hemorheological abnormalities—including an increase in blood viscosity—that cause a decreased blood flow. OCT angiography is a novel technology that can detect very mild capillary circulation disorders, which can be an early predictor of hyperviscosity syndrome in these subjects. A better identification of patients with decreased circulation could prevent the different complications of hyperviscosity syndrome, such as bleeding disorders, vision-threatening complications, and neurological deficits. Moreover, the earlier detection of microcirculatory disorders may allow closer monitoring for the further progression of the condition.

We acknowledge that our study has some limitations, including its small sample size and the cross-sectional nature of the work, with a lack of follow-up to define accuracy measures in the patients with monoclonal gammopathy. In addition, it would have been noteworthy to analyze the association between the blood parameters, visual acuity, and OCTA parameters simultaneously. In the future, larger prospective studies will be needed to confirm our results, in order to highlight the role of OCT angiography in disease monitoring and therapeutic follow-up.

5. Conclusions

In summary, a decreased superficial retinal vessel density measured using OCT angiography in patients with monoclonal gammopathy suggests the presence of a sluggish blood flow, reduced capillary circulation, and consequent tissue hypoperfusion due to an increased blood viscosity. An OCT angiographic examination of the retinal blood flow in monoclonal gammopathy—taking into account the influence of the image quality on the OCTA parameters—can be a sensitive method for the non-invasive detection and follow-up of early microcirculatory disorders caused by hyperviscosity.

Author Contributions: Conceptualization, I.K. and N.S.; methodology, C.C., K.K., I.K. and N.S.; formal analysis, D.G., K.K., K.K.-K., O.N., G.T., G.L.S., A.C., A.L., Z.Z.N., G.V., L.G., G.M., I.K. and N.S.; investigation, D.G., K.K., K.K.-K., O.N., G.T., G.L.S., A.C., A.L., Z.Z.N., G.V., L.G., G.M., I.K. and N.S.; resources, G.M., I.K. and N.S.; data curation, C.C., D.G. and K.K.; writing—original draft preparation, C.C.; writing—review and editing, D.G., K.K., K.K.-K., O.N., G.T., G.L.S., A.C., A.L., Z.Z.N., G.V., L.G., G.M., I.K. and N.S.; visualization, C.C. and D.G.; supervision, G.M, G.V., I.K. and N.S.; project administration, C.C., D.G. and N.S. All authors have read and agreed to the published version of the manuscript.

Funding: This research received no external funding.

Institutional Review Board Statement: The study was conducted according to the Declaration of Helsinki, with respect to relevant national and local requirements, and was approved by the National Drug Agency's Ethical Review Board for Human Research (OGYÉI/50115/2018).

Informed Consent Statement: Written informed consent has been obtained from the patients to publish this paper.

Data Availability Statement: Data will be available on request from the corresponding author.

Conflicts of Interest: The authors declare no conflict of interest.

References

1. Kyle, R.A. Monoclonal gammopathy of undetermined significance. Natural history in 241 cases. *Am. J. Med.* **1978**, *64*, 814–826. [CrossRef]
2. Kyle, R.A.; Therneau, T.M.; Rajkumar, S.V.; Larson, D.R.; Plevak, M.F.; Offord, J.R.; Dispenzieri, A.; Katzmann, J.A.; Melton, J.L. Prevalence of monoclonal gammopathy of undetermined significance. *N. Engl. J. Med.* **2006**, *354*, 1362–1369. [CrossRef] [PubMed]
3. Rajkumar, S.V.; Dimopoulos, M.A.; Palumbo, A.; Blade, J.; Merlini, G.; Mateos, M.V.; Kumar, S.; Hillengass, J.; Kastritis, E.; Richardson, P.; et al. International Myeloma Working Group updated criteria for the diagnosis of multiple myeloma. *Lancet Oncol.* **2014**, *15*, 538–548. [CrossRef] [PubMed]
4. Kyle, R.A.; Larson, D.R.; Therneau, T.M.; Dispenzieri, A.; Kumar, S.; Cerhan, J.R.; Rajkumar, S.V. Long-Term Follow-up of Monoclonal Gammopathy of Undetermined Significance. *N. Engl. J. Med.* **2018**, *378*, 241–249. [CrossRef] [PubMed]
5. Omoti, A.E.; Omoti, C.E. Ophthalmic manifestations of multiple myeloma. *West Afr. J. Med.* **2007**, *26*, 265–268.
6. Agorogiannis, E.I.; Kotamarthi, V. Paraproteinemia and central retinal vein occlusion. *Hippokratia* **2015**, *19*, 92.
7. Kormányos, K.; Kovács, K.; Németh, O.; Tóth, G.; Sándor, G.L.; Csorba, A.; Czakó, C.N.; Langenbucher, A.; Nagy, Z.Z.; Varga, G.; et al. Ocular Signs and Ocular Comorbidities in Monoclonal Gammopathy: Analysis of 80 Subjects. *J. Ophthalmol.* **2021**, *2021*, 9982875. [CrossRef]
8. Kormányos, K.; Kovács, K.; Németh, O.; Tóth, G.; Sándor, G.L.; Csorba, A.; Czakó, C.N.; Módis, L., Jr.; Langenbucher, A.; Nagy, Z.Z.; et al. Corneal Densitometry and In Vivo Confocal Microscopy in Patients with Monoclonal Gammopathy-Analysis of 130 Eyes of 65 Subjects. *J. Clin. Med.* **2022**, *11*, 1848. [CrossRef]
9. Menke, M.N.; Feke, G.T.; McMeel, J.W.; Branagan, A.; Hunter, Z.; Treon, S.P. Hyperviscosity-related retinopathy in waldenstrom macroglobulinemia. *Arch. Ophthalmol.* **2006**, *124*, 1601–1606. [CrossRef]
10. Eton, E.A.; Abrams, G.; Khan, N.W.; Fahim, A.T. Autoimmune retinopathy associated with monoclonal gammopathy of undetermined significance: A case report. *BMC Ophthalmol.* **2020**, *20*, 153. [CrossRef]

11. Garibaldi, D.C.; Gottsch, J.; de la Cruz, Z.; Haas, M.; Green, W.R. Immunotactoid keratopathy: A clinicopathologic case report and a review of reports of corneal involvement in systemic paraproteinemias. *Surv. Ophthalmol.* **2005**, *50*, 61–80. [CrossRef]
12. Smith, S.J.; Johnson, M.W.; Ober, M.D.; Comer, G.M.; Smith, B.D. Maculopathy in Patients with Monoclonal Gammopathy of Undetermined Significance. *Ophthalmol. Retin.* **2020**, *4*, 300–309. [CrossRef]
13. Coscas, F.; Sellam, A.; Glacet-Bernard, A.; Jung, C.; Goudot, M.; Miere, A.; Souied, E.H. Normative data for vascular density in superficial and deep capillary plexuses of healthy adults assessed by optical coherence tomography angiography. *Investig. Ophthalmol. Vis. Sci.* **2016**, *57*, 211–223. [CrossRef]
14. Watson, J.A.; Olson, D.J.; Zhang, A.Y. Hyperviscosity Retinopathy Due to Waldenström Macroglobulinemia: A Case Report and Literature Review. *J. VitreoRetinal Dis.* **2021**, *5*, 520–524. [CrossRef]
15. Li, J.; Zhang, R.; Gu, F.; Liu, Z.L.; Sun, P. Optical coherence tomography angiography characteristics in Waldenström macroglobulinemia retinopathy: A case report. *World J. Clin. Cases* **2020**, *8*, 6071–6079. [CrossRef]
16. Dursun, M.E.; Erdem, S.; Karahan, M.; Ava, S.; Hazar, L.; Dursun, B.; Karakas, A.; Demircan, V.; Keklikci, U. Retinal Microvascular Changes in Patients with Multiple Myeloma: A Study Based on Optical Coherence Tomography Angiography. *Curr. Eye Res.* **2022**, *47*, 874–881. [CrossRef] [PubMed]
17. Kwaan, H.C. Hyperviscosity in plasma cell dyscrasias. *Clin. Hemorheol. Microcirc.* **2013**, *55*, 75–83. [CrossRef]
18. Dumas, G.; Merceron, S.; Zafrani, L.; Canet, E.; Lemiale, V.; Kouatchet, A.; Azoulay, E. Syndrome d'hyperviscosité plasmatique [Hyperviscosity syndrome]. *Rev. Med. Interne* **2015**, *36*, 588–595. [CrossRef] [PubMed]
19. Caimi, G.; Hopps, E.; Carlisi, M.; Montana, M.; Gallà, E.; Lo Presti, R.; Siragusa, S. Hemorheological parameters in Monoclonal Gammopathy of Undetermined Significance (MGUS). *Clin. Hemorheol. Microcirc.* **2018**, *68*, 51–59. [CrossRef]
20. Uggla, B.; Nilsson, T.K. Whole blood viscosity in plasma cell dyscrasias. *Clin. Biochem.* **2015**, *48*, 122–124. [CrossRef] [PubMed]
21. Kashani, A.H.; Chen, C.L.; Gahm, J.K.; Zheng, F.; Richter, G.M.; Rosenfeld, P.J.; Shi, Y.; Wang, R.K. Optical coherence tomography angiography: A comprehensive review of current methods and clinical applications. *Prog. Retin. Eye Res.* **2017**, *60*, 66–100. [CrossRef] [PubMed]
22. Tokayer, J.; Jia, Y.; Dhalla, A.H.; Huang, D. Blood flow velocity quantification using split-spectrum amplitude-decorrelation angiography with optical coherence tomography. *Biomed. Opt. Express* **2013**, *4*, 1909–1924. [CrossRef] [PubMed]
23. Pascual-Prieto, J.; Burgos-Blasco, B.; Ávila Sánchez-Torija, M.; Fernández-Vigo, J.I.; Arriola-Villalobos, P.; Barbero Pedraz, M.A.; García-Feijoo, J.; Martínez-de-la-Casa, J.M. Utility of optical coherence tomography angiography in detecting vascular retinal damage caused by arterial hypertension. *Eur. J. Ophthalmol.* **2020**, *30*, 579–585. [CrossRef] [PubMed]
24. Tan, W.; Yao, X.; Le, T.T.; Tan, A.C.S.; Cheung, C.Y.; Chin, C.W.L.; Schmetterer, L.; Chua, J. The Application of Optical Coherence Tomography Angiography in Systemic Hypertension: A Meta-Analysis. *Front. Med.* **2021**, *8*, 778330. [CrossRef]
25. Czakó, C.; Sándor, G.; Ecsedy, M.; Récsán, Z.; Horváth, H.; Szepessy, Z.; Nagy, Z.Z.; Kovács, I. Decreased retinal capillary density is associated with a higher risk of diabetic retinopathy in patients with diabetes. *Retina* **2019**, *39*, 1710–1719. [CrossRef]
26. István, L.; Czakó, C.; Benyó, F.; Élő, Á.; Mihály, Z.; Sótonyi, P.; Varga, A.; Nagy, Z.Z.; Kovács, I. The effect of systemic factors on retinal blood flow in patients with carotid stenosis: An optical coherence tomography angiography study. *Geroscience* **2022**, *44*, 389–401. [CrossRef]
27. Lee, C.W.; Cheng, H.C.; Chang, F.C.; Wang, A.G. Optical Coherence Tomography Angiography Evaluation of Retinal Microvasculature Before and After Carotid Angioplasty and Stenting. *Sci. Rep.* **2019**, *9*, 14755. [CrossRef]
28. Lahme, L.; Storp, J.J.; Marchiori, E.; Esser, E.; Eter, N.; Mihailovic, N.; Alnawaiseh, M. Evaluation of Ocular Perfusion in Patients with End-Stage Renal Disease Receiving Hemodialysis Using Optical Coherence Tomography Angiography. *J. Clin. Med.* **2023**, *12*, 3836. [CrossRef]
29. Sampson, D.M.; Dubis, A.M.; Chen, F.K.; Zawadzki, R.J.; Sampson, D.D. Towards standardizing retinal optical coherence tomography angiography: A review. *Light Sci. Appl.* **2022**, *11*, 63. [CrossRef]
30. Rakusiewicz, K.; Kanigowska, K.; Hautz, W.; Ziółkowska, L. Usefulness of retinal optical coherence tomography angiography evolution in cases of systemic diseases. *Klin. Oczna.* **2021**, *123*, 166–172. [CrossRef]
31. Czakó, C.; István, L.; Ecsedy, M.; Récsán, Z.; Sándor, G.; Benyó, F.; Horváth, H.; Papp, A.; Resch, M.; Borbándy, Á.; et al. The effect of image quality on the reliability of OCT angiography measurements in patients with diabetes. *Int. J. Retin. Vitr.* **2019**, *5*, 46. [CrossRef] [PubMed]
32. Czakó, C.; István, L.; Benyó, F.; Élő, Á.; Erdei, G.; Horváth, H.; Nagy, Z.Z.; Kovács, I. The Impact of Deterministic Signal Loss on OCT Angiography Measurements. *Transl. Vis. Sci. Technol.* **2020**, *9*, 10. [CrossRef]
33. Greipp, P.R.; San Miguel, J.; Durie, B.G.; Crowley, J.J.; Barlogie, B.; Bladé, J.; Boccadoro, M.; Child, J.A.; Avet-Loiseau, H.; Kyle, R.A.; et al. International staging system for multiple myeloma. *J. Clin. Oncol.* **2005**, *23*, 3412–3420. [CrossRef] [PubMed]
34. Palumbo, A.; Avet-Loiseau, H.; Oliva, S.; Lokhorst, H.M.; Goldschmidt, H.; Rosinol, L.; Richardson, P.; Caltagirone, S.; Lahuerta, J.J.; Facon, T.; et al. Revised International Staging System for Multiple Myeloma: A Report from International Myeloma Working Group. *J. Clin. Oncol.* **2015**, *33*, 2863–2869. [CrossRef] [PubMed]

Disclaimer/Publisher's Note: The statements, opinions and data contained in all publications are solely those of the individual author(s) and contributor(s) and not of MDPI and/or the editor(s). MDPI and/or the editor(s) disclaim responsibility for any injury to people or property resulting from any ideas, methods, instructions or products referred to in the content.

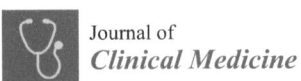

Article

Normative Data for Macular Thickness and Volume for Optical Coherence Tomography in a Diabetic Population without Maculopathies

Carolina Arruabarrena [1,*], Antonio Rodríguez-Miguel [2], Fernando de Aragón-Gómez [1], Purificación Escámez [1], Ingrid Rosado [1] and Miguel A. Teus [1,3]

1. Retina Unit, Department of Ophthalmology, University Hospital "Príncipe de Asturias", 28805 Alcalá de Henares, Madrid, Spain
2. Department of Biomedical Sciences, University of Alcalá (IRYCIS), 28805 Alcalá de Henares, Madrid, Spain
3. Department of Medical Sciences (Ophthalmology), University of Alcalá, 28805 Alcalá de Henares, Madrid, Spain
* Correspondence: carruabarrenas@gmail.com; Tel.: +34-9-1887-8100

Abstract: Purpose: The purpose was to establish normative data for the macular thicknesses and volume using spectral-domain optical coherence tomography (SD-OCT) in a diabetic population without maculopathies for use as a reference in diabetic retinopathy (DR) and diabetic macular edema screening programs. Methods: This was an observational study nested in a cohort of diabetics from a telemedicine DR screening program. Each patient underwent SD-OCT centered on the fovea. Macular thickness and volume were described and compared using the built-in normative database of the device. Quantile regression models for the 97.5% percentile were fitted to evaluate the predictors of macular thickness and volume. Results: A total of 3410 eyes (mean age, 62.25 (SD, 0.22) years) were included. Mean (SD) central subfield thickness (CST) was 238.2 (23.7) µm, while center thickness (CT), average thickness (AT), and macular volume (MV) were 205.4 (31.6) µm, 263.9 (14.3) µm, and 7.46 (0.40) mm^3, respectively. Para- and perifoveal thicknesses were clinically and statistically significantly thinner in our population than in the normative reference database. The 97.5% percentile of the thickness of all sectors was increased in males and in the para- and perifovea among those with DR. Conclusions: All ETDRS sectors were thinner in patients with diabetes than in the reference population, except for the CST, which was the most stable parameter that only changed with sex. The upper cutoff limit to detect diabetic macular edema (DME) was different from that of the reference population and was influenced by conditions related to diabetes, such as DR. Therefore, specific normative data for diabetic patients should be used for the screening and diagnosis of DME using SD-OCT.

Keywords: diabetic macular edema; diabetic retinopathy; normative macular thickness; optical coherence tomography; screening

Citation: Arruabarrena, C.; Rodríguez-Miguel, A.; de Aragón-Gómez, F.; Escámez, P.; Rosado, I.; Teus, M.A. Normative Data for Macular Thickness and Volume for Optical Coherence Tomography in a Diabetic Population without Maculopathies. *J. Clin. Med.* **2023**, *12*, 5232. https://doi.org/10.3390/jcm12165232

Academic Editor: José Ignacio Fernández-Vigo

Received: 30 June 2023
Revised: 6 August 2023
Accepted: 9 August 2023
Published: 11 August 2023

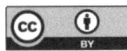

Copyright: © 2023 by the authors. Licensee MDPI, Basel, Switzerland. This article is an open access article distributed under the terms and conditions of the Creative Commons Attribution (CC BY) license (https://creativecommons.org/licenses/by/4.0/).

1. Introduction

Optical coherence tomography (OCT) is a non-invasive technique that obtains images of the macula with histological resolution [1,2]. Nowadays, it has become the gold standard for the diagnosis and follow-up of maculopathies because of its high sensitivity, good reliability, and reproducibility [3]. The first temporal domain devices (TD-OCT) have been replaced by spectral domain OCT (SD-OCT) devices that have higher scanning speed, fewer artifacts [4], better axial resolutions, and an acceptable cost. Almost all OCT devices provide similar retinal thickness parameters based on the Early Treatment of Diabetic Retinopathy Study (ETDRS) maps [5]. The central subfield (CST) is the most widely used inclusion and retreatment criteria in clinical trials and practice, including diabetic macular edema (DME) [6], and the other are four inner and outer sectors of the ETDRS map (para and perifovea areas, Figure 1), center thickness (CT), average thickness (AT), and macular volume (MV) [5].

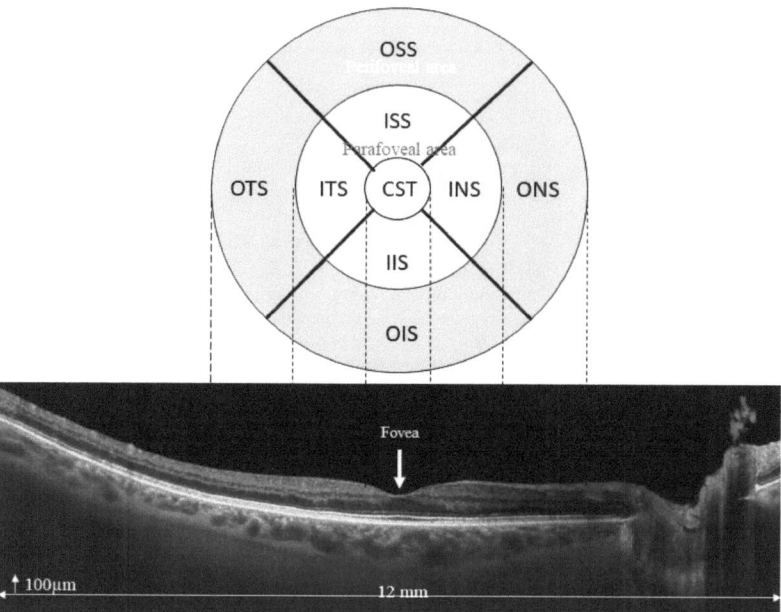

Figure 1. ETDRS map showing CT, CST, inner sectors or parafoveal area (inner temporal sector (ITS), inner nasal sector (INS), inner superior sector (ISS) and inner inferior sector (IIS)), and outer sectors or perifoveal area (outer temporal sector (OTS), outer nasal sector (ONS), outer superior sector (OSS), and outer inferior sector (OIS)).

Currently, the thicknesses are calculated using an automatic segmentation software that sets the inner and outer limits and calculates the AT in each of the nine sectors of the ETDRS map. All SD-OCT devices use the internal limiting membrane as the internal limit, but each device uses a different external limit to obtain different thicknesses for the same B-scan [4,7]. Therefore, due to this and other factors such as the refractive index mismatch, resolution, scan numbers used for 2D or 3D scans, dispersion correction methods used to match the system performance, laser power, bandwidth, and central wavelength used for different OCT systems, the macular thickness varies depending on the OCT device employed and the scanning protocol used [7–9].

The thicknesses have been measured in a healthy population with different OCT instruments to create a normative database for each instrument. They were compared with each other and with initial TD-OCT in healthy populations [5,7,9] and patients with macular diseases [4,8] to measure reproducibility and create conversion tables [9–11].

Macular thickness in healthy people varies according to age [5,12–16], sex [5,13–16], refractive error [1–19], and race [16], but it is not clear if in patients with DM, it also changes with the severity of diabetic retinopathy (DR) and the duration of DM [5]. Some studies found no difference between DM patients without retinopathy and healthy subjects, although both studies used TD-OCT and a SD-OCT prototype, with limited resolution [18,19]. However, a decrease in the macular thickness in diabetic patients even without DR, due to diabetic neurodegenerative retinopathy, has recently been described using modern OCT technology [20–24]. Based on the observations from OCT scans of diabetic patients without DR, it seems that some kind of neurodegeneration occurs before DR. Specifically, a reduction in inner retinal layers (ganglion cell layer and nerve fiber layer) in the macular and peripapillary regions has been clearly detected [20–25]. In addition, it has been hypothesized that these changes in OCT may be an early marker of systemic ischemic damage [26]. However, there is controversy regarding the influence of DM on total retinal thickness in both old [27] and modern studies [22]. This is due, at least in part, because of the heterogeneity of the study designs, which include type 1 and type 2 diabetics, patients with and without DR, and the different OCT devices used [26]. In addition, there are differences in the duration of DM within subgroups. Nevertheless, it seems that patients with diabetes for more than 10 years may experience an increase in global retinal thickness despite a decrease in the inner retina [22,28].

The Topcon 3SD-OCT Maestro 1 (Topcon Medical Systems, Inc., Oakland, NJ, USA) is a suitable device for screening DR, as it combines a non-mydriatic camera and SD-OCT. Introduced in 2013, it has an analysis software (OCT Data Collector) that obtains the AT in each sector of the ETDRS map, in addition to the MV and overall AT. It uses a reference normative database of macular thicknesses from healthy subjects (published elsewhere) [12,17] in the internal literature. However, at present, there is a lack of specific data on the thicknesses in the diabetic population [12,17].

Specific normality data for individuals with DM are crucial since they establish the threshold for diagnosing DME. If the threshold differs from that of the healthy population, it may lead to misdiagnosis among these patients. Our group conducted a previous study [29] to identify the best DME diagnostic criteria in SD-OCT within a DR screening program. Our research revealed that using as a cutoff either an MV >8 mm^3 or a thickness of the parafoveal area beyond two standard deviations (SD) of the mean normal value resulted in numerous false positives and a low positive predictive value.

Therefore, we aimed to create a normative database for diabetic patients with different degrees of retinopathy (excluding proliferative diabetic retinopathy (PDR)), without maculopathies or neuropathies, and to evaluate whether other characteristics such as age, sex, DM duration, and degree of retinopathy could act as predictors. Finally, we compared our data with the built-in normative database of the Topcon 3SD-OCT Maestro.

2. Materials and Methods

2.1. Design and Subject Selection

This observational study was nested in a cohort of diabetics from a telemedicine DR screening program. A randomly sampled eye from one visit of patients with DM referred for ophthalmological screening between 2016 to 2019 was included.

Eligible participants were 18 years old or older with type 1 or type 2 DM sent by their referring doctor for community DR screening. Exclusion criteria were as follows: (1) retinal thickening or thinning due to any macular disease based on fundus photography examination or OCT, (2) macular laser photocoagulation, proliferative DR, or pan-photocoagulation based on grading of fundus photographs, (3) prior treatment for macular edema, (4) glaucoma or other neuropathy based on fundus photography or OCT, (5) OCT scans with artifacts, and (6) OCT scans with a signal strength of less than Top Q 40 [30].

2.2. OCT Measurements Procedures and Main Outcomes

An experienced optometrist imaged all patients with a Topcon 3D SD-OCT Maestro 1, with a lateral and axial resolution of 20 and 6 μm, respectively, using a 6 × 6 mm^2 3D macular cube protocol (Figure 2).

For consistent clinical practice, OCT measurements were performed using the default axial length (24.46 mm) and refractive error (0.0 diopters). After acquisition, all macular images were manually checked to ensure that they were free of artifacts (boundary errors and off-centering), and complete cross-sectional images were obtained for all individual line scans. All OCT measurements were performed under non-mydriatic conditions. In cases of poor image quality, the patients were dilated with tropicamide (10 mg/mL) and reimaged.

The instrument software automatically determined the retinal thickness of the macula as the distance between the internal limiting membrane and the signal from the anterior boundary of the retinal pigment epithelium–choriocapillaris region.

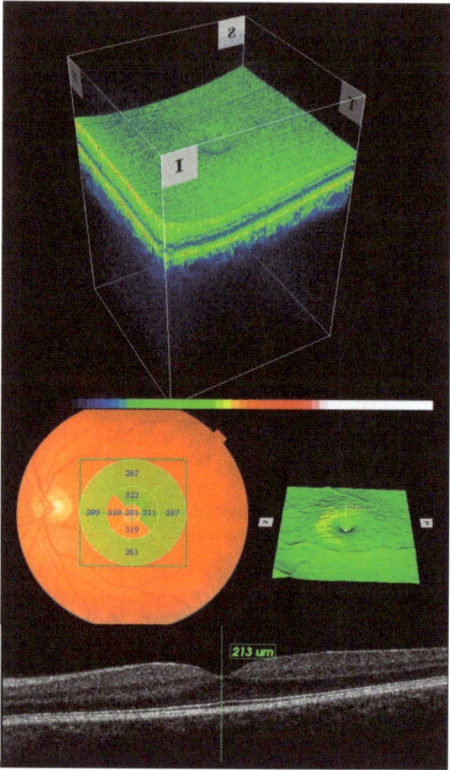

Figure 2. The figure shows a composite image of the 6 × 6 mm cube in 3D, with a 2D B-scan centered in the fovea, a superficial topographic macular map, and fundus photography with the ETDRS map superimposed.

The main outcomes (CT, CST, AT, inner and outer ETDRS map sector thicknesses, and MV) were automatically measured on the 6 mm macular thickness map analysis (6 × 6 3D macular cube) and displayed through the OCT data collector software.

2.3. Statistical Analysis

Quantitative variables are expressed as mean (±SD) or median and interquartile range (IQR) for non-normally distributed data as well as the range. Qualitative variables are expressed as frequencies and percentages. Differences in quantitative variables between two groups were compared using the Student's t-test, and one-way ANOVA or Kruskal–Wallis tests (for parametric or non-parametric evaluation, respectively) were used for comparisons of three or more groups. Differences in frequencies were compared using the chi-square test or Fisher's exact test when the assumptions needed for the former were not met. Absolute standardized differences for quantitative and qualitative variables were calculated as measures of imbalance between populations, and a value > 0.40 was considered a high imbalance.

Stratified analyses were performed according to age, sex, type of DM, presence of DR, and time since DM diagnosis.

Quantile regression models were fitted for the 97.5% percentile to evaluate the predictors of macular thickness and volume, and fully adjusted coefficients with their 95% confidence intervals (95%CI) were obtained.

Statistical significance was set at $p < 0.05$ but was adjusted for multiple comparisons when necessary. All analyses were performed using STATA/MP v.17 (Stata Corp LLC., College Station, TX, USA, 2017).

2.4. Ethics

The Ethics Committee of the University Hospital Príncipe de Asturias (Alcalá de Henares, Madrid, Spain) approved this study, which was conducted in accordance with the Declaration of Helsinki (Fortaleza 2013).

3. Results

3.1. Selection of Eyes, Baseline Clinical Characteristics of the Eyes Included, Overall and by Other Comorbidities

From 2016 to 2019, 7275 screens met the eligibility criteria (Figure 3), and 1 eye from each patient was randomly selected; thus, finally, 3410 eyes were included in the study.

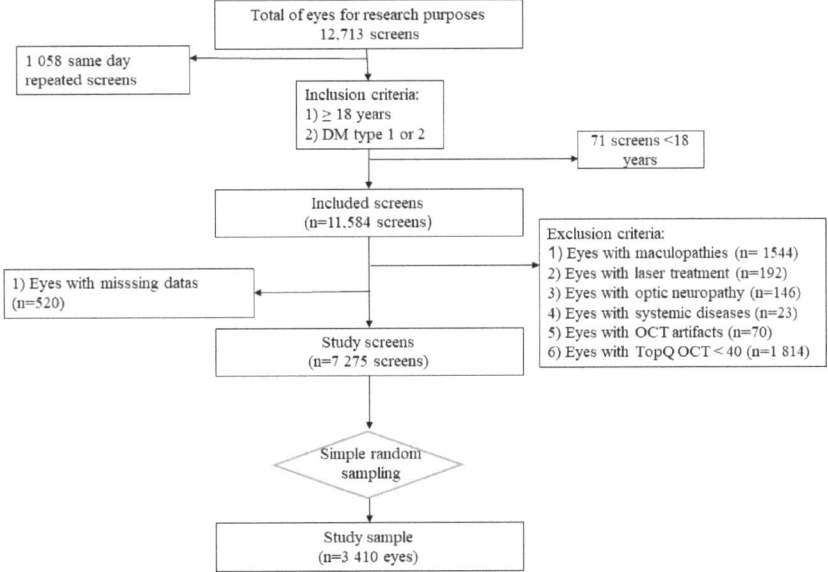

Figure 3. Flowchart of study sample inception.

The patients were 57.7% males, with a mean age of 62.2 ± 12.8 years (range, 18–93 years), and 3078 (90.2%) patients had a BCVA ≥ 6/12. Most patients were diagnosed with type 2 DM with a time from the diagnosis lower than 15 years. Among the patients, 2849 (83.5%) had no DR, and 14 eyes (0.5%) had severe non-proliferative DR. More than 60% (2137) of the patients had hypertension and hypercholesterolemia (2292). A total of 684 (20%) patients were current smokers, 396 (11.6%) had a history of acute myocardial infarction, 20 (0.6%) had a history of stroke, and 391 eyes (11.5%) were reimaged after pharmacological mydriasis (Table 1).

Table 1. Clinical and sociodemographic characteristics of the population.

	Overall ($n = 3410$)
Age. mean (SD)	62.25 (0.22)
Gender male n, (%)	1968 (57.7%)
Right eye n, (%)	1668 (48.9%)
CV risk factors, n (%):	
Current smoker	684 (20.0%)
Hypertension	2137 (62.7%)
Dyslipidemia	2292 (67.2%)
History of acute myocardial infarction	396 (11.6%)
History of stroke	20 (0.59%)

Table 1. *Cont.*

	Overall (n = 3410)
VA categorized by groups, n, (%)	
≤0.3	1237 (36.3%)
0.4–0.5	253 (7.42%)
≥0.5	1920 (56.3%)
Duration of diabetes, in years, n (%):	
≤15	2552 (74.8%)
>15	858 (25.2%)
DM type 2, n (%)	3135 (91.9%)
Diabetic retinopathy, * n (%):	
No abnormalities	2849 (83.5%)
Mild non-proliferative	362 (10.6%)
Moderate non-proliferative	185 (5.42%)
Severe non-proliferative	14 (0.47%)
Sight-threatening DR, n (%):	
No abnormalities	2849 (83.5%)
ST-DR	14 (0.47%)
No ST-DR	547 (16.0%)
Dilated, n (%)	391 (11.5%)

DM: diabetes mellitus, SD. Standard deviation, CV: Cardiovascular, VA: Visual acuity, DR: diabetic retinopathy, ST-DR: Sight-threatening diabetic retinopathy. * According to ICO grading system.

3.2. Macular Thickness and Volume Measured with SD-OCT in DM Patients without Maculopathies

Mean (SD) CST, CT, AT, and MV were 238.2 (23.7) µm, 205.4 (31.6) µm, 263.9 (14.3) µm, and 7.46 (0.40) mm³, respectively (Table 2). Overall thickness was greater within the inner macula, nasal was the thickest (299.0 µm; SD: 17.4), followed by superior, inferior, and temporal, which were 296.6 (18.4) µm, 292.9 (18.1) µm, and 285.1 (16.8) µm, respectively. Within the outer macula, the order was similar, but mean (SD) thicknesses were thinner: 272.0 (16.1) µm, 255.0 (16.3) µm, 253.2 (16.2) µm, and 244.0 (17.5) µm (Table 2). As Figure 1 displayed, our study showed a distinct topography where the retinal thickness is thinnest in the fovea and thicker in the parafoveal area.

Table 2. Normative Data for ETDRS Macular Thickness (in µm) and Volume (in mm³) measured by Spectral-Domain Optical Coherence Tomography (Topcon 3SD OCT Master).

n = 3410	Center Macula		Inner Macula				Outer Macula				Average Thickness	Total Volume
	CST	Center	Temporal	Superior	Nasal	Inferior	Temporal	Superior	Nasal	Inferior		
Median	237.3	200	285.6	297.6	299.3	293.4	244.8	255.5	272.4	253.0	264.3	7.47
IQR	222.6–252.7	183–222	274.6–296.3	286.0–308.2	287.9–310.6	282.0–304.7	235.1–254.4	245.1–265.2	261.4–282.9	243.2–263.5	254.9–273.2	7.21–7.72
Mean	238.2	205.4	285.1	296.6	299.0	292.9	244.0	255.0	272.0	253.2	263.9	7.46
SD	23.7	31.6	16.8	18.4	17.4	18.1	17.5	16.3	16.1	16.2	14.3	0.40
Min–Max	165.8–336.1	117–345	128.5–368	107.7–388.6	227.2–382.3	185.9–350.0	178.5–314.0	133.2–310.9	153.2–331.4	166.0–317.0	190.9–313.4	5.40–8.86
95%CI	237.4–239.0	204.3–206.4	284.5–285.7	295.9–297.2	298.5–299.6	292.3–293.5	243.4–244.6	254.4–255.5	271.4–272.6	252.7–253.8	263.4–264.3	7.44–7.47

ETDRS: Early treatment Diabetic retinopathy study; CST: Central subfield thickness; SD: standard deviation; IQR: Interquartile range; CI: confidence interval; min: minimum; and max: maximum.

3.3. Comparison of the Macular Thickness Measured with SD-OCT in DM Patients without Maculopathies with the Reference Normative Database of Topcon 3SD Maestro

The parafoveal area was thinner in our population than in the reference: ITS, 285.1 (16.8) μm vs. 296.59 (16.62) μm; ISS, 296.6 (18.4) μm vs. 308.98 (16.19) μm; INS, 299.0 (17.4) μm vs. 309.33 (16.68) μm; IIS, 292.9 (18.1) μm vs. 305.73 (16.32) μm; and even thinner in DM without DR. The absolute standardized difference was >0.59 for all sectors, meaning a high imbalance between populations (Table 3). Similar results were observed within the perifovea, with an absolute standardized difference ≥ 0.52 for all sectors except the OIS, which was 0.33 (Table 3). In contrast, CST was statistically significantly thicker in our population than in the reference: the mean (SD) was 238.2 (23.7) μm vs. 234 (20.65) μm, respectively, and even thicker in our population with DR: the mean (SD) was 239.0 (25.4) μm, although the standardized absolute difference was 0.18 (Table 3).

Table 3. Comparison between Topcon normative database of healthy people and our normative database of diabetic people without maculopathies.

		Mean (SD), μm				Absolute Standardized Difference	p Value
		Arruabarrena et al. n = 3410	Arruabarrena et al. no DR n = 2849	Arruabarrena et al. DR n = 561	Chaglasian et al. [12] + Normative Topcon 3D SD-OCT Maestro N = 395		
Center macula	CST	238.2 (23.7)	238.0 (23.4)	239.0 (25.4)	234 (20.65)	0.18 [1] 0.17 [2] 0.21 [3]	<0.001 [1] <0.001 [2] <0.001 [3]
Inner macula	Temporal	285.1 (16.8)	284.9 (16.6)	286.0 (17.7)	296.59 (16.62)	0.68 [1] 0.70 [2] 0.61 [3]	<0.001 [1] <0.001 [2] <0.001 [3]
Inner macula	Superior	296.6 (18.4)	296.5 (18.2)	296.8 (19.5)	308.98 (16.19)	0.68 [1] 0.69 [2] 0.67 [3]	<0.001 [1] <0.001 [2] <0.001 [3]
Inner macula	Nasal	299.0 (17.4)	299.0 (17.2)	298.8 (18.3)	309.33 (16.68)	0.59 [1] 0.60 [2] 0.60 [3]	<0.001 [1] <0.001 [2] <0.001 [3]
Inner macula	Inferior	292.9 (18.1)	292.8 (17.8)	293.5 (19.5)	305.73 (16.32)	0.72 [1] 0.74 [2] 0.67 [3]	<0.001 [1] <0.001 [2] <0.001 [3]
Outer macula	Temporal	244.0 (17.5)	243.6 (17.2)	246.1 (18.5)	252.93 (13.94)	0.52 [1] 0.55 [2] 0.41 [3]	<0.001 [1] <0.001 [2] <0.001 [3]
Outer macula	Superior	255.0 (16.3)	254.5 (16.0)	257.2 (17.4)	269.50 (15.16)	0.90 [1] 0.94 [2] 0.74 [3]	<0.001 [1] <0.001 [2] <0.001 [3]
Outer macula	Nasal	272.0 (16.1)	271.8 (16.5)	273.1 (18.1)	284.15 (16.42)	0.75 [1] 0.75 [2] 0.63 [3]	<0.001 [1] <0.001 [2] <0.001 [3]
Outer macula	Inferior	253.2 (16.2)	252.9 (16.0)	254.6 (17.2)	258.58 (14.90)	0.33 [1] 0.35 [2] 0.24 [3]	<0.001 [1] <0.001 [2] <0.001 [3]

[1] Arruabarrena vs. Chaglasian; [2] Arruabarrena No DR vs. Chaglasian (statistically significant p-value = 0.025); [3] Arruabarrena DR vs. Chaglasian (statistically significant p-value = 0.025). SD: standard deviation; DR: diabetic retinopathy; SD-OCT: spectral-domain optical coherence tomography; CST: central subfield thickness; CI: confidence interval.

3.4. Baseline Characteristics and Comorbidities Associated with Macular Thickness and Volume in DM Patients without Maculopathies

Regarding the 97.5% percentile of CT, male sex, age > 60 years, history of stroke, and dyslipidemia were associated with increased thickness, while image quality and the need for pupil dilation were associated with decreased thickness (Table 4). The 97.5% percentile of the CST was associated with an increased thickness among males and a decrease depending on the quality of the images (Table 4). In contrast, the 97.5% percentile of the para- and perifoveal areas increased in males and among those with DR, while age showed a trend toward decreased thickness, especially among those older than 71 years (Table 4). The 97.5% cutoff value of MV was influenced only by sex and age > 71 years (Table 4).

Table 4. Factors associated with macular thickness and volume in 97.5% percentile, by quantile regression.

	CT, CST, and Volume		
	Fully Adjusted Coefficients (95%CI)		
97.5% Percentile	CT µm	CST µm	MV mm^3
Gender: Females Males	Ref. 9.80 (2.35, 17.2)	Ref. 10.7 (4.51, 17.0)	Ref. 0.13 (0.06, 0.20)
Age, years: ≤60 61–70 ≥71	Ref. 13.4 (4.43, 22.4) 15.6 (5.68, 25.5)	Ref. 2.16 (−5.34, 9.66) 7.38 (−0.92, 15.7)	Ref. 0.09 (−0.18, 0.003) −0.17 (−0.27, −0.07)
Laterality: Left eye Right eye	Ref. −7.00 (−14.3, 0.33)	Not a predictor	Not a predictor
Time since DM diagnosis, in years: ≤5 6–10 ≥10	Not a predictor	Not a predictor	Ref. −0.03 (−0.13, 0.07) −0.05 (−0.14, 0.04)
TopQ, quartiles	−5.40 (−8.86, −1.94)	−4.97 (−7.85, −2.08)	Not a predictor
Visual acuity, decimal Snellen: 0.02–0.4 0.5–1	Not a predictor	Not a predictor	Not a predictor
Pupil dilation: No Yes	Ref. −12.4 (−24.1, −0.68)	Ref. −7.31 (−17.1, 2.50)	Not a predictor
DR: No abnormalities ST and non-ST	Not a predictor	Not a predictor	Ref. 0.09 (−0.01, 0.19)
Antecedents of: * Hypertension Acute myocardial infarction Stroke Dyslipidemia Current exmoker	Not a predictor Not a predictor 54.2 (6.29, 102.1) 8.20 (0.18, 16.2) Not a predictor	Not a predictor Not a predictor 39.9 (−0.16, 80.0) 5.25 (−1.46, 12.0) Not a predictor	−0.07 (−0.14, 0.01) Not a predictor Not a predictor Not a predictor Not a predictor

Table 4. Cont.

	Average parafoveal and perifoveal area	
	Fully Adjusted Coefficients (95%CI), μm	
97.5% Percentile	Parafoveal Area	Perifoveal Area
Gender: Females Males	Ref. 5.80 (3.19, 8.42)	Ref. 5.11 (2.84, 7.37)
Age, years: ≤60 61–70 ≥71	Ref. −1.08 (−4.18, 2.02) −4.65 (−7.98, −1.32)	Ref. −4.68 (−7.36, −2.00) −8.02 (−10.9, −5.13)
Laterality: Left eye Right eye	Not a predictor	Ref. −3.13 (−5.34, −0.92)
Time since DM diagnosis, in years: ≤5 6–10 ≥10	Not a predictor	Not a predictor
TopQ, quartiles	Not a predictor	Not a predictor
Visual acuity, decimal Snellen: 0.02–0.4 0.5–1	Not a predictor	Not a predictor
Pupil dilation: No Yes	Not a predictor	Not a predictor
DR: No abnormalities ST and non-ST	Ref. 5.50 (2.03, 8.96)	Ref. 3.85 (0.87, 6.83)
Antecedents of: * Hypertension Acute myocardial infarction Stroke Dyslipidemia Current smoker	−4.72 (−7.51, −1.94) Not a predictor Not a predictor Not a predictor Not a predictor	−1.59 (−4.00, 0.83) −2.70 (−6.24, 0.85) Not a predictor Not a predictor Not a predictor

CI: confidence interval; μM: microns; DM: diabetes mellitus; TopQ: quality of the scan; DR: diabetic retinopathy; ST: sight-threatening; and Ref.: reference. * The category of reference is no presence of the disease.

Similar results were observed when stratifying by type of DM: males were associated with an increased thickness in all sectors and volume for the 97.5% percentile, across both strata, except for CT in type 1 DM, which did not reach statistical significance, while age, especially among those with type 2 DM ≥ 71 years was associated with a decreased 97.5% percentile (Table 5).

Table 5. Factors associated with 97.5% cutoff level of macular central thickness and volume, by DM type. Factors associated with 97.5% cutoff level of parafoveal and perifoveal thickness, by DM type.

	97.5% Cutoff Level, Fully Adjusted Coefficient (95%CI)					
	CT, μm		CST, μm		Macular Volume, mm³	
	DM Type 1	DM Type 2	DM Type 1	DM Type 2	DM Type 1	DM Type 2
Gender:						
Males	22.00 (−12.23, 56.23)	9.80 (1.13, 18.47)	20.21 (3.56, 36.85)	11.10 (4.55, 17.65)	0.36 (0.23, 0.49)	0.12 (0.05, 0.19)
Age, years:						
61–70	−9.00 (−97.93, 79.93)	12.00 (1.60, 22.40)	22.59 (−21.26, 66.44)	2.16 (−5.72, 10.04)	−0.20 (−0.54, 0.13)	−0.06 (−0.14, 0.02)
≥71	53.00 (−90.05, 196.05)	11.80 (0.33, 23.27)	35.91 (−33.39, 105.21)	7.02 (−1.63, 15.67)	−1.04 (−1.58, −0.51)	−0.14 (−0.23, −0.05)
Time since DM diagnosis, in years:						
6–10	Not a predictor		Not a predictor		0.13 (−0.11, 0.38)	−0.02 (−0.11, 0.07)
≥10					0.17 (−0.02, 0.36)	−0.05 (−0.13, 0.03)

Table 5. Cont.

	97.5% Cutoff Level, Fully Adjusted Coefficient (95%CI)					
	CT, μm		CST, μm		Macular Volume, mm³	
	DM Type 1	DM Type 2	DM Type 1	DM Type 2	DM Type 1	DM Type 2
TopQ, quartiles	1.00 (−16.56, 18.56)	−5.40 (−9.39, −1.41)	−4.16 (−12.81, 4.49)	−4.85 (−7.86, −1.83)	Not a predictor	
Visual acuity, Snellen decimal:						
0.5–1	−4.00 (−131.86, 123.86)	−13.00 (−32.15, 6.15)	Not a predictor		Not a predictor	
Pupil dilation:					Not a predictor	
Yes	−3.00 (−118.01, 112.01)	−14.00 (−27.14, −0.85)	6.49 (−50.19, 63.17)	−8.21 (−18.17, 1.76)		
DR:						
ST and non-ST	Not a predictor		Not a predictor		0.08 (−0.05, 0.22)	0.07 (−0.03, 0.17)
Antecedents of:						
Hypertension	Not a predictor	Not a predictor	Not a predictor	Not a predictor	0.17 (−0.02, 0.36)	−0.06 (−0.13, 0.01)
Acute myocardial infarction	Not a predictor	Not a predictor	Not a predictor	Not a predictor	Not a predictor	Not a predictor
Stroke	Not a predictor	54.00 (0.79, 107.21)	Not a predictor	Not a predictor	Not a predictor	Not a predictor
Dyslipidemia	−3.00 (−42.21, 36.21)	8.20 (−1.23, 17.63)	4.11 (−15.21, 23.43)	39.57 (−0.78, 79.92)	Not a predictor	Not a predictor
Current smoker	Not a predictor	Not a predictor	Not a predictor	6.01 (−1.15, 13.16)	−0.02 (−0.16, 0.11)	0.04 (−0.05, 0.13)

	97.5% Cutoff Level, Fully Adjusted Coefficients (95%CI), μm			
	Average Parafoveal Area		Average Perifoveal Area	
	DM Type 1	DM Type 2	DM Type 1	DM Type 2
Gender: Males	**16.53 (11.28, 21.78)**	**5.39 (2.53, 8.24)**	**6.51 (0.13, 12.89)**	**3.69 (1.24, 6.15)**
Age, years:				
61–70	2.95 (−11.17, 17.08)	−0.77 (−4.15, 2.60)	−1.72 (−18.66, 15.23)	**−4.52 (−7.41, −1.64)**
≥71	−14.16 (−36.66, 8.35)	**−4.40 (−8.00, −0.81)**	−26.00 (−54.87, 2.87)	**−7.32 (−10.41, −4.23)**
Time since DM diagnosis, in years: 6–10 ≥10	Not a predictor		Not a predictor	
TopQ, quartiles	Not a predictor		Not a predictor	
Visual acuity, Snellen decimal:				
0.5–1	Not a predictor		Not a predictor	
Pupil dilation: Yes	Not a predictor		Not a predictor	
DR: ST and non-ST	−0.61 (−6.07, 4.84)	**5.86 (1.93, 9.80)**	1.04 (−5.48, 7.57)	1.33 (−2.02, 4.69)
Antecedents of:				
Hypertension	6.26 (−1.00, 13.52)	**−4.87 (−7.91, −1.83)**	2.64 (−6.13, 11.42)	−2.10 (−4.71, 0.52)
Acute myocardial infarction	Not a predictor	Not a predictor	−11.05 (−34.47, 12.36)	−2.06 (−5.75, 1.63)
Stroke	Not a predictor	Not a predictor	Not a predictor	Not a predictor
Dyslipidemia	Not a predictor	Not a predictor	Not a predictor	Not a predictor
Current smoker	Not a predictor	Not a predictor	Not a predictor	Not a predictor

CI: confidence interval; μM: microns; DM: diabetes mellitus; TopQ: quality of the scan; DR: diabetic retinopathy; ST: sight-threatening. Reference categories: Gender: female; Age: <60 years; Time since DM diagnosis: <5 years; Visual acuity: <0.5; Pupil dilatation: no; DR: No abnormalities; Antecedent of: no presence of the disease.

The median (IQR) thickness of the ETDRS sectors stratified by age showed a decreasing trend (nasal > superior > inferior > temporal), remained stable until 60 years of age, and then decreased. CST, CT, and MV increased after 40 years, reached a maximum at 51–60 years, and decreased thereafter (Figure 4). Therefore, the comparison between those younger and those older than 60 years was statistically significant for MV and all thicknesses, except for CST (Supplementary Table S1).

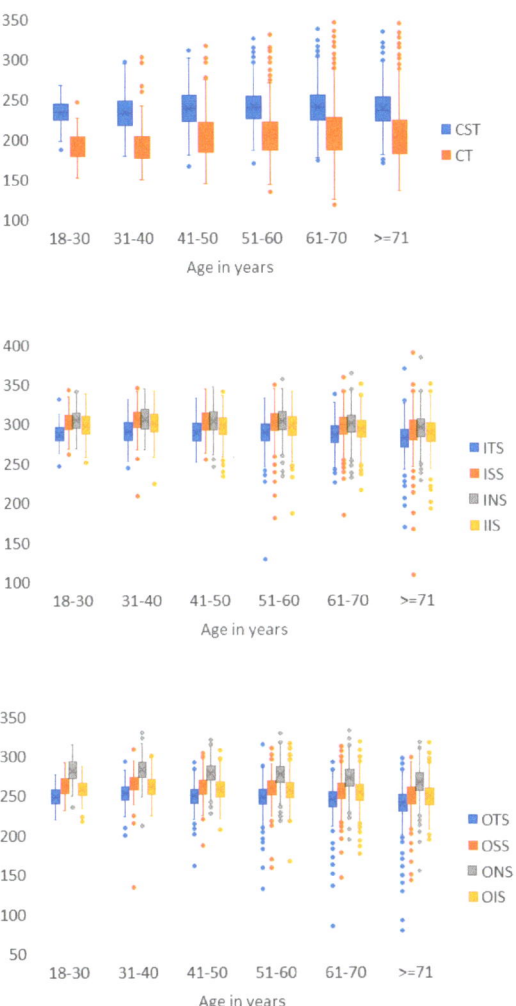

Figure 4. Median ETDRS map sector thickness by groups of age. The horizontal line (_) within the box represents the median, and the cross within the box (X) represents the mean.

We found statistically significant differences according to sex; they were lower in females (Supplementary Table S2). Among eyes with DR, we found a slight but statistically significant increase in MV, perifoveal thickness, and AT compared to those without (Supplementary Table S3).

The main outcomes were statistically significantly thinner among subjects with Type 2 DM than in type 1 and in those with ≥15 years of DM follow-up, except CST and CT, which were related to greater values in type 2 DM Supplementary Tables S4 and S5).

4. Discussion

We found that the cutoff values at the upper limit of normal macular thicknesses are not only influenced by some characteristics, such as sex and age, in diabetic patients without maculopathies, as well as in the general population, but also depend on image quality [30] and pupil dilation. Moreover, the cutoff thickness of the para- and perifoveal sectors increases in diabetics who present with DR. These data could explain the high percentage of false positives that we found in a previous study [29] for DR when we used an increase beyond 2SD from the mean of the reference population in the fovea and parafovea as a detection criterion. In the current study, we found that 45.3% of the false positives [29] when using the foveal and parafoveal thickening criteria were in patients with a normal macular profile that exceeded the thickness beyond 2SD from the mean of the reference population. If we use the new normative values for the healthy diabetic population, the number of false positives in the DR screening program would decrease, and the diagnostic profile of this quantitative criterion, which is simple to obtain, easy, and quick to evaluate, would improve. Apart from the CST, healthy patients with DM differ significantly from healthy patients and should use a special normative database for SD-OCT.

The thickness of the CST and CT is the least influenced by DM, not presenting statistically significant differences either by the type of DM, the time since the diagnosis of DM, or the presence of DR. CST only showed statistically significant differences according to sex, as shown in other studies in DM patients without maculopathy [14,15,18]. This means that CST is probably the most reliable parameter for evaluating the changes induced by treatments or interventions, but it must be considered with different limits for each sex; males have significantly thicker parameters on OCT, not only in DM patients [18,22] but also in healthy patients [12–15,17,19]. Invernizzi et al. [16] attributed this difference to the thicker inner and outer nuclear layers present in males.

Topographically, there is a pattern of thickness distribution: the foveal center is the thinnest in patients with DM without maculopathy, and the parafoveal area is the thickest. In our study, we found that the nasal sector was the thickest of the para- and perifoveal regions, followed by the superior, inferior, and temporal sectors (Table 2). These patterns were maintained in both sexes and all age groups (Supplementary Material Tables S1 and S2). Previous studies [14,15] using different types of OCT or retinal thickness analyzers in healthy populations and patients with DM (without maculopathy) [14] also reported a similar pattern of macular thickness that might be related to the crowding of nerve fibers in the parafoveal region and along the papillomacular bundle in the perifovea [15,16].

The effect of aging on macular thickness measured through OCT has revealed controversial results [13,15,19] that motivated a systematic review of the literature [31]. In our study, a characteristic pattern of changes in OCT thickness with age has been demonstrated in the DM population. The thicknesses of the peri- and parafovea remained stable until 51–60 years and decreased progressively thereafter. While the CST and CT remained stable between the ages of 18 and 40 years, they increased progressively until the age range of 61 to 70 years and then began to decrease (Figure 3). Similar data have been reported in healthy populations [13–16,31]. It is believed that cells in the foveal area (cones and RPE cells) remain stable until old age, when metabolic and phagocytic processes increase and RPE cells become thicker. However, the para- and perifoveal regions are composed of more cell layers, especially ganglion cells and nerve fiber layers, which diminish with age.

Although initial studies in patients with DM without DR did not show differences from healthy subjects [18,19], other studies have revealed differences in the OCT thicknesses of patients with DM (without maculopathy) [22,28]. This is probably due to the lower precision of the first OCT instrument (TD-OCT), which did not allow small differences to be detected. Our normative database of patients with DM without maculopathies, as in other previous studies [22–25], showed leaner parameters than the Topcon 3SD OCT1-Maestro normative database for healthy subjects [12,17] (Table 3). An increase in the CST in the group of healthy DM patients compared to the Topcon normative base was statistically significant ($p < 0.025$), both for DM patients without DR and, more importantly, for healthy DM patients with DR. Similar data have been found in other study [22] that describes an increase in the total macular thickness, especially at the central area in DM patients with DR, and a decrease in the thickness of the internal retina, which would mainly affect the para- and perifoveal area. We also found a decrease in the thickness in all sectors of the peri- and parafovea in patients with DM without maculopathies that were both clinically relevant (standardized absolute differences greater than 0.5) and statistically significant ($p < 0.025$) in DM eyes with and without DR. Neuronal degeneration is a likely explanation for the differential macular thinning in patients with diabetes because the most affected layer in this neurodegeneration is the nerve fiber layer [20–25]. This layer is almost absent in the central macula and thicker in the parafovea, thus making this area more sensitive to reflect changes in the nerve fiber thickness. There is a study that suggests that neurodegeneration and a decrease in nerve fiber layer thickness appear early in the disease. Later, the retina may show an increase in the total retinal thickness over time due to the vascular injury and the increased vascular permeability and edema that the DM may cause in the retina [22].

Other factors to consider are that the different types of DM [23,24] and duration of the disease [22,28] present differences in the distribution of some characteristics, which could bias the results, and that there may be thinning of the macula due to ischemia that could interfere with the results [24] that we cannot analyze in this study since we have not performed Fluorescein angiography or Angio-OCT to evaluate it.

When we analyzed the different characteristics related to DM that can influence thickness, we only found clinically relevant and statistically significant differences in general parameters between type 1 and type 2 DM (Supplementary Table S4). Differences between patients with and without DR (Supplementary Table S3), or with more or less than 15 years of DM evolution (Supplementary Table S5), although statistically significant, have little clinical relevance.

The strength of the current study is that it is the first to provide normative macular thickness data using the Topcon 3SD-OCT1 Maestro device in a large sample of patients with DM without maculopathy. Furthermore, the wide age range of our sample provides a good representation of older and younger adults in clinical practice. Therefore, our data provide a benchmark for clinicians to assess and compare macular changes in patients with DM, particularly those with DME. The normative database with which the Topcon 3D- OCT Maestro was marketed was based on a sample of 115 healthy patients. In 2018, a new normative database for the instrument was established using a sample of 399 subjects studied in 2015 [13]. This sample included only 35 subjects over 70 years of age and a sparse representation of patients with DM, although the macular thicknesses used by the instrument to set the cutoff limits for DME detection were based on these data.

Our study has some limitations: we used the default axial length (24.46 mm) and refraction (0.0 diopters) to capture the scans, although this should not affect the thickness values apart from a slight overestimation in the perifovea. Refractive errors and axial length were not measured, although eyes with high myopia, which seem to induce most artifacts [30], were excluded. Finally, our patients were Caucasians, and it would be interesting to include patients of other ethnicities.

Supplementary Materials: The following supporting information can be downloaded at: https://www.mdpi.com/article/10.3390/jcm12165232/s1, Supplementary Table S1. Normative Data for ETDRS Macular Thickness (in µm) and volume (in mm^3) measured through Spectral-Domain Optical Coherence Tomography (Topcon 3SD OCT Master), by age; Supplementary Table S2. Normative Data for Macular Thickness (in µm) and volume (in mm^3) measured through Spectral-Domain Optical Coherence Tomography (Topcon 3SD OCT Master), by gender; Supplementary Table S3. Normative Data for Macular Thickness (in µm) and volume (in mm^3) measured through Spectral-Domain Optical Coherence Tomography (Topcon 3SD OCT Master), by DR existence; Supplementary Table S4. Normative Data for Macular Thickness (in µm) and volume (in mm^3) measured through Spectral-Domain Optical Coherence Tomography (Topcon 3SD OCT Master), by type of DM; Supplementary Table S5. Normative Data for Macular Thickness (in µm) and volume (in mm^3) measured through Spectral-Domain Optical Coherence Tomography (Topcon 3SD OCT Master), by the years since DM diagnosis.

Author Contributions: The author contributions were as follows: Conceptualization, C.A. and M.A.T.; methodology, A.R.-M. and F.d.A.-G.; software, A.R.-M.; validation, P.E., C.A. and I.R.; formal analysis, C.A. and P.E.; investigation, C.A. and M.A.T.; resources, F.d.A.-G. and M.A.T.; data curation, IR, P.E. and F.d.A.-G.; writing—original draft preparation, C.A.; writing—review and editing, C.A., A.R.-M. and M.A.T.; visualization, A.R.-M.; supervision, M.A.T.; project administration, C.A.; funding acquisition, C.A. All authors have read and agreed to the published version of the manuscript.

Funding: The APC was funded by the Biomedical Investigation Foundation of the Principe de Asturias University Hospital.

Institutional Review Board Statement: The study was conducted in accordance with the Declaration of Helsinki and approved by the Institutional Review Board (or Ethics Committee) of Príncipe de Asturias University Hospital (protocol code OE10/2018 and date of approval May 2018).

Informed Consent Statement: Patient consent was waived due to the huge number of participants included in the sample and the ambispective character of the study.

Data Availability Statement: The data presented in this study are available in the article or Supplementary Material here.

Conflicts of Interest: The authors declare no conflict of interest. The funders had no role in the design of the study; in the collection, analyses, or interpretation of data; in the writing of the manuscript; or in the decision to publish the results.

References

1. Huang, D.; Swanson, E.A.; Lin, C.P.; Schuman, J.S.; Stinson, W.G.; Chang, W.; Hee, M.R.; Flotte, T.; Gregory, K.; Puliafito, C.A.; et al. Optical coherence tomography. *Science* **1991**, *254*, 1178–1181. [CrossRef] [PubMed]
2. Puliafito, C.A.; Hee, M.R.; Lin, C.P.; Reichel, E.; Schuman, J.S.; Duker, J.S.; Izatt, J.A.; Swanson, E.A.; Fujimoto, J.G. Imaging of Macular Diseases with Optical Coherence Tomography. *Ophthalmology* **1995**, *102*, 217–229. [CrossRef]
3. Virgili, G.; Menchini, F.; Casazza, G.; Hogg, R.; Das, R.R.; Wang, X.; Michelessi, M. Optical coherence tomography (OCT) for detection of macular oedema in patients -with diabetic retinopathy. *Cochrane Database Syst. Rev.* **2015**, *1*, CD008081. [CrossRef] [PubMed]
4. Ho, J.; Sull, A.C.; Vuong, L.N.; Chen, Y.; Liu, J.; Fujimoto, J.G.; Schuman, J.S.; Duker, J.S. Assessment of Artifacts and Reproducibility across Spectral- and Time-Domain Optical Coherence Tomography Devices. *Ophthalmology* **2009**, *116*, 1960–1970. [CrossRef]
5. Liu, T.B.; Hu, A.Y.; Kaines, A.; Yu, F.; Schwartz, S.D.; Hubschman, J.-P. A Pilot Study of Normative Data for Macular Thickness and Volume Measurements Using Cirrus High-Definition Optical Coherence Tomography. *Retina* **2011**, *31*, 1944–1950. [CrossRef]
6. Goebel, W.; Franke, R. Retinal thickness in diabetic retinopathy: Comparison of optical coherence tomography, the retinal thickness analyzer, and fundus photography. *Retina* **2006**, *26*, 49–57. [CrossRef]
7. Giani, A.; Cigada, M.; Choudhry, N.; Deiro, A.P.; Oldani, M.; Pellegrini, M.; Staurenghi, G. Reproducibility of retinal thickness measurements on normal and pathologic eyes by different optical coherence tomography instruments. *Am. J. Ophthalmol.* **2011**, *151*, 737, Erratum in *Am. J. Ophthalmol.* **2010**, *150*, 815–824.. [CrossRef]
8. Bahrami, B.; Ewe, S.Y.P.; Hong, T.; Zhu, M.; Ong, G.; Luo, K.; Chang, A. Influence of Retinal Pathology on the Reliability of Macular Thickness Measurement: A Comparison Between Optical Coherence Tomography Devices. *Ophthalmic Surg. Lasers Imaging Retin.* **2017**, *48*, 319–325. [CrossRef]
9. Pierro, L.; Giatsidis, S.M.; Mantovani, E.; Gagliardi, M. Macular Thickness Interoperator and Intraoperator Reproducibility in Healthy Eyes Using 7 Optical Coherence Tomography Instruments. *Am. J. Ophthalmol.* **2010**, *150*, 199–204.e1. [CrossRef] [PubMed]
10. Diabetic Retinopathy Clinical Research Network Writing Committee; Edwards, A.R.; Chalam, K.V.; Bressler, N.M.; Glassman, A.R.; Jaffe, G.J.; Melia, M.; Saggau, D.D.; Plous, O.Z. Reproducibility of spec-tral-domain optical coherence tomography retinal thickness measurements and conversion to equivalent time-domain metrics in diabetic macular edema. *JAMA Ophthalmol.* **2014**, *132*, 1113–1122.
11. Leung, C.K.-S.; Cheung, C.Y.-L.; Weinreb, R.N.; Lee, G.; Lin, D.; Pang, C.P.; Lam, D.S.C. Comparison of Macular Thickness Measurements between Time Domain and Spectral Domain Optical Coherence Tomography. *Investig. Opthalmology Vis. Sci.* **2008**, *49*, 4893–4897. [CrossRef] [PubMed]
12. Chaglasian, M.; Fingeret, M.; Davey, P.G.; Huang, W.-C.; Leung, D.; Ng, E.; Reisman, C. The development of a reference database with the Topcon 3D OCT-1 Maestro. *Clin. Ophthalmol.* **2018**, *12*, 849–857. [CrossRef]
13. Ooto, S.; Hangai, M.; Sakamoto, A.; Tomidokoro, A.; Araie, M.; Otani, T.; Kishi, S.; Matsushita, K.; Maeda, N.; Shirakashi, M.; et al. Three-Dimensional Profile of Macular Retinal Thickness in Normal Japanese Eyes. *Investig. Opthalmology Vis. Sci.* **2010**, *51*, 465–473. [CrossRef] [PubMed]
14. Von Hanno, T.; Lade, A.C.; Mathiesen, E.B.; Peto, T.; Njølstad, I.; Bertelsen, G. Macular thickness in healthy eyes of adults (N = 4508) and relation to sex, age and refraction: The Tromsø Eye Study (2007–2008). *Acta Ophthalmol.* **2017**, *95*, 262–269. [CrossRef]

15. Duan, X.R.; Liang, Y.B.; Friedman, D.S.; Sun, L.P.; Wong, T.Y.; Tao, Q.S.; Bao, L.; Wang, N.L.; Wang, J.J. Normal Macular Thickness Measurements Using Optical Coherence Tomography in Healthy Eyes of Adult Chinese Persons: The Handan Eye Study. *Ophthalmology* **2010**, *117*, 1585–1594. [CrossRef]
16. Invernizzi, A.; Pellegrini, M.; Acquistapace, A.; Benatti, E.; Erba, S.; Cozzi, M.; Staurenghi, G. Normative Data for Retinal-Layer Thickness Maps Generated by Spec-tral-Domain OCT in a White Population. *Ophthalmol. Retin.* **2018**, *2*, 808–815.e1. [CrossRef] [PubMed]
17. Topcon 3DSD-OCT Normative Database. Published 24 October 2020. Available online: https://es.scribd.com/document/478708713/3D-OCT-Series-Normative-Summary (accessed on 2 January 2023).
18. Bressler, N.M.; Edwards, A.R.; Antoszyk, A.N.; Beck, R.W.; Browning, D.J.; Ciardella, A.P.; Danis, R.P.; Elman, M.J.; Friedman, S.M.; Glassman, A.R.; et al. Retinal Thickness on Stratus Optical Coherence Tomography in People with Diabetes and Minimal or No Diabetic Retinopathy. *Am. J. Ophthalmol.* **2008**, *145*, 894–901.e1. [CrossRef]
19. Massin, P.; Erginay, A.; Haouchine, B.; Ben Mehidi, A.; Paques, M.; Gaudric, A. Retinal Thickness in Healthy and Diabetic Subjects Measured Using Optical Coherence Tomography Mapping Software. *Eur. J. Ophthalmol.* **2002**, *12*, 102–108. [CrossRef]
20. Clerck, E.E.B.D.; Schouten, J.S.A.G.; Berendschot, T.T.J.M.; Kessels, A.G.H.; Nuijts, R.M.M.; Beckers, H.J.M.; Schram, M.T.; Stehouwer, C.D.; Webers, C.A.B. New ophthalmologic imaging techniques for detection and monitoring of neurodegenerative changes in diabetes: A systematic review. *Lancet Diabetes Endocrinol.* **2015**, *3*, 653–663. [CrossRef]
21. Jia, X.; Zhong, Z.; Bao, T.; Wang, S.; Jiang, T.; Zhang, Y.; Li, Q.; Zhu, X. Evaluation of Early Retinal Nerve Injury in Type 2 Diabetes Patients Without Diabetic Retinopathy. *Front. Endocrinol.* **2020**, *11*, 475672. [CrossRef]
22. Oshitari, T.; Hanawa, K.; Adachi-Usami, E. Changes of macular and RNFL thicknesses measured by Stratus OCT in patients with early stage diabetes. *Eye* **2008**, *23*, 884–889. [CrossRef] [PubMed]
23. Mohd-Ilham, I.; Tai, E.L.M.; Suhaimi, H.; Shatriah, I. Evaluation of Macular and Retinal Nerve Fiber Layer Thickness in Children with Type 1 Diabetes Mellitus without Retinopathy. *Korean J. Ophthalmol.* **2021**, *35*, 287–294. [CrossRef]
24. Satue, M.; Cipres, M.; Melchor, I.; Gil-Arribas, L.; Vilades, E.; Garcia-Martin, E. Ability of Swept source OCT technology to detect neurodegeneration in patients with type 2 diabetes mellitus without diabetic retinopathy. *Jpn. J. Ophthalmol.* **2020**, *64*, 367–377. [CrossRef]
25. Vujosevic, S.; Midena, E. Retinal Layers Changes in Human Preclinical and Early Clinical Diabetic Retinopathy Support Early Retinal Neuronal and Müller Cells Alterations. *J. Diabetes Res.* **2013**, *2013*, 905058. [CrossRef] [PubMed]
26. Ciprés, M.; Satue, M.; Melchor, I.; Gil-Arribas, L.; Vilades, E.; Garcia-Martin, E. Retinal neurodegeneration in patients with type 2 diabetes mellitus without diabetic retinopathy. *Arch. Soc. Española Oftalmol.* **2022**, *97*, 205–218. [CrossRef]
27. Schaudig, U.H.; Glaefke, C.; Scholz, F.; Richard, G. Optical Coherence Tomography for Retinal Thickness Measurement in Diabetic Patients without Clinically Significant Macular Edema. *Ophthalmic Surg. Lasers Imaging Retin.* **2000**, *31*, 182–186. [CrossRef]
28. Niestrata-Ortiz, M.; Fichna, P.; Stankiewicz, W.; Stopa, M. Determining the Effect of Diabetes Duration on Retinal and Choroidal Thicknesses in Children with Type 1 Diabetes Mellitus. *Retina* **2020**, *40*, 421–427. [CrossRef] [PubMed]
29. Arruabarrena, C.; Rodríguez-Miguel, A.; Allendes, G.; Vera, C.; Son, B.; Teus, M.A. Evaluation of the Inclusion of Spectral-Domain Optical Coherence Tomography in a Telemedicine Diabetic Retinopathy Screening Program: A Real Clinical Practice. *Retina* **2023**, *43*, 1308–1316. [CrossRef]
30. Huang, J.; Liu, X.; Wu, Z.; Sadda, S. Image quality affects macular and retinal nerve fiber layer thickness measurements on fouri-er-domain optical coherence tomography. *Ophthalmic Surg. Lasers Imaging Retin.* **2011**, *42*, 216–221. [CrossRef]
31. Subhi, Y.; Forshaw, T.; Sørensen, T.L. Macular thickness and volume in the elderly: A systematic review. *Ageing Res. Rev.* **2016**, *29*, 42–49. [CrossRef]

Disclaimer/Publisher's Note: The statements, opinions and data contained in all publications are solely those of the individual author(s) and contributor(s) and not of MDPI and/or the editor(s). MDPI and/or the editor(s) disclaim responsibility for any injury to people or property resulting from any ideas, methods, instructions or products referred to in the content.

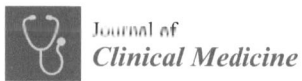

Article

Agreement and Reproducibility of Anterior Chamber Angle Measurements between CASIA2 Built-In Software and Human Graders

Gustavo Espinoza [1,2,3,*], Katheriene Iglesias [2], Juan C. Parra [2,3], Ignacio Rodriguez-Una [4], Sergio Serrano-Gomez [3], Angelica M. Prada [1,2,3] and Virgilio Galvis [1,2,3]

[1] Centro Oftalmológico Virgilio Galvis, Floridablanca 681004, Santander, Colombia; angieropra@hotmail.com (A.M.P.)
[2] Fundación Oftalmológica de Santander, Floridablanca 681004, Santander, Colombia
[3] Facultad de Ciencias de la Salud, Universidad Autónoma de Bucaramanga, Bucaramanga 680002, Santander, Colombia
[4] Instituto Universitario Fernández-Vega, Fundación de Investigación Oftalmológica, Universidad de Oviedo, 33012 Oviedo, Spain; irodriguezu@fernandez-vega.com
* Correspondence: drgustavoespinoza@hotmail.com; Tel.: +57-316-222-5620

Abstract: Purpose: This study evaluated the agreement and reproducibility of ACA measurements obtained using the built-in software of the CASIA2 (Version 3G.1) and the measurements derived from expert clinicians. Methods: Healthy volunteers underwent ophthalmological evaluation and AS-OCT examination. ACA measurements derived from automated and manual SS location were obtained using the CASIA2 automated software and clinician identification, respectively. The intraobserver, interobserver reproducibility, CASIA2–human grader reproducibility and CASIA2 repeatability were assessed using intraclass correlation coefficients (ICCs). Results: The study examined 58 eyes of 30 participants. The CASIA2 software showed excellent repeatability for all ACA parameters (ICC > 0.84). Intraobserver, interobserver, and CASIA2–human grader reproducibility were also excellent (ICC > 0.87). Interobserver agreement was high, except for nasal TISA500, differing between observers 1 and 2 ($p < 0.05$). The agreement between CASIA2 measurements and human graders was high, except for nasal TISA500, where observer 1 values were smaller ($p < 0.05$). Conclusion: The CASIA2 built-in software reliably measures ACA parameters in healthy individuals, demonstrating high consistency. Although a small difference was observed in nasal TISA500 measurements, interobserver and CASIA2–human grader reproducibility remained excellent. Automated SS detection has the potential to facilitate evaluation and monitoring of primary angle closure disease.

Keywords: agreement; anterior chamber angle; AS-OCT; optical coherence tomography; primary angle closure glaucoma; reproducibility

1. Introduction

Primary angle closure glaucoma (PACG) is a major cause of glaucoma-related blindness globally [1]. Angle closure is characterized by appositional approximation or contact between the iris and trabecular meshwork.

Visualization of the anterior chamber angle (ACA) is crucial for diagnosing glaucoma, especially angle closure variants. Although gonioscopy is the gold standard, it has limitations such as subjectivity, dependence on clinician expertise and patient cooperation. In fact, previous studies conducted in the United States showed that many ophthalmologists do not include gonioscopy in their routine examination or even in the examination of glaucoma patients [2,3].

New anterior segment imaging tools, such as anterior segment optical coherence tomography (AS-OCT), offer objective and quantitative ACA analysis [4]. The CASIA2 (Tomey Corporation, Nagoya, Japan) is the second generation of swept-source AS-OCT with a wavelength of 1310 nm and an acquisition speed of 50,000 A-scans/s which allows to perform cross-sections of the anterior chamber 16 mm wide.

The trabecular iris space area (TISA) and angle opening distance (AOD) are some of the measurements used to evaluate the dimensions of the ACA. Previous studies have confirmed a strong relationship between these measurements and gonioscopic angle closure [5–7]. The accuracy of these parameters depends on the location of the scleral spur (SS). The CASIA2 incorporates the possibility of automatic detection of the SS. However, the location of the SS is usually edited by a human grader to achieve a more precise location. Therefore, we consider it important to assess the accuracy of the built-in software to adequately measure these parameters and compare it with the measurements derived from the semi-automated SS location.

The aim of this study was to evaluate the agreement between the ACA measurements obtained by the built-in software of the CASIA2 and the measurements derived from expert clinicians. Furthermore, we evaluated the intraobserver, interobserver reproducibility, CASIA2–human grader reproducibility, and CASIA2 built-in software repeatability of these measurements.

2. Materials and Methods

This study included healthy volunteers evaluated at the Fundación Oftalmológica de Santander "Carlos Ardila Lülle" (FOSCAL), Colombia. This study was approved by the ethics committee board of Fundación Oftalmológica de Santander (reference: 002338) and adhered to the tenets of the Declaration of Helsinki. Informed consent was obtained from each participant.

2.1. Participants

The inclusion criteria were age $\geq$18 years, normal ophthalmological evaluation, intraocular pressure <21 mmHg, open angles confirmed by gonioscopy with the Shaffer classification $\geq$3, best-corrected visual acuity using the Snellen chart $\geq$20/40, refractive error between +3 diopters and −6 diopters of spherical equivalent and cylinder $\leq$3 diopters, normal visual field with a glaucoma hemifield test, and mean deviation within normal limits. The exclusion criteria were a history of laser procedures, intraocular surgery, use of topical medications that could modify the pupil size, unreliable visual field tests (false-negative and/or false-positive rates $\geq$33% and/or fixation losses $\geq$20%), and poor quality AS-OCT images.

All participants underwent ophthalmological evaluation by a single evaluator (G.E.) that included refraction, slit-lamp biomicroscopy, Goldmann applanation tonometry, gonioscopy under low-light conditions, and fundoscopy. The computerized visual field examination was performed using the Humphrey Field Analyzer® (Carl Zeiss Meditec, Dublin, CA, USA) under the SITA Standard strategy using a Goldmann III stimulus. Retinal nerve fiber layer OCT was also performed using a swept-source OCT device (DRI OCT Triton; Topcon, Tokyo, Japan) after pharmacological pupil dilation.

2.2. Sample Size Calculation

A sample size of 30 individuals was determined to observe a correlation coefficient of 0.6, with a type I error of 5%, type II error of 20%, and a 20% rate of data loss (Muestreo, Epidat Version 4.2).

2.3. AS-OCT Image Acquisition

After confirming that the ophthalmological evaluation was normal, the AS-OCT examination was performed at least 24 h after the initial assessment to avoid changes in the ACA that could induce modifications in the cornea during clinical examination. Each subject underwent examination of both eyes. After a 5 min adaptation period to standardized low-light conditions at 0 cd/m^2 (measured with a luxmeter), two AS-OCT captures of adequate quality were obtained for each eye by a single operator. During the examination, subjects were instructed to fixate their gaze on the internal fixation system of the equipment. The upper eyelid was gently raised, and a gentle traction of the lower eyelid was made by the operator taking care to avoid inadvertent pressure on the eyeball. The sulcus 0 + 90 measurement protocol was used for each capture. The image across the horizontal meridian was used for the analysis.

2.4. AS-OCT Image Analysis

Initially, a masked observer recorded the data of the nasal and temporal TISA500, TISA750, AOD500, and AOD750 parameters, derived from the automatic identification of SS performed with the CASIA2. The definition of AOD is the distance between the cornea and iris along a line perpendicular to the cornea at a specified distance (in μm) from the SS [8]. TISA, which can be tested and evaluated as well as AOD at several distances from the SS, is defined as the trapezoidal area with the following boundaries: anteriorly, the AOD; posteriorly, the line perpendicular to the plane of the inner corneoscleral wall drawn from the scleral spur to the opposing iris; superiorly, the inner corneoscleral wall; and inferiorly, the anterior iris surface [9]. The CASIA2 software utilizes a basic edge detection technique to identify the location of the scleral spur–uvea edge line, enabling SS detection. After obtaining the CASIA2 automatic ACA measurements, the masked observer intentionally relocated the SS to an incorrect position and saved the scan to minimize observer interpretation biases (Figure 1). Subsequently, the manual localization of the SS was carried out using the CASIA2 software tools (Version 3G.1) to obtain the measurements of these same parameters. The ciliary muscle and the bump method were used to identify the SS (Figure 2) [10]. This evaluation was performed by one glaucoma specialist with experience analyzing AS-OCT (G.E.) and one trained glaucoma fellow (K.I.). The evaluators were masked to the origin of the image data to ensure the anonymity of the eyes and participants. Each examiner evaluated each group of images independently (116 images/examiner). The second evaluation of the set of images per eye was performed 2 weeks after the first analysis.

The repeatability of the ACA parameters of the automated software was evaluated by comparing the data from capture 1 and capture 2 of each eye. For intraobserver reproducibility, evaluation 1 of capture 1 and 2 was compared with evaluation 2 of the same captures. For interobserver agreement analysis, evaluation 1 of capture 1 and 2 of G.E. was compared to evaluation 1 of capture 1 and 2 of K.I. Finally, to compare the agreement between each observer and the CASIA2 automatic parameters, evaluation 1 of capture 1 and 2 was compared to the readings of capture 1 and 2 obtained from the CASIA2 automated software.

2.5. Statistical Analysis

A univariate analysis was conducted to examine the sociodemographic and ophthalmological variables. Quantitative variables were analyzed using measures of central tendency and dispersion, such as mean and standard deviation. Qualitative variables were assessed using absolute and relative frequencies.

For the bivariate analysis, a comparison of means for the ACA parameters was performed among the different captures, evaluations, and evaluators. Additionally, an absolute intraclass correlation coefficient (ICC) was calculated to assess the reproducibility among the observers, both within and between different AS-OCT captures. Additionally, CASIA2–human grader agreement of measurements was assessed with an ICC and Bland–Altman plots with mean difference and limits of agreement (LoA).

A significance level (alpha) of 0.05 was employed for all analyses, and the statistical software Stata 16.0 was used to conduct the calculations. It is important to note that an ICC value of less than 0.4 indicates poor reproducibility, while a value between 0.4 and 0.75 suggests fair to good reproducibility. A value exceeding 0.75 indicates excellent reproducibility.

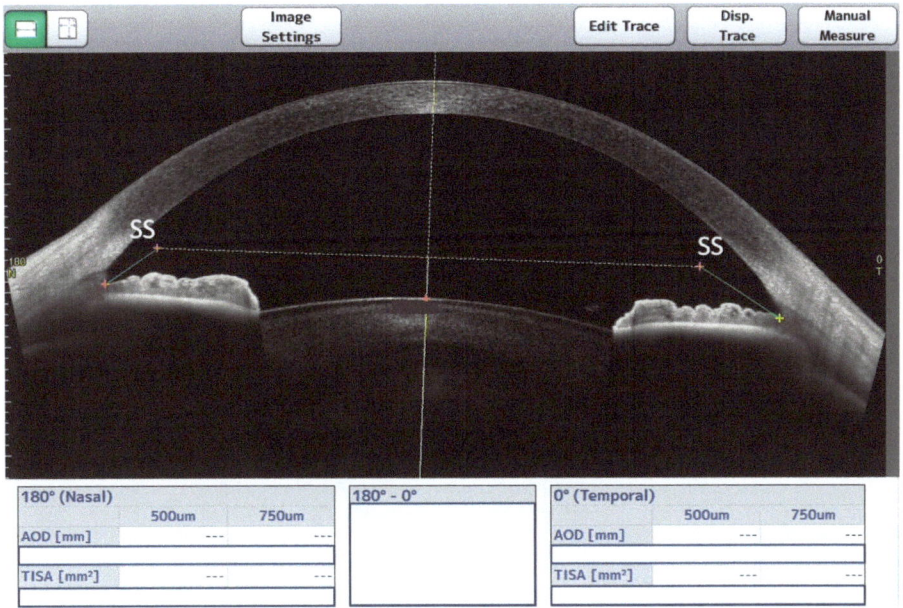

Figure 1. CASIA2 anterior segment OCT display after obtaining the automatic anterior chamber angle measurements and intentional relocation of the scleral spur (SS) that was performed by the masked observer. Nasal and temporal angle opening distance (AOD) and trabecular iris space area (TIA) are not available due to incorrect positioning of the SS.

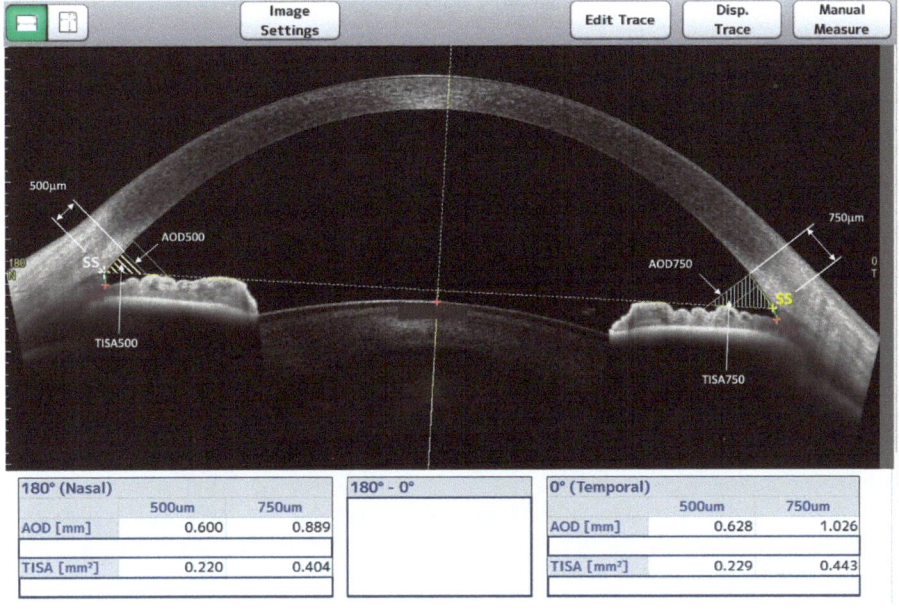

Figure 2. CASIA2 anterior segment OCT display after manual localization of the scleral spur (SS) was carried out by the human grader using the CASIA2 software tools to obtain the measurements of the anterior chamber angle parameters. Nasal and temporal angle opening distance (AOD) and trabecular iris space area (TISA) are shown in the image.

3. Results

A total of 60 eyes of 30 healthy volunteers were evaluated. Furthermore, 2 eyes of 2 participants were excluded due to missing images, leaving a total of 58 eyes in the final analysis. Among the 30 subjects, 16 (53.3%) were women and 14 (46.7%) were male. The mean age was 30.4 ± 9.05 years (range 21–64 years).

3.1. Repeatability of CASIA2 Automated Software

There were no significant differences ($p > 0.68$) between mean ACA measurements of capture 1 and 2 of the nasal and the temporal TISA500, TISA750, AOD500, and AOD750 (Table 1). Furthermore, repeatability was excellent for each of the parameters evaluated (ICC > 0.84).

Table 1. CASIA2 automated software ACA parameters' repeatability.

	Mean Capture 1	Mean Capture 2	*p*-Value	Mean Diff	ICC	ICC 95% CI
Temporal parameters						
AOD500 (mm)	0.490 ± 0.152	0.492 ± 0.152	0.94	−0.001	0.90	0.83–0.94
AOD750 (mm)	0.684 ± 0.212	0.690 ± 0.211	0.88	−0.005	0.88	0.80–0.93
TISA500 (mm^2)	0.168 ± 0.057	0.166 ± 0.050	0.89	0.001	0.84	0.73–0.90
TISA750 (mm^2)	0.316 ± 0.100	0.316 ± 0.093	0.99	0.000	0.87	0.78–0.92
Nasal parameters						
AOD500 (mm)	0.510 ± 0.156	0.497 ± 0.166	0.68	0.012	0.92	0.87–0.95
AOD750 (mm)	0.684 ± 0.186	0.679 ± 0.212	0.89	0.005	0.93	0.89–0.96
TISA500 (mm^2)	0.180 ± 0.057	0.178 ± 0.060	0.88	0.001	0.91	0.85–0.95
TISA750 (mm^2)	0.332 ± 0.097	0.328 ± 0.109	0.81	0.004	0.92	0.87–0.95

ICC = intraclass correlation coefficient; CI = confidence interval; ACA = anterior chamber angle; AOD = angle opening distance; TISA = trabecular iris space area.

3.2. Intraobserver ACA Measurements' Reproducibility

There were no significant differences of mean ACA measurements of the nasal or temporal parameters between the first and the second evaluation of images for both evaluators (range $p = 0.38$ to $p = 0.71$). There was also excellent intraobserver reproducibility of all parameters for both evaluators. The ICCs ranged from 0.96 to 0.98 for observer 1 (G.E.) and from 0.97 to 0.98 for observer 2 (K.I.) (Table 2).

Table 2. Intraobserver ACA measurements' reproducibility.

	Mean Evaluation 1	Mean Evaluation 2	*p*-Value	Mean Diff	ICC	ICC 95% CI
Observer 1						
Temporal parameters						
AOD500 (mm)	0.487 ± 0.190	0.478 ± 0.185	0.71	0.008	0.97	0.96–0.98
AOD750 (mm)	0.685 ± 0.267	0.671 ± 0.271	0.70	0.013	0.96	0.95–0.97
TISA500 (mm^2)	0.166 ± 0.073	0.162 ± 0.071	0.67	0.004	0.96	0.95–0.98
TISA750 (mm^2)	0.314 ± 0.129	0.308 ± 0.125	0.68	0.006	0.97	0.95–0.97
Nasal parameters						
AOD500 (mm)	0.469 ± 0.176	0.459 ± 0.171	0.66	0.009	0.97	0.96–0.98
AOD750 (mm)	0.656 ± 0.209	0.643 ± 0.206	0.61	0.013	0.97	0.96–0.98
TISA500 (mm^2)	0.161 ± 0.067	0.157 ± 0.065	0.61	0.004	0.98	0.97–0.98
TISA750 (mm^2)	0.303 ± 0.113	0.296 ± 0.110	0.61	0.007	0.98	0.97–0.98
Observer 2						
Temporal parameters						
AOD500 (mm)	0.522 ± 0.180	0.537 ± 0.188	0.54	−0.014	0.98	0.97–0.98
AOD750 (mm)	0.713 ± 0.242	0.742 ± 0.261	0.38	−0.028	0.97	0.96–0.98
TISA500 (mm^2)	0.182 ± 0.064	0.187 ± 0.068	0.51	−0.005	0.97	0.96–0.98
TISA750 (mm^2)	0.337 ± 0.113	0.349 ± 0.123	0.42	−0.012	0.97	0.96–0.98

Table 2. Cont.

	Mean Evaluation 1	Mean Evaluation 2	p-Value	Mean Diff	ICC	ICC 95% CI
Nasal parameters						
AOD500 (mm)	0.505 ± 0.151	0.515 ± 0.160	0.61	−0.010	0.97	0.96–0.98
AOD750 (mm)	0.681 ± 0.189	0.698 ± 0.202	0.50	−0.017	0.98	0.97–0.99
TISA500 (mm^2)	0.179 ± 0.057	0.183 ± 0.061	0.57	−0.004	0.97	0.96–0.98
TISA750 (mm^2)	0.330 ± 0.097	0.338 ± 0.103	0.53	−0.008	0.98	0.97–0.98

ICC = intraclass correlation coefficient; CI = confidence interval; ACA = anterior chamber angle; AOD = angle opening distance; TISA = trabecular iris space area.

3.3. Interobserver ACA Measurements' Agreement

The nasal TISA500 was smaller for observer 1 compared to the measurement of observer 2 with a mean of 0.161 ± 0.067 mm^2 and 0.179 ± 0.057 mm^2, respectively ($p < 0.05$). For all the other ACA measurements, there were no significant differences between the two observers (range $p = 0.06$ to 0.40).

Interobserver reproducibility was excellent for all parameters evaluated. ICC values ranged from 0.90 (nasal TISA500) to 0.96 (temporal AOD750), as shown in Table 3.

Table 3. Interobserver ACA measurements' agreement.

	Mean Evaluation 1 Observer 1	Mean Evaluation 1 Observer 2	p-Value	Mean Diff	ICC	ICC 95% CI
Temporal parameters						
AOD500 (mm)	0.487 ± 0.190	0.522 ± 0.180	0.14	−0.035	0.95	0.93–0.96
AOD750 (mm)	0.685 ± 0.267	0.713 ± 0.242	0.40	−0.028	0.96	0.95–0.97
TISA500 (mm^2)	0.166 ± 0.073	0.182 ± 0.064	0.08	−0.015	0.95	0.93–0.96
TISA750 (mm^2)	0.314 ± 0.129	0.337 ± 0.113	0.16	−0.022	0.95	0.93–0.97
Nasal parameters						
AOD500 (mm)	0.469 ± 0.176	0.505 ± 0.151	0.09	−0.035	0.91	0.87–0.93
AOD750 (mm)	0.656 ± 0.209	0.681 ± 0.189	0.34	−0.024	0.94	0.92–0.96
TISA500 (mm^2)	0.161 ± 0.067	0.179 ± 0.057	<0.05 *	−0.017	0.90	0.85–0.93
TISA750 (mm^2)	0.303 ± 0.113	0.330 ± 0.097	0.06	−0.026	0.91	0.88–0.94

ICC = intraclass correlation coefficient; CI = confidence interval; ACA = anterior chamber angle; AOD = angle opening distance; TISA = trabecular iris space area. The asterisk (*) in the table indicates significant differences ($p < 0.05$).

3.4. Agreement of ACA Measurements between CASIA2 and Both Observers

There were no significant differences with the mean measurements derived from the CASIA2 automated software and observer 2 (range $p = 0.05$ to 0.99). However, nasal TISA500 was smaller for observer 1 compared to the CASIA2 with mean values of 0.161 ± 0.067 mm^2 and 0.179 ± 0.060 mm^2, respectively ($p < 0.05$). All the other parameters did not show any significant difference (range $p = 0.06$ to 0.95).

Reproducibility of CASIA2 measurements and those corresponding to observer 1 and 2 was excellent. CASIA2 measurements showed ICC values that ranged from 0.87 to 0.93 and from 0.90 to 0.96 compared to observer 1 and 2, respectively (Table 4). Bland–Altman figures illustrating the agreement between CASIA2 and both observers for the nasal and temporal ACA parameters can be found in Figure 3. A high level of agreement was observed with minimal variability among the measurements conducted by each of the observers and the CASIA2. The agreement between observer 1 and CASIA2 exhibited a slightly lower level of concordance compared to that observed between observer 2 and CASIA2.

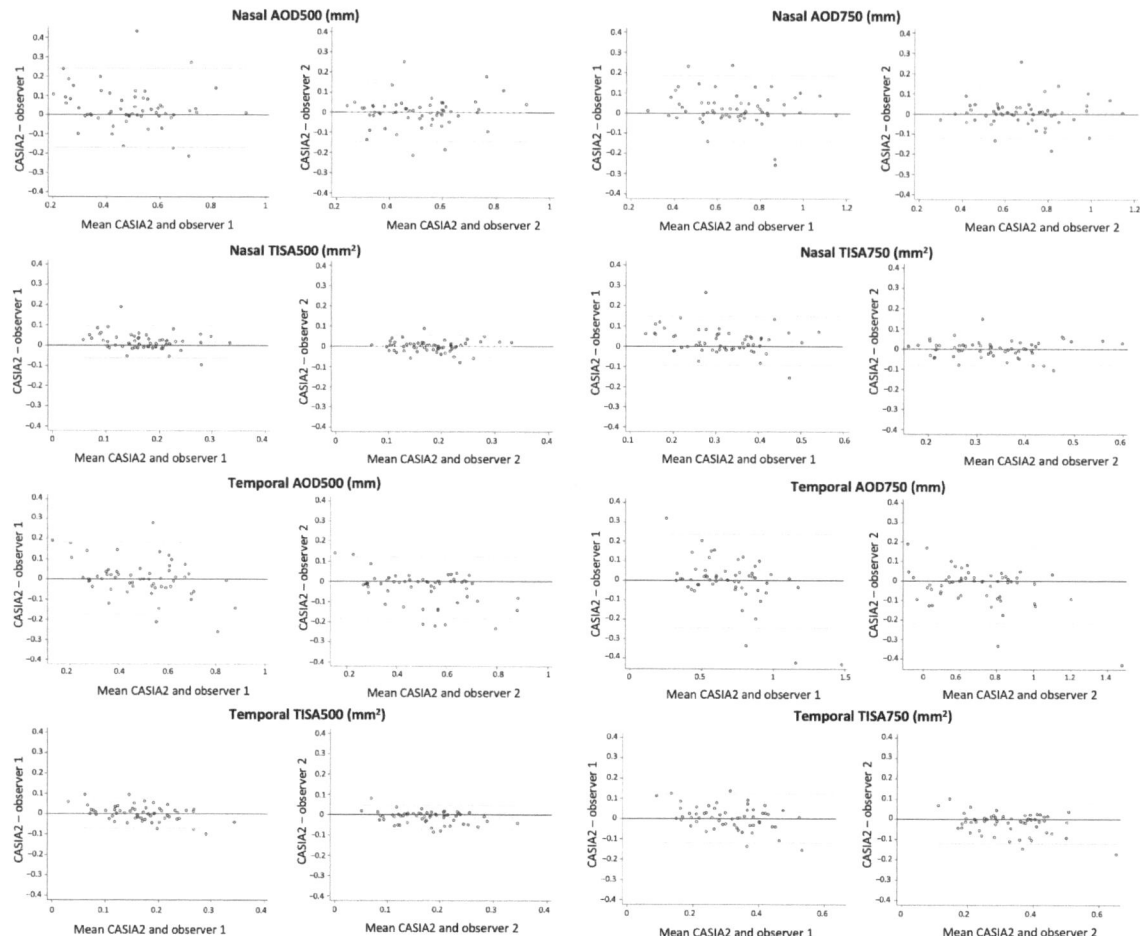

Figure 3. Bland–Altman plot: comparison of nasal and temporal ACA parameters between CASIA2 and both observers.

Table 4. Agreement of ACA measurements between CASIA2 and both observers.

	Mean Observer Measurements	Mean CASIA2 Measurements	p-Value	Mean Diff	ICC	ICC 95% CI
Observer 1						
Temporal parameters						
AOD500 (mm)	0.487 ± 0.190	0.491 ± 0.151	0.86	0.003	0.90	0.85–0.93
AOD750 (mm)	0.685 ± 0.267	0.687 ± 0.211	0.95	0.001	0.90	0.86–0.93
TISA500 (mm^2)	0.166 ± 0.073	0.167 ± 0.054	0.08	0.001	0.88	0.82–0.91
TISA750 (mm^2)	0.314 ± 0.129	0.316 ± 0.096	0.92	0.001	0.89	0.84–0.92
Nasal parameters						
AOD500 (mm)	0.469 ± 0.176	0.504 ± 0.160	0.11	0.034	0.88	0.81–0.92
AOD750 (mm)	0.656 ± 0.209	0.681 ± 0.199	0.35	0.025	0.93	0.90–0.95
TISA500 (mm^2)	0.161 ± 0.067	0.179 ± 0.060	<0.05 *	0.017	0.87	0.77–0.92
TISA750 (mm^2)	0.303 ± 0.113	0.330 ± 0.009	0.06	0.026	0.89	0.81–0.93

Table 4. Cont.

	Mean Observer Measurements	Mean CASIA2 Measurements	p-Value	Mean Diff	ICC	ICC 95% CI
Observer 2						
Temporal parameters						
AOD500 (mm)	0.522 ± 0.180	0.491 ± 0.151	0.15	−0.031	0.92	0.88–0.95
AOD750 (mm)	0.713 ± 0.242	0.687 ± 0.211	0.37	−0.026	0.93	0.90–0.95
TISA500 (mm^2)	0.182 ± 0.064	0.167 ± 0.054	0.05	−0.014	0.90	0.83–0.94
TISA750 (mm^2)	0.337 ± 0.113	0.316 ± 0.096	0.13	−0.021	0.92	0.87–0.95
Nasal parameters						
AOD500 (mm)	0.505 ± 0.151	0.504 ± 0.160	0.96	−0.001	0.93	0.91–0.95
AOD750 (mm)	0.681 ± 0.189	0.681 ± 0.199	0.98	0.000	0.96	0.94–0.97
TISA500 (mm^2)	0.179 ± 0.057	0.179 ± 0.060	0.99	0.000	0.92	0.89–0.94
TISA750 (mm^2)	0.330 ± 0.097	0.330 ± 0.009	0.96	0.000	0.94	0.91–0.95

ICC = intraclass correlation coefficient; CI = confidence interval; ACA = anterior chamber angle; AOD = angle opening distance; TISA = trabecular iris space area. The asterisk (*) in the table indicates significant differences ($p < 0.05$).

4. Discussion

This study evaluated the ability of the built-in CASIA2 software to obtain ACA measurements and compared them with measurements obtained by ophthalmologists. The CASIA2 measurements not only demonstrated excellent repeatability for all parameters, but also when compared with the measurements obtained by the human graders, an excellent degree of agreement was also observed, except for nasal TISA500. To our knowledge, this is the first study evaluating the capability of the CASIA2 built-in software to obtain ACA measures derived from automatic SS location. Although previous studies suggested that SS placement should be conducted by a human grader, our study demonstrates that CASIA2 software can achieve consistent measurements in healthy subjects with high reliability.

The importance of automated SS detection lies in its potential to facilitate the evaluation and monitoring of patients with primary angle closure disease. In this study, we were able to demonstrate that the measurements derived from the automatic SS location of the CASIA2 were comparable to those of the human graders. However, nasal TISA500 measurements showed a significant difference compared to measurements obtained from the most experienced evaluator. In fact, this difference was also observed between the expert in AS-OCT analysis and the less experienced trained fellow. This might be explained by a small difference in the nasal SS location during the AS-OCT analysis. Previous studies have shown that a small change in the position of the SS mainly affects the parameters that measure size or angle configuration such as TISA500 and TISA750 [10]. However, even though there was a difference with the nasal TISA500 measurement in our study, the interobserver reproducibility and the CASIA2 vs. human graders reproducibility was excellent (ICC > 0.87). Interestingly, Tan et al. also evaluated the reproducibility of ACA measurements between expert and non-expert observers in AS-OCT analysis with the Visante OCT (Carl Zeiss, Meditec Inc., Dublin, CA, USA). They were able to demonstrate that the reproducibility of nasal and temporal ACA parameters between 2 experts and 23 non-experts was high. All the parameters showed excellent reproducibility with ICC means of 0.875, 0.942, and 0.906 for expert 1, expert 2, and non-expert observers, respectively. Nonetheless, the range of the coefficient of variation of ACA measurements was larger in the non-expert group [11].

In our study, we were also able to show that the reproducibility of the ACA measurements using the CASIA2 software tools to manually locate the SS was excellent for both evaluators (ICC > 0.96). In the past, to obtain the ACA measurements with some AS-OCT devices, it was necessary to export the images to an external software for the analysis. Nowadays, these machines have quite efficient software that allows an adequate location of the SS and the parameters derived from it. Xu et al. found that using the CASIA2 software to manually locate the SS, the reproducibility for AOD750, and TISA750 in healthy subjects was excellent with an ICC of 0.98 and 0.94, respectively [12]. Chan et al. evaluated the test–retest variabilities of different ACA parameters including AOD500 and TISA500 in healthy and primary angle closure subjects using two swept-source AS-OCTs, the CASIA2 and the ANTERION (Heidelberg Engineering, Heidelberg, Germany). They found that the CASIA2 repeatability coefficient for AOD500 and TISA500 were 0.035 mm and 0.014 mm^2, respectively. Moreover, these repeatability coefficients measured with CASIA2 were found to be statistically significantly different, albeit slightly smaller, compared to those obtained from the ANTERION ($p \leq 0.001$) [13]. In a multicenter study, Liu et al. evaluated the repeatability of ACA measurements in 116 healthy subjects with 171 eyes with primary angle closure disease. In their study, one single observer marked the nasal and temporal SS position of 18 evenly spaced B-scans over the 360° area of each eye. Repeatability coefficients for AOD750 and TISA750 were 0.058 mm and 0.030 mm^2, respectively [14].

Recently, artificial intelligence has been used to obtain the location of the SS and subsequently be able to obtain the parameters derived from this. Xu et al. evaluated a deep neural network model for automatic SS detection using the CASIA SS-1000. These authors found that the distributions of prediction errors for the artificial intelligence model and intraobserver variability for the reference grader were similar. In fact, these prediction errors were significantly smaller than the interobserver variability seen between human expert graders [15]. Similarly, Pham et al. evaluated a deep convolutional neural network model for the location of the SS and found excellent agreement between the human grader and the artificial intelligence model. They also found that the ACA measurements repeatability for the artificial intelligence model was higher than the human graders [16]. Liu et al. used a deep learning model in the CASIA2 that allowed the automatic location of the SS and compared it with the manual location of an observer, finding that the deep learning model achieved a repeatability similar to that obtained by the human grader for TISA750 and AOD750 parameters. In fact, the authors report that the repeatability of these values was better with the deep learning model compared to the manual method with a higher mean absolute difference for the latter (0.0167 ± 0.0188 mm vs. 0.0210 ± 0.0212 mm, p = 0.003 for AOD750; 0.0093 ± 0.0093 mm^2 vs. 0.0109 ± 0.0110 mm^2, p = 0.018 for TISA750) [14]. One of the main advantages described for these artificial intelligence models is the ability to determine the location of the SS in less than 2 s, which is much faster than a human observer [14,16]. However, even though these models have shown a high repeatability in the measurement of the ACA parameters, they also have the limitation that they are trained on data that was originally labeled by human graders. This means that the models are likely to inherit any errors or biases that were present in the original data.

There is skepticism as to whether ACA measurements can be interchangeable between different platforms. Xu et al. evaluated the reproducibility and agreement of ACA measurements between the CASIA2 and Heidelberg Spectralis OCT2 AS-OCT (Heidelberg Engineering, Heidelberg, Germany). Their study showed good correlation for TISA750 and AOD750 (ICC = 0.78). However, there was poor agreement for anterior chamber (ICC = 0.20). These authors suggested that even though there was good agreement between both devices, the data from these two AS-OCTs should not be used interchangeably for clinical purposes [12]. Similarly, Chan et al. evaluated the agreement of ACA measurements between the CASIA2 and the ANTERION and found poor agreement for TISA500 and AOD500 (p < 0.001), suggesting that the measures of these devices may not be interchangeable [13]. Pardeshi et al. described that the differences between platforms could be related to poor image resolution or different wavelength when comparing the CASIA2 with the time domain and spectral domain AS-OCT. In their study, they evaluated the repeatability and agreement between two swept-source AS-OCTs, the CASIA SS-1000 and the ANTERION. They found that ACA measurements for both were nearly interchangeable [17,18]. However, differences between the CASIA2 and the ANTERION suggested that caution should be exercised when comparing ACA measurements across different OCT platforms, even if they share similar technology.

Our study has some limitations which should be considered. Firstly, the sample predominantly comprised individuals of Latin descent and only one type of AS-OCT scan. Therefore, caution should be exercised when extrapolating the results of our study to other populations or when using different types of AS-OCT scans. Secondly, our study focused solely on evaluating normal eyes, and it remains uncertain whether the reproducibility of our results could be replicated in eyes with glaucoma, primary angle closure, or other abnormalities affecting the angle geometry or structures. Finally, our study excluded individuals with a history of laser procedures, intraocular surgery, and use of topical medications that could modify the pupil size, among others. While these exclusion criteria were relevant for this specific study, they may limit the generalizability of the findings to broader populations. Therefore, further investigations are needed to assess the performance and reliability of the CASIA2 software in different populations and clinical scenarios.

In summary, this study demonstrates excellent repeatability in ACA measurements obtained through automatic SS detection using the CASIA2 built-in software. Furthermore, strong agreement was observed between these measurements and those provided by the two clinicians. However, despite the built-in software's capability to accurately locate the SS and derive parameters from it, it is still suggested that human examiner supervision is needed to confirm the SS location. These findings highlight the potential value of parameters derived from the CASIA2 built-in software for clinical practice, particularly in assessing healthy individuals.

Author Contributions: Conceptualization, G.E., I.R.-U. and K.I.; methodology, S.S.-G., G.E. and A.M.P.; validation, G.E., I.R.-U., J.C.P. and V.G.; formal analysis, S.S.-G.; investigation, G.E. and K.I.; resources, G.E. and K.I.; writing—original draft preparation, G.E. and K.I.; writing—review and editing, G.E. and I.R.-U.; visualization, G.E.; supervision, G.E., I.R.-U., J.C.P. and V.G.; project administration, G.E. All authors have read and agreed to the published version of the manuscript.

Funding: This research received no external funding.

Institutional Review Board Statement: This study was conducted in accordance with the Declaration of Helsinki and approved by the Ethics Committee of FOSCAL in June 2020 (reference: 002338).

Informed Consent Statement: Informed consent was obtained from all subjects involved in this study.

Data Availability Statement: All the obtained data used to support the findings of this study are available from the corresponding author upon reasonable request.

Conflicts of Interest: The authors declare no conflict of interest.

References

1. Tham, Y.C.; Li, X.; Wong, T.Y.; Quigley, H.A.; Aung, T.; Cheng, C.Y. Global prevalence of glaucoma and projections of glaucoma burden through 2040: A systematic review and meta-analysis. *Ophthalmology* **2014**, *121*, 2081–2090. [CrossRef] [PubMed]
2. Coleman, A.L.; Yu, F.; Evans, S.J. Use of gonioscopy in Medicare beneficiaries before glaucoma surgery. *J. Glaucoma* **2006**, *15*, 427–432. [CrossRef] [PubMed]
3. Quigley, H.A.; Friedman, D.S.; Hahn, S.R. Evaluation of Practice Patterns for the Care of Open-angle Glaucoma Compared with Claims Data. *Ophthalmology* **2007**, *114*, 1599–1606. [CrossRef] [PubMed]
4. Radhakrishnan, S.; Rollins, A.M.; Roth, J.E.; Yazdanfar, S.; Westphal, V.; Bardenstein, D.S.; Izatt, J.A. Real-time optical coherence tomography of the anterior segment at 1310 nm. *Arch. Ophthalmol.* **2001**, *119*, 1179–1185. [CrossRef] [PubMed]
5. Narayanaswamy, A.; Sakata, L.M.; He, M.G.; Friedman, D.S.; Chan, Y.H.; Lavanya, R.; Baskaran, M.; Foster, P.J.; Aung, T. Diagnostic performance of anterior chamber angle measurements for detecting eyes with narrow angles: An anterior segment OCT study. *Arch. Ophthalmol.* **2010**, *128*, 1321–1327. [CrossRef] [PubMed]
6. Xu, B.Y.; Burkemper, B.; Lewinger, J.P.; Jiang, X.; Pardeshi, A.A.; Richter, G.; Torres, M.; McKean-Cowdin, R.; Varma, R. Correlation between Intraocular Pressure and Angle Configuration Measured by OCT. *Ophthalmol. Glaucoma* **2018**, *1*, 158–166. [CrossRef] [PubMed]
7. Bao, Y.K.; Xu, B.Y.; Friedman, D.S.; Cho, A.; Foster, P.J.; Jiang, Y.; Porporato, N.; Pardeshi, A.A.; Jiang, Y.; Munoz, B.; et al. Biometric Risk Factors for Angle Closure Progression after Laser Peripheral Iridotomy. *JAMA Ophthalmol.* **2023**, *141*, 516–524. [CrossRef] [PubMed]

8. Pavlin, C.J.; Harasiewicz, K.; Foster, F.S. Ultrasound biomicroscopy of anterior segment structures in normal and glaucomatous eyes. *Am. J. Ophthalmol.* **1992**, *113*, 381–389. [CrossRef] [PubMed]
9. Radhakrishnan, S.; Huang, D.; Smith, S.D. Optical coherence tomography imaging of the anterior chamber angle. *Ophthalmol. Clin. North Am.* **2005**, *18*, 375–381. [CrossRef] [PubMed]
10. Seager, F.E.; Wang, J.; Arora, K.S.; Quigley, H.A. The effect of scleral spur identification methods on structural measurements by anterior segment optical coherence tomography. *J. Glaucoma* **2014**, *23*, e10–e15. [CrossRef] [PubMed]
11. Tan, A.N.; Sauren, L.D.; de Brabander, J.; Berendschot, T.T.; Passos, V.L.; Webers, C.A.; Nuijts, R.M.; Beckers, H.J. Reproducibility of anterior chamber angle measurements with anterior segment optical coherence tomography. *Investig. Ophthalmol. Vis. Sci.* **2011**, *52*, 2095–2099. [CrossRef] [PubMed]
12. Xu, B.Y.; Mai, D.D.; Penteado, R.C.; Saunders, L.; Weinreb, R.N. Reproducibility and Agreement of Anterior Segment Parameter Measurements Obtained Using the CASIA2 and Spectralis OCT2 Optical Coherence Tomography Devices. *J. Glaucoma* **2017**, *26*, 974–979. [CrossRef] [PubMed]
13. Chan, P.P.; Lai, G.; Chiu, V.; Chong, A.; Yu, M.; Leung, C.K. Anterior chamber angle imaging with swept-source optical coherence tomography: Comparison between CASIAII and ANTERION. *Sci. Rep.* **2020**, *10*, 18771. [CrossRef] [PubMed]
14. Liu, P.; Higashita, R.; Guo, P.Y.; Okamoto, K.; Li, F.; Nguyen, A.; Sakata, R.; Duan, L.; Aihara, M.; Lin, S.; et al. Reproducibility of deep learning based scleral spur localisation and anterior chamber angle measurements from anterior segment optical coherence tomography images. *Br. J. Ophthalmol.* **2023**, *107*, 802–808. [CrossRef] [PubMed]
15. Xu, B.Y.; Chiang, M.; Pardeshi, A.A.; Moghimi, S.; Varma, R. Deep Neural Network for Scleral Spur Detection in Anterior Segment OCT Images: The Chinese American Eye Study. *Transl. Vis. Sci. Technol.* **2020**, *9*, 18. [CrossRef] [PubMed]
16. Pham, T.H.; Devalla, S.K.; Ang, A.; Soh, Z.-D.; Thiery, A.H.; Boote, C.; Cheng, C.-Y.; A Girard, M.J.; Koh, V. Deep learning algorithms to isolate and quantify the structures of the anterior segment in optical coherence tomography images. *Br. J. Ophthalmol.* **2021**, *105*, 1231–1237. [CrossRef] [PubMed]
17. Pardeshi, A.A.; Song, A.E.; Lazkani, N.; Xie, X.; Huang, A.; Xu, B.Y. Intradevice Repeatability and Interdevice Agreement of Ocular Biometric Measurements: A Comparison of Two Swept-Source Anterior Segment OCT Devices. *Transl. Vis. Sci. Technol.* **2020**, *9*, 14. [CrossRef] [PubMed]
18. Chansangpetch, S.; Nguyen, A.; Mora, M.; Badr, M.; He, M.; Porco, T.C.; Lin, S.C. Agreement of Anterior Segment Parameters Obtained from Swept-Source Fourier-Domain and Time-Domain Anterior Segment Optical Coherence Tomography. *Investig. Ophthalmol. Vis. Sci.* **2018**, *59*, 1554–1561. [CrossRef] [PubMed]

Disclaimer/Publisher's Note: The statements, opinions and data contained in all publications are solely those of the individual author(s) and contributor(s) and not of MDPI and/or the editor(s). MDPI and/or the editor(s) disclaim responsibility for any injury to people or property resulting from any ideas, methods, instructions or products referred to in the content.

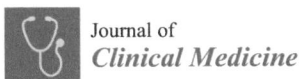

Article

Normative Database of the Superior–Inferior Thickness Asymmetry for All Inner and Outer Macular Layers of Adults for the Posterior Pole Algorithm of the Spectralis SD-OCT

Ana Palazon-Cabanes [1], Begoña Palazon-Cabanes [2], Jose Javier Garcia-Medina [3,4,5,6,*], Aurora Alvarez-Sarrion [4] and Monica del-Rio-Vellosillo [7,8]

1. Department of Ophthalmology, Hospital Virgen del Castillo, 30510 Murcia, Spain; a.palazoncabanes@gmail.com
2. Department of Neurology, Hospital de la Vega Lorenzo Guirao, 30530 Murcia, Spain; abega_ct@hotmail.com
3. Department of Ophthalmology, General University Hospital Morales Meseguer, 30008 Murcia, Spain
4. Department of Ophthalmology and Optometry, University of Murcia, 30120 Murcia, Spain; aurora.alvarezopt@gmail.com
5. Ophthalmic Research Unit "Santiago Grisolia", 46010 Valencia, Spain
6. Spanish Net of Inflammatory Diseases RICORS, Institute of Health Carlos III, 28029 Madrid, Spain
7. Department of Anesthesiology, University Hospital Virgen de la Arrixaca, 30120 Murcia, Spain; monica.delrio@um.es
8. Department of Surgery, Obstetrics and Gynecology and Pediatrics, University of Murcia, 30120 Murcia, Spain
* Correspondence: jj.garciamedina@um.es

Abstract: Background: This study aims to establish a reference for the superior–inferior hemisphere asymmetry in thickness values for all macular layers for the posterior pole algorithm (PPA) available for the Spectralis SD-OCT device. Methods: We examined 300 eyes of 300 healthy Caucasian volunteers aged 18–84 years using the PPA, composed of a grid of 64 (8 × 8) cells, to analyze the thickness asymmetries of the following automatically segmented macular layers: retinal nerve fiber layer (RNFL); ganglion cell layer (GCL); inner plexiform layer (IPL); inner nuclear layer (INL); outer plexiform layer (OPL); outer nuclear layer (ONL); retinal pigment epithelium (RPE); inner retina; outer retina; complete retina. Mean ± standard deviation and the 2.5th and 97.5th percentiles of the thickness asymmetry values were obtained for all the corresponding cells. Results: All the macular layers had significant superior–inferior thickness asymmetries. GCL, IPL, INL, ONL and RPE showed significantly greater thicknesses in the superior than the inferior hemisphere, whereas RNFL and OPL were thicker in the inferior hemisphere. The largest differences between hemispheres were for RNFL and ONL. Conclusions: This is the first normative database of macular thickness asymmetries for the PPA and should be considered to distinguish normal from pathological values when interpreting superior–inferior macular asymmetries.

Keywords: normative database; asymmetry; hemispheres; thickness; macula; layer; posterior pole algorithm; optical coherence tomography; glaucoma; neuro-ophthalmology

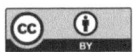

1. Introduction

Asymmetry in the macular structure due to changes in different macular layer thicknesses has been demonstrated in several diseases [1–6], especially in glaucoma [7–11]. Glaucoma is a leading cause of irreversible blindness worldwide and its incidence is increasing over time [12]. Glaucoma is a multifactorial disease characterized by the progressive apoptosis of retinal ganglion cells and the degeneration of their axons. This leads to the asymmetric thinning of the innermost macular layers, accompanied by corresponding visual field defects that initially tend to respect the horizontal midline [7,8]. It has also been suggested that the thickness of the inner nuclear layers and the different outer macular layers can also change in glaucoma, although the findings of previous studies are still controversial [8–11]. As this condition remains asymptomatic until advanced stages, regular screening examinations are essential, mainly in high-risk populations. However, the sensitivity and specificity of the glaucoma screening tests available today are low [13,14]. Therefore, the early detection of thickness asymmetry of the different macular layers between the superior and inferior hemispheres could constitute a novel strategy to improve the early diagnosis and treatment of glaucoma [15].

The Spectralis spectral domain optical coherence tomography (SD-OCT) device has several exploration protocols for the macula. One of them, the posterior pole algorithm (PPA), was specifically designed to follow-up patients with suspected or diagnosed glaucoma [16]. This protocol allows the automatic segmentation of the different macular layers and is able to detect retinal thickness differences of up to 30 microns between the corresponding points of the superior and inferior hemispheres of the macula [16]. However, previous studies have reported that thickness asymmetry is also present in healthy subjects [7,17]. Hence, a simple thickness asymmetry analysis is not specific enough to distinguish the physiological asymmetries from those that can be early signs of glaucoma.

The aim of the present study was to determine the normal range of asymmetries of the macular thicknesses between the corresponding points of the superior and inferior hemispheres in a healthy Caucasian population using the PPA of the Spectralis SD-OCT. To the best of our knowledge, such a normative database has not yet been published.

2. Materials and Methods

This is an observational cross-sectional study that included 300 eyes of 300 healthy Caucasian adults. Only one eye per patient was randomly selected. Volunteers were recruited in the Department of Ophthalmology at the University General Hospital Reina Sofia in Murcia, Spain. They were chosen proportionally according to gender and age to obtain a representative sample population, and included 50 people (25 males, 25 females) in all six established age groups (18–29, 30–39, 40–49, 50–59, 60–69 and 70–85 years). The inclusion criteria were as follows: aged 18–85 years, Caucasian ethnicity, normal ophthalmological examination and normal peripapillary retinal nerve fiber layer (pRNFL) thickness. The exclusion criteria were as follows: adjusted intraocular pressure (IOP) > 21 mmHg, cup-to-disc ratio > 0.4, sphere ≥ 5 diopters and/or cylinder ≥ 2 diopters, any ocular surgery within the last 6 months, any previous or current ocular disease (glaucoma, diabetic retinopathy, uveitis, amblyopia, etc.), any neuropsychiatric diseases or any media opacities leading to a signal strength of the OCT images below 25.

The study protocol adhered to the ethical principles of the Declaration of Helsinki and was approved by the Local Ethics Committee at the University General Hospital Reina Sofia in Murcia, Spain (protocol number 03/19). Subjects were informed about the study and informed consent was obtained from them all before enrollment.

A comprehensive ophthalmologic examination was carried out on all the participants, including autorefractometry (NIDEK ARK-710A; NIDEK, Aichi, Japan), visual acuity, IOP determination pneumatic tonometry, slit-lamp biomicroscopy and fundus examination, as well as measurement of axial length, keratometry (IOL Master; Carl Zeiss Meditec Inc., Dublin, CA, USA) and pachymetry (Specular Microscope EM-3000; Tomey; Phoenix, AZ, USA). The PPA and the optic disk circle protocols of the Spectralis (Heidelberg Engineering, Heidelberg, Germany; software version 6.0) were employed to acquire OCT images of the macula and optic disk, respectively. All the OCT examinations were performed by the same experienced ophthalmologist (A.P.C).

The PPA scans a macular cube measuring $30° \times 25°$, centered on the fovea and oriented using fovea–disk alignment [16]. The results are shown on a macular grid that is divided into 64 cells, each measuring $3° \times 3°$, which are distributed in eight rows and eight columns (8×8 PPA). Cell numbering is established from inferior to superior and from temporal to nasal. Thus, the nomenclature is specular between eyes. Cell 1.1 is the most inferior—temporal cell and cell 8.8 is the most superior–nasal, both in right and left eyes. Using the automatic segmentation tool of this protocol, for each cell, we obtained the thickness values of the following macular layers: retinal nerve fiber layer (RNFL); ganglion cell layer (GCL); inner plexiform layer (IPL); inner nuclear layer (INL); outer plexiform layer (OPL); outer nuclear layer (ONL); retinal pigment epithelium (RPE). We also obtained the joint automatic segmentation of the different retinal layers: from RNFL to ONL or inner retina (INNER); photoreceptors and RPE or outer retina (OUTER); all the retinal layers or the complete retina (RETINA).

Every scan was inspected by the same ophthalmologist (A.P.C) to detect segmentation errors and other issues, such as misalignments, decentration or motion artifacts. No manual adjustments were made. Because of the specular nomenclature of the macular grid, we represent the left eye data in the right eye format.

Statistical Analysis

All the statistical analyses were run using the SPSS software (version 26.0; SPSS Inc., Chicago, IL, USA). We assessed the normal distribution of all thickness values using the Kolmogorov–Smirnov test. We analyzed the thickness differences between the mean thickness of the 32 inferior cells and the mean thickness of the 32 superior cells of all the macular layers using Student's *t*-test for paired samples. We also compared the thickness of each cell in the inferior hemisphere to the thickness of the corresponding cells in the superior hemisphere using Student's *t*-test for paired samples (Figure 1). We expressed the results as the mean ± standard deviation (SD) of the thickness differences. Heatmaps depicting half the mean thickness difference between corresponding cells were plotted to highlight the inferior–superior asymmetry. Finally, we calculated the 2.5th and the 97.5th percentiles of the thickness differences in the 64 cells of all the macular layers. A *p* value < 0.05 was considered statistically significant.

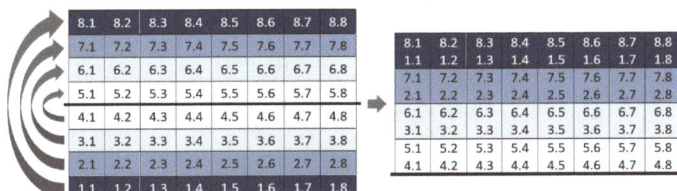

Figure 1. Corresponding cells of the 8 × 8 macular grid. All cells on the same-colored line in the superior and inferior hemispheres are corresponding cells. For example, cell 1.1 and cell 8.1 are corresponding cells.

3. Results

In total, 300 eyes of 300 subjects were included in this study, of which 152 were right eyes (51%) and 147 were left eyes (49%). The mean age of the men (50%) and women (50%) enrolled in this study was 49.78 ± 17.41 years (range 18–84). The mean axial length was 23.64 ± 0.90 mm (range 21.25–25.95). The mean keratometry was 44.14 ± 1.45 diopters for the steepest meridian and 43.25 ± 1.40 diopters for the flattest. The mean pachymetry was 530.40 ± 36.87 microns, and the mean adjusted IOP was 15.60 ± 2.94 mmHg.

When comparing the mean thickness values between hemispheres (Table 1, see below), we observed that the thickness of the OUTER and complete RETINA was significantly thicker in the superior than in the inferior hemisphere, whereas the thickness of the INNER retina was similar between hemispheres. The thickness of RNFL and OPL was significantly thicker in the inferior than in the superior hemisphere. Conversely, the thickness of IPL, ONL and RPE was significantly thinner in the inferior than in the superior hemisphere. The thickness of GCL and INL did not show any significant differences between hemispheres.

The results of the comparison of the thicknesses between the corresponding cells of the inferior and superior hemispheres of the different macular layers, and of the 2.5th and 97.5th percentiles of these thickness differences, are shown in Tables S1–S10.

Table 1. Analysis of the retinal layer thickness between the superior and inferior hemispheres of the macula using Student's test for paired samples (n = 300). The superior hemisphere was considered the mean of the 32 superior cells and the inferior hemisphere was taken as the mean of the 32 inferior cells of the 8 × 8 grid. Abbreviations: RNFL: retinal nerve fiber layer; GCL: ganglion cell layer; IPL: inner plexiform layer; INL: inner nuclear layer; OPL: outer plexiform layer; ONL: outer nuclear layer; RPE: retinal pigmentary epithelium; INNER: inner retina; OUTER: outer retina; RETINA: complete retina.

Layer	Hemisphere	Mean ± SD	p Value
RNFL	Superior	38.76 ± 25.03	<0.001
	Inferior	46.33 ± 30.36	
GCL	Superior	33.05 ± 10.34	0.333
	Inferior	32.89 ± 10.88	
IPL	Superior	27.79 ± 8.21	<0.001
	Inferior	26.77 ± 8.66	
INL	Superior	31.61 ± 5.88	0.054
	Inferior	31.43 ± 6.39	
OPL	Superior	26.20 ± 5.12	<0.001
	Inferior	27.14 ± 6.26	
ONL	Superior	55.54 ± 11.08	<0.001
	Inferior	51.98 ± 11.74	
RPE	Superior	13.03 ± 2.49	<0.001
	Inferior	12.57 ± 2.22	
INNER	Superior	215.92 ± 33.27	0.066
	Inferior	216.62 ± 33.58	
OUTER	Superior	78.61 ± 3.65	<0.001
	Inferior	77.00 ± 3.81	
RETINA	Superior	294.53 ± 34.46	<0.001
	Inferior	293.61 ± 34.96	

In order to better visually understand the differences between corresponding cells, Figure 2 provides heatmaps illustrating the asymmetry in thickness for each macular layer in relation to the horizontal midline. As depicted, significantly greater thicknesses were observed in most of the inferior cells on RNFL than in the corresponding superior cells, with larger differences in the peripheral cells than in the central cells. GCL and INL displayed a similar asymmetric pattern: significantly thicker cells were detected in most superior cells than in the corresponding inferior cells, but the temporal inferior cells near the horizontal midline were significantly thicker than their corresponding superior cells. However, significant differences were detected in fewer corresponding cells in INL than in GCL. IPL showed significantly thicker cells in the superior hemisphere, except in the central and nasally paracentral cells, where the pattern was the inverse. All the superior cells in ONL and most of the superior cells in RPE were significantly thicker than their corresponding inferior cells, while OPL had significantly higher thickness values in the inferonasal cells. We detected significantly thicker cells in the paracentral superonasal cells in the INNER and complete RETINA layers, while the peripheral superonasal cells and central superotemporal cells were significantly thinner than their corresponding cells on these layers. Finally, we observed that the OUTER layer was thicker in the superior hemisphere.

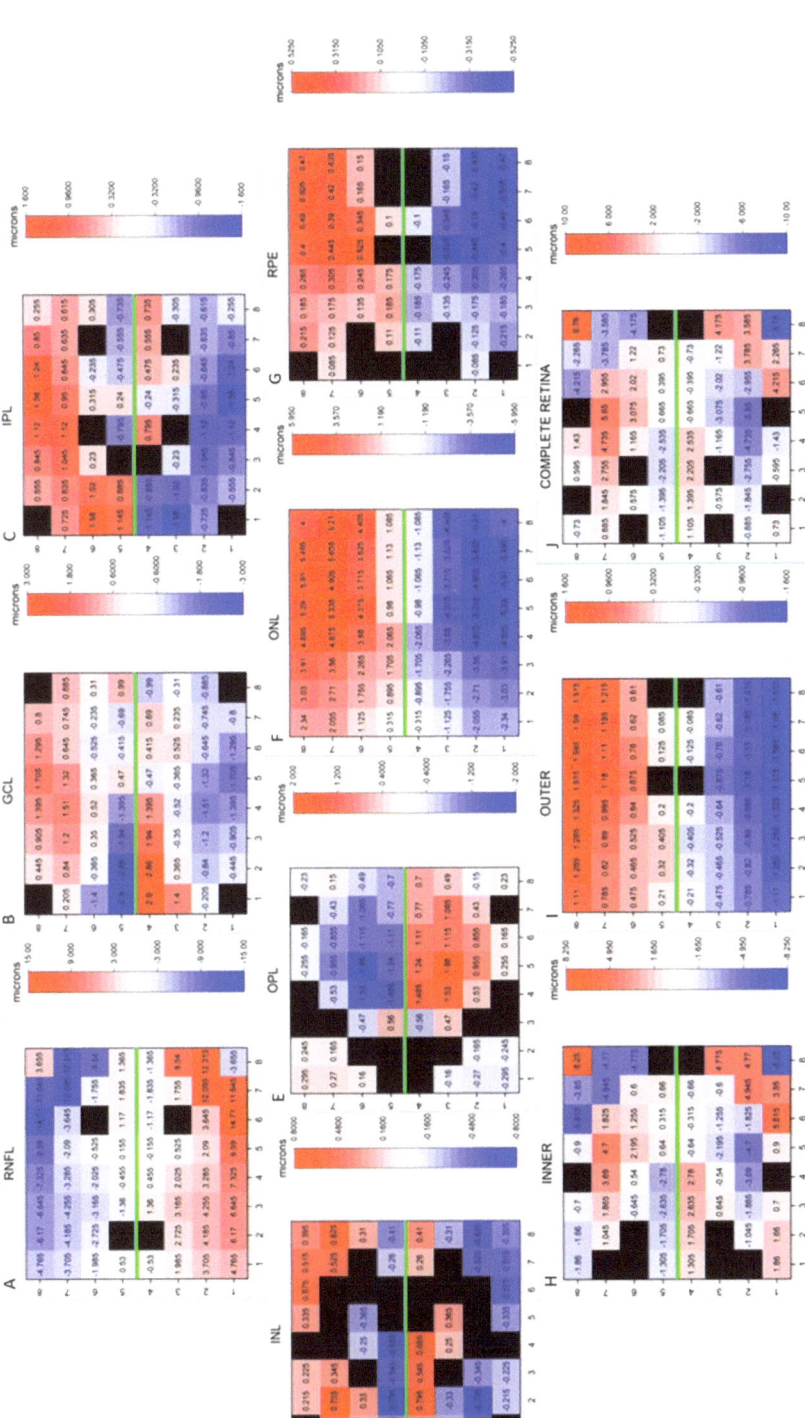

Figure 2. Asymmetry thickness heatmaps of the different retinal layers. Note that half the mean thickness differences between corresponding cells are plotted when significant differences are found. Red represents thickening, and blue depicts thinning. Corresponding cells with no statistically significant difference are shown in black. The horizontal midline is represented in green. All segmentations are represented as if all eyes were right eyes. Abbreviations: (**A**) RNFL: retinal nerve fiber layer; (**B**) GCL: ganglion cell layer; (**C**) IPL: inner plexiform layer; (**D**) INL: inner nuclear layer; (**E**) OPL: outer plexiform layer; (**F**) ONL: outer nuclear layer; (**G**) RPE: retinal pigmentary epithelium; (**H**) INNER: inner retina; (**I**) OUTER: outer retina; (**J**) RETINA: complete retina.

4. Discussion

The PPA was designed in 2011 as a novel tool for the diagnosis and follow-up of glaucoma [16]. This protocol is based on the asymmetric nature of this disease, and it establishes comparisons between the thickness value of a given cell in the inferior macular hemisphere and the thickness value of its corresponding superior cell in the same eye. The results are then displayed on a gray-colored asymmetric thickness map. Unlike the Early Treatment Diabetic Retinopathy Study (ETDRS) map, which is usually employed for macular explorations, the 8×8 PPA provides thickness values at 64 different points of the macula, is oriented along the fovea–disk axis and respects the horizontal midline. Therefore, this protocol seems more appropriate to analyze macular thickness asymmetries than the ETDRS.

Research works into the presence of intraocular physiological macular thickness asymmetry are limited [17–21]. According to previous studies [17–21], the results of the present study showed that the thickness asymmetries between the superior and inferior hemispheres of the macula are present in healthy eyes. This finding highlights the need to develop a normative database that allows improvements to be made to the interpretation of tomography images and to identify incipient pathological asymmetries of macular thicknesses secondary to glaucoma [8] or to other retinal or neuropsychiatric diseases [1–6].

Altemir et al. [22] established that the normal range of ocular thickness asymmetries corresponds to the 95th central percentiles values that, in turn, correspond to the values between the 2.5th and 97.5th percentiles of the thickness asymmetry detected in a healthy population with normal distribution. Thus asymmetric thickness values below the 2.5th percentile or above the 97.5th percentile should be considered likely to be pathological asymmetric thickness values.

A previous study [17] reported similar mean thickness values of the 32 cells of the superior macular hemisphere and of the 32 cells of the inferior macular hemisphere of the total retina to the results of this study when analyzing a healthy Caucasian adult population. However, conversely to our results, these authors did not find any significant statistical thickness differences between hemispheres, likely due to their smaller sample size (n = 105) than herein (n = 300). We detected that the standard deviation of the mean thickness values, which represents the inter-individual variability of macular thickness, was lower when analyzing individual cells than when clustering several cells (mean ± SD thickness). This finding agrees with other previous studies [17,23]. Therefore, the analysis of the thickness asymmetry for each couple of corresponding cells of the different macular layers could constitute a more sensitive test than those that analyze sectors, like the peripapillary retinal nerve layer thickness analysis or the macular ganglion cell layer analysis [15]. Furthermore, a previous study [21] demonstrated that age, gender and axial length have less impact on the intraocular retinal thickness asymmetry than on the quantitative retinal thickness values.

Two previous research works [19,20] also employed the PPA of the Spectralis to analyze the presence of the thickness asymmetries of the total retina in each couple of corresponding cells of the macular grid. One of them [20] showed significant thickness asymmetries in some of the peripheral and nasal cells of the macular grid, while our results revealed statistically significant differences in most of the couples of the corresponding cells of the complete RETINA. These differences could be explained by the higher statistical power in our study due to its bigger sample size.

We can also see that the absolute values of the thickness asymmetries of the complete RETINA in our study and other previous studies [19,20] differ, likely due to the distinct sample populations' demographic and ophthalmological characteristics. So the normative database shown in our study should be employed mainly to analyze Caucasian populations.

Through the thickness asymmetry analysis of each couple of the corresponding cells between the inferior and superior hemispheres on different macular layers, we observed that the magnitude of the thickness asymmetries was not homogeneously distributed. We found larger significant intraocular thickness asymmetries on RNFL and ONL, while the

RPE displayed a minimal significant thickness asymmetry between hemispheres. Other authors [21] also indicate more intraocular variations in RNFL thickness than on GCL and IPL when analyzing the physiological intraocular thickness asymmetries of the inner retinal layers. Conversely to all these findings, a previous study [17] did not show any significant asymmetries thickness on GCL, likely because these authors analyzed grouped cells instead of individual ones.

As we can see, most of the thickness asymmetry values included within the normal ranges (Tables S1–S10) are lower than 30 microns. Thus, the PPA should be able to detect pathological thickness asymmetries because it is able to represent differences of up to 30 microns [16]. However, we also note that the 2.5th and 97.5th percentile values of the thickness asymmetries are larger than 30 microns in some couples of the corresponding cells on RNFL, and in three couples of the corresponding cells on ONL that could be considered physiological. Another remarkable finding in our study is that GCL did not show either 2.5th or 97.5th percentile values of thickness asymmetries larger than 30 micros. Furthermore, a previous study [21] demonstrated less physiological variation in the intraocular thickness asymmetry for GCL than for RNFL. This means that the analysis of the intraocular thickness asymmetries of GCL using the PPA could constitute the most sensitive and specific test for the screening and follow-up of glaucoma.

Limitations

Our study has some limitations. First of all, the PPA is only able to detect intraocular macular thickness differences up to 30 microns, while physiological thickness asymmetries can exceed 30 in some macular layers. As we included only Caucasian adult subjects and we excluded eyes with high refractive errors, this normative database should be employed to analyze populations with the same characteristics. Finally, one may argue that the sample size of the studied group of subjects is relatively small (n = 300). However, we should keep in mind that other commercial normative databases have a smaller sample size than ours [24].

5. Conclusions

This study demonstrates that there are physiological macular thickness asymmetries in healthy eyes between the superior and inferior hemispheres. This study provides the first normative database of the thickness asymmetries on each macular layer to improve the classification of OCT images into normal or pathological findings when analyzing macular thickness asymmetries.

Supplementary Materials: The following supporting information can be downloaded at: https://www.mdpi.com/article/10.3390/jcm12247609/s1, Table S1. Mean ± SD of the thickness difference between corresponding cells of the inferior and superior hemispheres of the retinal nerve fiber layer (RNFL) and its statistical significance (p value) (Student's test for paired samples). Positive values indicate that thicker thicknesses are detected in the inferior cells than in its corresponding cells in the superior hemisphere. Negative values indicate that inferior cell show thinner thicknesses than its corresponding cells in the superior hemisphere. 2.5th and 97.5th percentiles of the asymmetry thickness in each cell of the 8×8 grid for the RNFL are also shown; Table S2. Table S2. Mean ± SD of the thickness difference between corresponding cells of the inferior and superior hemispheres of the ganglion cell layer (GCL) and its statistical significance (p value) (Student's test for paired samples). Positive values indicate that thicker thicknesses are detected in the inferior cells than in its corresponding cells in the superior hemisphere. Negative values indicate that inferior cell show thinner thicknesses than its corresponding cells in the superior hemisphere. 2.5th and 97.5th percentiles of the asymmetry thickness in each cell of the 8×8 grid for the GCL are also shown; Table S3. Mean ± SD of the thickness difference between corresponding cells of the inferior and superior hemispheres of the inner plexiform layer (IPL) and its statistical significance (p value) (Student's test for paired samples). Positive values indicate that thicker thicknesses are detected in the inferior cells than in its corresponding cells in the superior hemisphere. Negative values indicate that inferior cell show thinner thicknesses than its corresponding cells in the superior hemisphere. 2.5th and

97.5th percentiles of the asymmetry thickness in each cell of the 8 × 8 grid for the IPL are also shown; Table S4. Mean ± SD of the thickness difference between corresponding cells of the inferior and superior hemispheres of the inner nuclear layer (INL) and its statistical significance (p value) (Student's test for paired samples). Positive values indicate that thicker thicknesses are detected in the inferior cells than in its corresponding cells in the superior hemisphere. Negative values indicate that inferior cell show thinner thicknesses than its corresponding cells in the superior hemisphere. 2.5th and 97.5th percentiles of the asymmetry thickness in each cell of the 8x8 grid for the INL are also shown; Table S5. Mean ± SD of the thickness difference between corresponding cells of the inferior and superior hemispheres of the outer plexiform layer (OPL) and its statistical significance (p value) (Student's test for paired samples). Positive values indicate that thicker thicknesses are detected in the inferior cells than in its corresponding cells in the superior hemisphere. Negative values indicate that inferior cell show thinner thicknesses than its corresponding cells in the superior hemisphere. 2.5th and 97.5th percentiles of the asymmetry thickness in each cell of the 8 × 8 grid for the OPL are also shown; Table S6. Mean ± SD of the thickness difference between corresponding cells of the inferior and superior hemispheres of the outer nuclear layer (ONL) and its statistical significance (p value) (Student's test for paired samples). Positive values indicate that thicker thicknesses are detected in the inferior cells than in its corresponding cells in the superior hemisphere. Negative values indicate that inferior cell show thinner thicknesses than its corresponding cells in the superior hemisphere. 2.5th and 97.5th percentiles of the asymmetry thickness in each cell of the 8 × 8 grid for the ONL are also shown; Table S7. Mean ± SD of the thickness difference between corresponding cells of the inferior and superior hemispheres of the retinal pigmentary epithelium (RPE) and its statistical significance (p value) (Student's test for paired samples). Positive values indicate that thicker thicknesses are detected in the inferior cells than in its corresponding cells in the superior hemisphere. Negative values indicate that inferior cell show thinner thicknesses than its corresponding cells in the superior hemisphere. 2.5th and 97.5th percentiles of the asymmetry thickness in each cell of the 8 × 8 grid for the RPE are also shown; Table S8. Mean ± SD of the thickness difference between corresponding cells of the inferior and superior hemispheres of the inner retina (INNER) and its statistical significance (p value) (Student's test for paired samples). Positive values indicate that thicker thicknesses are detected in the inferior cells than in its corresponding cells in the superior hemisphere. Negative values indicate that inferior cell show thinner thicknesses than its corresponding cells in the superior hemisphere. 2.5th and 97.5th percentiles of the asymmetry thickness in each cell of the 8 × 8 grid for the INNER are also shown: Table S9. Mean ± SD of the thickness difference between corresponding cells of the inferior and superior hemispheres of the outer retina (OUTER) and its statistical significance (p value) (Student's test for paired samples). Positive values indicate that thicker thicknesses are detected in the inferior cells than in its corresponding cells in the superior hemisphere. Negative values indicate that inferior cell show thinner thicknesses than its corresponding cells in the superior hemisphere. 2.5th and 97.5th percentiles of the asymmetry thickness in each cell of the 8 × 8 grid for the OUTER are also shown; Table S10. Mean ± SD of the thickness difference between corresponding cells of the inferior and superior hemispheres of the complete retina (RETINA) and its statistical significance (p value) (Student's test for paired samples). Positive values indicate that thicker thicknesses are detected in the inferior cells than in its corresponding cells in the superior hemisphere. Negative values indicate that inferior cell show thinner thicknesses than its corresponding cells in the superior hemisphere. 2.5th and 97.5th percentiles of the asymmetry thickness in each cell of the 8 × 8 grid for the RETINA are also shown.

Author Contributions: Conceptualization and methodology, writing original draft preparation: All authors; validation, formal analysis, and investigation: A.P.-C., B.P.-C. and J.J.G.-M.; data curation A.P.-C.; critical review of the last draft of the paper: B.P.-C., J.J.G.-M. and M.d.-R.-V.; supervision: J.J.G.-M. All authors have read and agreed to the published version of the manuscript.

Funding: This research received no external funding.

Institutional Review Board Statement: The study protocol adhered to the ethical principles stated in the Declaration of Helsinki and was approved by the Local Ethics Committee at the University General Hospital Reina Sofia in Murcia, Spain (protocol number 03/19, approval date 29 January 2019).

Informed Consent Statement: Subjects were informed about the study and informed consent was obtained from them all before enrollment.

Data Availability Statement: Our data are shown in the main text or as Supplementary Materials.

Acknowledgments: We would like to thank José Manuel Tamarit (Heidelberg Engineering, Heidelberg, Germany) for his technical support with the SD-OCT Spectralis device.

Conflicts of Interest: The authors declare no conflict of interest.

References

1. Petzold, A.; Balcer, L.J.; Calabresi, P.A.; Costello, F.; Frohman, T.C.; Frohman, E.M.; Martinez-Lapiscina, E.H.; Green, A.J.; Kardon, R.; Outteryck, O.; et al. Retinal layer segmentation in multiple sclerosis: A systematic review and meta-analysis. *Lancet Neurol.* **2017**, *16*, 797–812. [CrossRef] [PubMed]
2. Chan, V.T.; Sun, Z.; Tang, S.; Chen, L.J.; Wong, A.; Tham, C.C.; Wong, T.Y.; Chen, C.; Ikram, M.K.; Whitson, H.E.; et al. Spectral-domain OCT measurements in Alzheimer's disease: A systematic review and meta-analysis. *Ophthalmology* **2019**, *126*, 497–510. [CrossRef] [PubMed]
3. Garcia-Martin, E.; Larrosa, J.M.; Polo, V.; Satue, M.; Marques, M.L.; Alarcia, R.; Seral, M.; Fuertes, I.; Otin, S.; Pablo, L.E. Distribution of retinal layer atrophy in patients with Parkinson disease and association with disease severity and duration. *Am. J. Ophthalmol.* **2014**, *157*, 470–478.e2. [CrossRef] [PubMed]
4. Almonte, M.T.; Capellàn, P.; Yap, T.E.; Cordeiro, M.F. Retinal correlates of psychiatric disorders. *Ther. Adv. Chronic. Dis.* **2020**, *11*, 2040622320905215. [CrossRef] [PubMed]
5. García-Medina, J.J.; García-Piñero, M.; Del-Río-Vellosillo, M.; Fares-Valdivia, J.; Ragel-Hernández, A.B.; Martínez-Saura, S.; Cárcel-López, M.D.; Zanon-Moreno, V.; Pinazo-Duran, M.D.; Villegas-Pérez, M.P. Comparison of Foveal, Macular, and Peripapillary Intraretinal Thicknesses Between Autism Spectrum Disorder and Neurotypical Subjects. *Investig. Ophthalmol. Vis. Sci.* **2017**, *58*, 5819–5826. [CrossRef] [PubMed]
6. Garcia-Medina, J.J.; Bascuñana-Mas, N.; Sobrado-Calvo, P.; Gomez-Molina, C.; Rubio-Velazquez, E.; De-Paco-Matallana, M.; Zanon-Moreno, V.; Pinazo-Duran, M.D.; Del-Rio-Vellosillo, M. Macular Anatomy Differs in Dyslexic Subjects. *J. Clin. Med.* **2023**, *12*, 2356. [CrossRef] [PubMed]
7. Unterlauft, J.D.; Rhak, M.; Böhm, M.R.R.; Rrauscher, F.G. Analyzing the impact of glaucoma on the macular architecture using spectral-domain optical coherence tomography. *PLoS ONE* **2018**, *13*, e0209610. [CrossRef] [PubMed]
8. García-Medina, J.J.; Del-Río-Vellosillo, M.; Palazón-Cabanes, A.; Pinazo-Duran, M.D.; Zanon-Moreno, V.; Villegas-Pérez, M.P. Glaucomatous Maculopathy: Thickness Differences on Inner and Outer Macular Layers between Ocular Hypertension and Early Primary Open-Angle Glaucoma Using 8 × 8 Posterior Pole Algorithm of SD-OCT. *J. Clin. Med.* **2020**, *9*, 1503. [CrossRef]
9. Fujihara, F.M.F.; De Arruda Mello, P.A.; Lindenmeyer, R.L.; Pakter, H.M.; Lavinsky, J.; Benfica, C.Z.; Castoldi, N.; Picetti, E.; Lavinsky, D.; Finkelsztejn, A.; et al. Individual Macular Layer Evaluation with Spectral Domain Optical Coherence Tomography in Normal and Glaucomatous Eyes. *Clin. Ophthalmol.* **2020**, *14*, 1591–1599. [CrossRef]
10. Cifuentes-Canorea, P.; Ruiz-Medrano, J.; Gutierrez-Bonet, R.; Peña-Garcia, P.; Saenz-Frances, F.; Garcia-Feijoo, J.; Martinez-De-La-Casa, J.M. Analysis of inner and outer retinal layers using spectral domain optical coherence tomography automated segmentation software in ocular hypertensive and glaucoma patients. *PLoS ONE* **2018**, *13*, e0196112. [CrossRef]
11. Vianna, J.R.; Butty, Z.; A Torres, L.; Sharpe, G.P.; Hutchison, D.M.; Shuba, L.M.; Nicolela, M.T.; Chauhan, B.C. Outer retinal layer thickness in patients with glaucoma with horizontal hemifield visual field defects. *Br. J. Ophthalmol.* **2019**, *103*, 1217–1222. [CrossRef] [PubMed]
12. Quigley, H.A.; Broman, A.T. The number of people with glaucoma worldwide in 2010 and 2020. *Br. J. Ophthalmol.* **2006**, *90*, 262–267. [CrossRef] [PubMed]
13. Vessani, R.M.; Moritz, R.; Batis, L.; Benetti-Zagui, R.; Bernardoni, S.; Susanna, R. Comparison of quantitative imaging devices and subjective optic nerve head assessment by general ophthalmologists to differentiate normal from glaucomatous eyes. *J. Glaucoma* **2009**, *18*, 253–261. [CrossRef] [PubMed]
14. Abrams, L.S.; Scott, I.U.; Spaeth, G.L.; Quigley, H.A.; Varma, R. Agreement among optometrists, ophthalmologists, and residents in evaluating the optic disc for glaucoma. *Ophthalmology* **1994**, *101*, 1662–1667. [CrossRef] [PubMed]
15. Um, T.W.; Sung, K.R.; Wollstein, G.; Yun, S.C.; Na, J.H.; Schuman, J.S. Asymmetry in hemifield macular thickness as an early indicator of glaucomatous change. *Investig. Ophthalmol. Vis. Sci.* **2012**, *53*, 1139–1144. [CrossRef] [PubMed]
16. Asrani, S.; Rosdahl, J.A.; Allingham, R.R. Novel software strategy for glaucoma diagnosis: Asymmetry analysis of retinal thickness. *Arch. Ophthalmol.* **2011**, *129*, 1205–1211. [CrossRef] [PubMed]
17. Altan, C.; Arman, B.H.; Arici, M.; Urdem, U.; Solmaz, B.; Pasaoglu, I.; Basarir, B.; Onmez, F.; Taskapili, M. Normative posterior pole asymmetry analysis data in healthy Caucasian population. *Eur. J. Ophthalmol.* **2019**, *29*, 386–393. [CrossRef]
18. Dave, P.; Jethani, J.; Shah, J. Asymmetry of retinal nerve fiber layer and posterior pole asymmetry analysis parameters of spectral domain optical coherence tomography in children. *Semin. Ophthalmol.* **2017**, *32*, 443–448. [CrossRef]
19. Yamashita, T.; Sakamoto, T.; Kakiuchi, N.; Tanaka, M.; Kii, Y.; Nakao, K. Posterior pole asymmetry analyses of retinal thickness of upper and lower sectors and their association with peak retinal nerve fiber layer thickness in healthy young eyes. *Investig. Ophthalmol. Vis. Sci.* **2014**, *55*, 5673–5678. [CrossRef]

20. Jacobsen, A.G.; Bendtsen, M.D.; Vorum, H.; Bogsted, M.; Hargitai, J. Normal value ranges for central retinal thickness asymmetry in healthy Caucasian adults measured by SPECTRALIS SD-OCT posterior pole asymmetry analysis. *Investig. Ophthalmol. Vis. Sci.* **2015**, *56*, 3875–3882. [CrossRef]
21. Choovuthayakorn, J.; Chokesuwattanaskul, S.; Phinyo, P.; Hansapinyo, L.; Pathanapitoon, K.; Chaikitmongkol, V.; Watanachai, N.; Kunavisarut, P.; Patikulsila, D. Reference Database of Inner Retinal Layer Thickness and Thickness Asymmetry in Healthy Thai Adults as Measured by the Spectralis Spectral Domain Optical Coherence Tomography. *Ophthalmic. Res.* **2022**, *65*, 668–677. [CrossRef] [PubMed]
22. Altemir, I.; Oros, D.; Elía, N.; Polo, V.; Larrosa, J.M.; Pueyo, V. Retinal asymmetry in children measured with optical coherence tomography. *Am. J. Ophthalmol.* **2013**, *156*, 1238–1243. [CrossRef]
23. Alluwimi, M.S.; Swanson, W.H.; Malinovsky, V.E. Between-subject variability in asymmetry analysis of macular thickness. *Optom. Vis. Sci.* **2014**, *91*, 484–490. [CrossRef] [PubMed]
24. Cirrus HD-OCT. *User Manual, 2660021162665 Rev. A*; Carl Zeiss Meditec: Jena, Germany, 2016.

Disclaimer/Publisher's Note: The statements, opinions and data contained in all publications are solely those of the individual author(s) and contributor(s) and not of MDPI and/or the editor(s). MDPI and/or the editor(s) disclaim responsibility for any injury to people or property resulting from any ideas, methods, instructions or products referred to in the content.

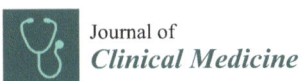 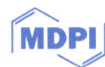

Article

Ocular Biometry Features and Their Relationship with Anterior and Posterior Segment Lengths among a Myopia Population in Northern China

Linbo Bian [1,2], Wenlong Li [1,2], Rui Qin [1,2], Zhengze Sun [1,2], Lu Zhao [1,2], Yifan Zhou [1,2], Dehai Liu [1,2], Yiyun Liu [1,2], Tong Sun [1,2] and Hong Qi [1,2,*]

1. Department of Ophthalmology, Peking University Third Hospital, Beijing 100191, China; linbobian@163.com (L.B.)
2. Beijing Key Laboratory of Restoration of Damaged Ocular Nerve, Beijing 100191, China
* Correspondence: doctorqihong@163.com

Abstract: Objectives: The study aims to explore the ocular biometry of a myopic population in Northern China, focusing specifically on anterior and posterior segment lengths. **Methods:** This is a cross-sectional study. The medical records of 3458 myopic patients who underwent refractive surgery were evaluated. Axial length (AL), anterior chamber depth (ACD), lens thickness (LT) and other biometric parameters were measured using the IOL Master 700. The study determined the anterior segment length (ASL = ACD + LT), the posterior segment length (PSL = AL − ASL) and the ratio of ASL to PSL (ASL/PSL). **Results:** This study included 3458 eyes from 3458 myopic patients (1171 men and 2287 women). The mean age was 27.38 ± 6.88, ranging from 16 to 48 years old. The mean ASL was 7.35 ± 0.27 mm, and the mean PSL was 18.39 ± 1.18 mm. The ASL and PSL trends demonstrate an age-related increase for both genders, with notable gender-specific variations. Across most age groups, males typically exhibited higher ASLs and PSLs than females, with the exception of the 35–40 and 40–45 age groups. The ASL and PSL consistently increased with a rising AL. The AL strongly correlates with the PSL and negatively correlates with the ASL/PSL ratio. The ACD and LT moderately correlate with the ASL, but an increased LT does not imply a longer posterior segment. The CCT and SE show little correlation with axial eye parameters. **Conclusions:** Among Chinese myopic patients, a longer ASL and PSL were correlated with older age and the male gender. The AL strongly correlates positively with the PSL and negatively correlates with the ASL/PSL ratio. An elongation of the posterior segment may primarily account for an eyeball's lengthening.

Keywords: anterior segment length; posterior segment length; IOL Master 700; myopic patients; axial length

Citation: Bian, L.; Li, W.; Qin, R.; Sun, Z.; Zhao, L.; Zhou, Y.; Liu, D.; Liu, Y.; Sun, T.; Qi, H. Ocular Biometry Features and Their Relationship with Anterior and Posterior Segment Lengths among a Myopia Population in Northern China. *J. Clin. Med.* **2024**, *13*, 1001. https://doi.org/10.3390/jcm13041001

Academic Editors: José Ignacio Fernández-Vigo and Edward Wylegala

Received: 5 December 2023
Revised: 29 January 2024
Accepted: 7 February 2024
Published: 9 February 2024

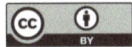

Copyright: © 2024 by the authors. Licensee MDPI, Basel, Switzerland. This article is an open access article distributed under the terms and conditions of the Creative Commons Attribution (CC BY) license (https:// creativecommons.org/licenses/by/ 4.0/).

1. Introduction

The increasing prevalence of myopia, especially in Asia, is a significant public health challenge. Recent research, such as a study conducted by Gao et al., has emphasized a noticeable rise in myopia rates among university students. At Tianjin Medical University, the occurrence of myopia increased from 93.5% in 2017 to 96.2% in 2020, suggesting a rising issue in educational environments [1]. Although the axial length (AL) is a crucial measurement when investigating eye growth, advances in ocular biometry have added supplementary measures that provide a more comprehensive viewpoint. Research into ocular biometry has shed light on the relationship between the AL and other biometry parameters in myopic eyes. An investigation conducted by Miao et al. concerning the biometry of the anterior segment in cases of high myopia unveiled that, in addition to cataractous eyes, high axial myopia was linked to corneal flattening, increased total corneal astigmatism and anterior segment enlargement [2]. The investigations' findings emphasize the complex correlation between anterior segment measures, the AL and the prevalence of myopia. This information provides insights for the formulation of therapeutic and public health policies targeted at tackling this pervasive disorder.

Two novel ocular biometric parameters, the anterior segment length (ASL) and the posterior segment length (PSL), have been applied to certain research in recent years [3]. The ASL is defined as the sum of the anterior chamber depth (ACD) and lens thickness (LT). It provides valuable insights into the structural components of the eye's anterior portion. Recent research has significantly advanced our understanding of the anterior segment, particularly in the context of myopia and cataract populations. In the realm of cataract research, studies like those by Pakuliene et al. and Lei et al. have explored the relationship between the ACD and ocular biometry parameters in cataract patients, revealing insights into anterior chamber angle anatomy and its correlation with lens position and the AL [4,5]. These findings are crucial for predicting narrow angles and understanding the biometric changes accompanying cataracts. Several studies have highlighted the associations between anterior segment biometry and high axial myopia [6–8]. Nevertheless, the overall anterior segment dimensions of the eyes have not been the focus of most studies.

The PSL represents the length of the vitreous chamber. It is derived by subtracting the ASL from the AL [9]. The PSL is instrumental in understanding the elongation of the eye. In myopia research, the PSL is especially relevant as it provides quantitative insights into the elongation patterns of the eye, a key factor in the progression of myopia. Paritala et al. conducted a study focusing on the vitreous chamber depth (VCD), which may also be referred to as the PSL, and its relationship with the AL (VCD/AL) and discovered a highly significant link between the AL and the VCD in individuals with high myopia [9]. This study underscores the importance of considering both the AL and PSL while comprehending the progression of myopia. In the field of cataracts, research by Qi et al. revealed that a longer ASL and a shorter PSL were associated with older age and the male gender, and the PSL correlated positively with the AL across the study population, indicating the importance of the PSL in the biometric assessment of cataractous eyes [3]. In the work of Jian et al., it was found that eyes that are more keratoconic may have a shorter AL and PSL but a deeper ACD [10]. Moreover, for the PSL, there was a clear distinction between the various retinopathy of prematurity (ROP) stages, whereas for the ACD, there was just a little difference [11]. Eyes afflicted by central retinal vein occlusion (CRVO) may have a reduced PSL compared to unaffected eyes. This anatomical characteristic might potentially lead to a higher likelihood of congestion in the central retinal vein and artery within the lamina cribrosa, therefore increasing the risk of developing CRVO [12].

The findings from these studies suggest that a comprehensive approach to measuring ocular biometry, including the ASL and PSL, could bring some new insights. Examining the diverse biometric patterns of the ASL and PSL within different populations can aid in our understanding of how the anterior and posterior segments grow, identify high-risk individuals and provide individualized care. However, there has been no comprehensive investigation conducted on the distribution of the ASL and PSL in the Chinese myopia population. Building upon the foundation laid by prior research, our study aims to comprehensively explore the ASL and PSL in the myopic population of Northern China. In this study, we measured the ocular biometry, including the AL, the central corneal thickness (CCT), the ACD, the LT, the keratometry (K), the total keratometry (TK), the keratometry spherical equivalent (SE), the corneal astigmatism based on keratometry (DeltaK), the total keratometry spherical equivalent (TSE), the corneal astigmatism based on total keratometry (DeltaTK) and the white-to-white distance (WTW), of myopic people who visited a refractive surgery center in Northern China using IOL Master 700 (Carl Zeiss Meditec AG, Jena, Germany). As we delved into the ASL and PSL measurements using advanced biometric tools, we anticipated uncovering novel correlations and contributing to the growing body of knowledge that shapes myopia management.

2. Methods

This cross-sectional comparative study was conducted at Peking University Third Hospital, Beijing, China. The study was approved by the Ethics Committee of the Peking University Third Hospital (M2023687) and was performed in accordance with the tenets of the Declaration of Helsinki. Informed written consent was obtained from all participants after a detailed explanation of the study.

2.1. Subjects

This study retrospectively reviewed medical records of refractive surgery, including corneal refractive surgery and implantable collamer lens (ICL) implantation, at the Peking University Third Hospital from November 2019 to September 2022. Patients with corneal opacity, lens dislocations, prior ocular trauma or operations or other ocular diseases that might influence the measurements were excluded. For each patient in this study, only one eye was counted. One eye was selected randomly for patients with both eyes eligible. In total, 3458 eyes of 3458 patients were included in this analysis.

The IOL Master 700 was used by skilled technicians to collect ocular biometric parameters. The technician visually verified the accurate fixation of the examinees on the fovea scan during each measurement. The standard deviation (SD) was automatically computed for each measurement of the AL, ACD and LT. If the SD for the AL exceeded 0.027 mm or for the ACD exceeded 0.021 mm, the device issued a warning indicating poor-quality findings. These data were discarded, and the measurements were repeated until consistent values were achieved.

The measurement of the AL was conducted by employing signals originating from the tear film and extending to the retinal pigment epithelium (RPE) of the fovea. The ACD was defined as the measurement of the distance between the anterior surface of the cornea and the anterior surface of the lens. The LT was defined as the measurement of the distance between the anterior and posterior surfaces of the lens. The ASL was determined by measuring the distance between the anterior surface of the cornea and the back surface of the lens. This value is obtained by adding the values of the LT and ACD. The PSL was determined as the difference between the AL and the ASL, representing the distance between the posterior lens surface and the RPE of the fovea. The ASL-to-PSL ratio (ASL/PSL) was also computed. In this study, we categorized all the eyes into six groups based on the AL measurements (19–22, 22–24, 24–26, 26–28, 28–30 and 30–32 mm) [5].

2.2. Statistical Analysis

The continuous data are shown as mean ± SD, while the categorical data are presented as the frequency for each category. The normality of the data for all ocular biometric parameters was assessed using the Kolmogorov–Smirnov (K-S) test. A skewed distribution was determined if $p < 0.05$. The Mann–Whitney U-test was used to analyze differences between two groups for continuous data, whereas the Kruskal–Wallis test was used to assess differences among more than two groups. The Pearson chi-squared test was used to compare differences in categorical data. The study used multiple linear regressions to analyze the relationship between the ASL and PSL, taking into account the AL, CCT, ACD, LT and SE as independent factors. Pearson's correlation was used to evaluate the associations between the lengths of the anterior and posterior segments and ocular biometric data. p-values below 0.05 were deemed to be statistically significant. The analyses and visualizations were conducted using IBM SPSS v27.0 (Chicago, IL, USA).

3. Results

3.1. Characteristics

Table 1 shows the general and ocular biometric characteristics of this study population. This study included 3458 eyes of 3458 myopic patients (1171 men and 2287 women). The mean age was 27.38 ± 6.88, ranging from 16 to 48 years old.

Table 1. General and ocular biometric characteristics in this study population.

	Total (n = 3458)
Age, years	27.38 ± 6.88
Sex, male/female	1171/2287
AL, mm	25.74 ± 1.18
ASL, mm	7.35 ± 0.27
PSL, mm	18.39 ± 1.18
ASL/PSL, %	0.40 ± 0.03
CCT, μm	539.23 ± 32.20
ACD, mm	3.67 ± 0.27
LT, mm	3.69 ± 0.27
SE, diopter	43.57 ± 1.45
DeltaK, diopter	−1.31 ± 0.78
TSE, diopter	43.56 ± 1.42
DeltaTK, diopter	−1.18 ± 0.72
WTW, mm	11.95 ± 0.42

AL, axial length; ASL, anterior segment length; PSL, posterior segment length; ASL/PSL, the ratio of ASL to PSL; CCT, central corneal thickness; ACD, anterior chamber depth; LT, lens thickness; SE, keratometry spherical equivalent; DeltaK, corneal astigmatism based on keratometry; TSE, total keratometry spherical equivalent; DeltaTK, corneal astigmatism based on total keratometry; WTW, white-to-white distance.

The mean ASL in this study population was 7.35 ± 0.27 mm, the mean PSL was 18.39 ± 1.18 mm and the mean ASL/PSL ratio was 40.0 ± 3.0%. The distributions of the ASL and the PSL among this study population are shown in Figure 1. The histograms suggested bell-shaped distributions for both the ASL and PSL, albeit with minor deviations from perfect normality (Kolmogorov–Smirnov test, both $p < 0.001$).

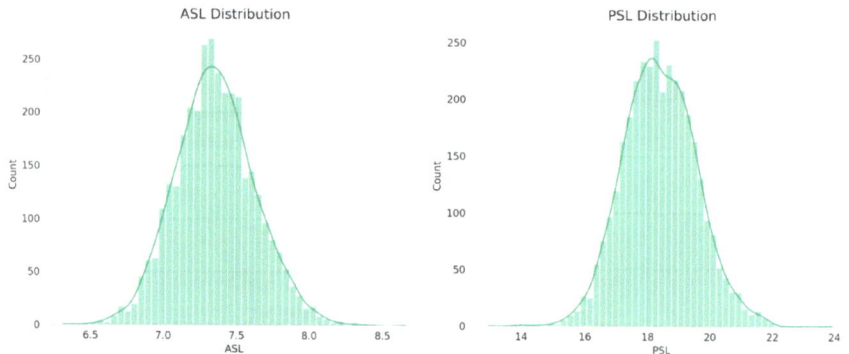

Figure 1. Distribution histograms for ASL and PSL.

3.2. Comparisons of ASL and PSL Stratified by Age and Sex

There is a general increase in the ASL with age for both genders. However, this increase is not linear across the age groups. Notably, the ASL for the females shows a significant increase in the 45–50 age group after a period of relative stability in the preceding age groups. On the other hand, the males exhibit a peak in the ASL in the 30–35 age group, followed by a decrease and then another increase in the 45–50 age group. Overall, the males tend to have a higher ASL compared to the females, except in the 35–40 and 40–45 age groups (Figure 2a).

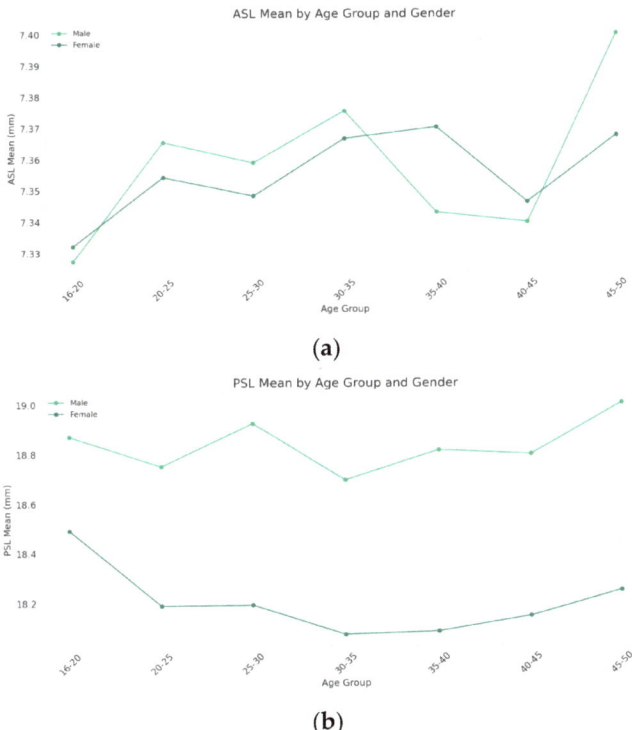

Figure 2. Comparisons of ASL and PSL stratified by age and sex. The (**a**) ASL and (**b**) PSL trends demonstrate an age-related increase for both genders, with notable gender-specific variations. Males generally exhibit higher ASLs and PSLs than females across age groups, except for the 35–40 and 40–45 groups. Males show consistent PSL growth, while females have a decrease until the 35–40 group, followed by a significant rise at 45–50.

While the PSL also increases with age for both genders, the males display a more consistent rise across age groups. In contrast, the females exhibit a decrease in the PSL from the 16–20 age group to the 35–40 age group, followed by an increase in the 45–50 age group. Throughout the age groups, the males have a higher PSL mean compared to the females, with the gap widening noticeably in the 45–50 age group. However, due to the limitations in sample size for certain age groups, the statistical significance of the differences between genders could not be determined (Figure 2b).

3.3. Changes in ASL and PSL with AL

The ASL presents a gradual increase as the AL extends from 19 mm to 32 mm. This relationship is not linear, as evidenced by a notable surge in the ASL for the AL 30–32 mm group. The variability within each AL group, represented by the error bars, suggests a consistent range of ASL measurements across most AL categories, with a pronounced increase in variability in the 30–32 mm group (Figure 3a). The PSL ascends steadily as the AL increases. This trend demonstrates a robust correlation, where a longer AL is associated with a greater PSL. The standard deviation within each AL category remains relatively uniform, implying a consistent relationship between the AL and PSL across the spectrum (Figure 3b). ANOVA test was conducted, indicating significant differences in the ASL and PSL measurements across the different AL groups (both $p < 0.001$).

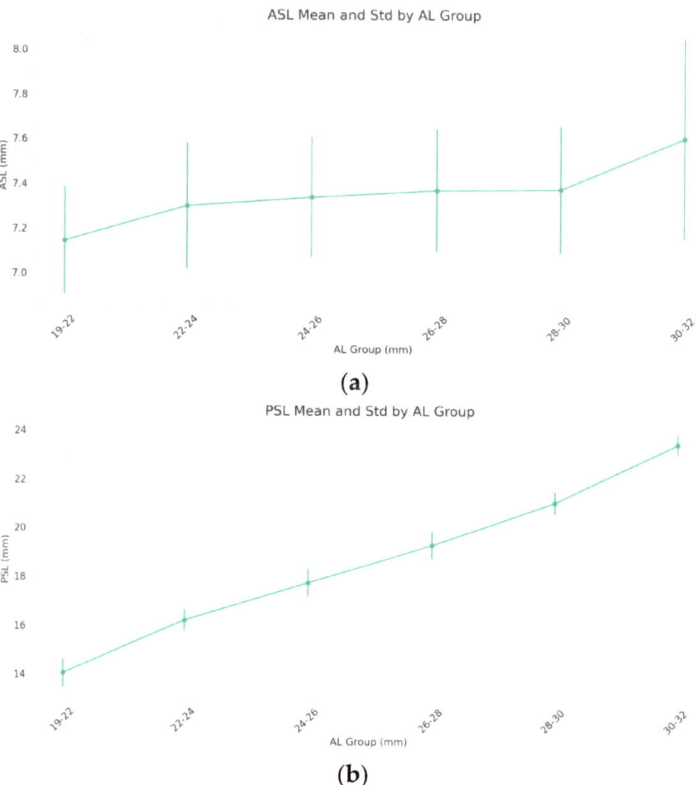

Figure 3. Changes in ASL and PSL with axial length (AL). The (**a**) anterior segment length (ASL) and (**b**) posterior segment length (PSL) consistently increased with rising AL.

3.4. Correlation Analysis of Various Eye Parameters

A correlation analysis was performed to identify the relationships between these parameters. A correlation matrix was generated using a heatmap to depict the strength and direction of the relationships. The heatmap provides a comprehensive overview of the correlation between various ocular measurements. Strong correlations are indicated by darker shades (Figure 4).

A strong positive correlation is observed between the AL and the PSL, as indicated by a coefficient close to one. Conversely, there is a strong negative correlation between the AL and the ASL/PSL ratio, denoted by a coefficient nearing −0.75. The ACD and LT both exhibit a moderate positive correlation with the ASL. The LT shows a strong negative correlation with the ASL/PSL ratio. As the LT increases, the anterior segment lengthens, but this does not necessarily translate to an increase in the posterior segment's length. The CCT shows very little to no correlation with the other parameters, implying that the corneal thickness is independent of axial dimensions and segment lengths within the eye. The SE does not exhibit significant correlations with the axial dimensions.

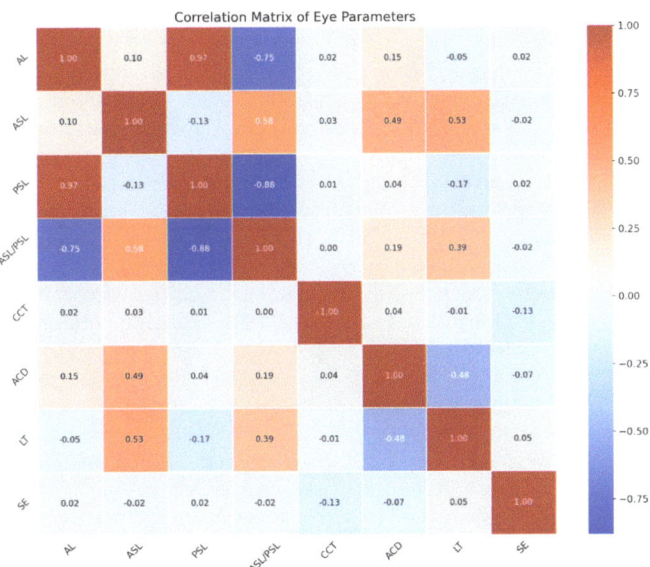

Figure 4. Correlations of ASL and PSL with other ocular biometric characteristics. AL strongly correlates with PSL and negatively correlates with the ASL/PSL ratio. ACD and LT moderately correlate with ASL, but an increased LT does not imply a longer posterior segment. CCT and SE show little correlation with axial eye dimensions. AL, axial length; ASL, anterior segment length; PSL, posterior segment length; ASL/PSL, the ratio of ASL to PSL; CCT, central corneal thickness; ACD, anterior chamber depth; LT, lens thickness; SE, keratometry spherical equivalent.

4. Discussion

In this comprehensive study, we explored the ocular biometry of a myopic population in Northern China, with a specific emphasis on the ASL and PSL. The study included a diverse sample of individuals aged from 16 to 48 years with varying degrees of myopia. This demographic representation is reflective of the broader population in the region, providing a robust basis for our analysis.

The eyeball is anatomically separated into two segments: the anterior segment and the posterior segment. The anterior segment consists of the cornea, anterior chamber, iris and lens. On the other hand, the posterior segment is filled with the vitreous body, retina, choroid and sclera. The IOLMaster 700, which is based on swept-source OCT, offers an image-based measurement that shows the entire longitudinal section of the eye. We conducted a thorough examination where we precisely measured the ASL and PSL using the IOLMaster 700 [13,14].

Our findings revealed that the distribution of the AL and the calculated ASL and PSL values align with previous studies conducted among East Asian populations. The mean ASL was 7.58 ± 0.39 mm and the mean PSL was 17.12 ± 2.64 mm in a cataractous population in Shanghai [3]. This consistency suggests that the myopic population in Northern China shares biometric characteristics with other East Asian cohorts. On the other hand, the ASL in our research group was comparatively short. This might be attributed to the generally lower thickness of the lens in young individuals. However, the discrepancy in the ASL also indicates a lesser decline in the ACD compared to the increase in the LT as individuals age [15]. Furthermore, it is possible for there to be variances caused by systematic errors and environmental factors. The measurements of the ASL and PSL contribute additional layers of information, allowing for a more nuanced understanding of ocular biometry. Comparisons with the existing literature, especially in the context of myopia, will enhance our comprehension of these parameters' significance in clinical practice.

The observed differences in the ASL and PSL as individuals age can be linked to physiological alterations in the anatomy of the eye throughout time. For both genders, the ASL and PSL trends show an increase with age. This could also be a reflection of how myopia develops in adulthood. Although myopia typically starts and progresses in childhood, it can also occur and develop during adulthood [16]. Myopia in adults needs to be continuously managed because a higher degree of myopia increases the absolute risk of myopia-related eye disorders and visual impairments. Sexually distinct characteristics can be explained by hormonal, genetic and environmental variables that affect the development and aging of the eyes [17]. The rise in the ASL with age, especially in females aged 45–50, may be attributed to hormonal effects on ocular structures, a notion that is substantiated by current evidence [18]. The gender disparities seen in the ASL and PSL distributions may suggest intrinsic anatomical and physiological variances, which are essential for tailored ophthalmic treatment [19]. These findings are consistent with research that indicates hormonal and biomechanical variables have a role in determining ocular dimensions.

Our analysis also revealed significant correlations between several eye parameters. The strong positive correlation between the AL and the PSL and the negative correlation between the AL and the ASL/PSL ratio highlight the interconnected nature of ocular biometry. The variations in the ASL and PSL across the different AL groups emphasize the need for individualized biometric assessments in refractive surgery and cataract management. This is particularly relevant for intraocular lens (IOL) power calculations, where accurate biometric data are essential for optimal visual outcomes [20,21]. The study's findings could inform the development of more precise biometric models for IOL power calculations, especially in patients with extreme ALs [22]. The correlation between the PSL and the AL, especially in cases of high myopia, underscores the role of posterior segment elongation in the progression of myopia. This finding is consistent with the notion that myopia involves structural changes in the eye, not just refractive errors [23]. The study by Paritala et al. on the correlation of the VCD with ocular biometry in high axial myopia provides foundational support for this understanding [9].

The independence of corneal parameters such as the CCT and SE from axial dimensions is an important finding, suggesting that corneal properties may be assessed independently of AL variations. This has implications for the diagnosis and management of corneal disorders and refractive errors, particularly in myopic patients. The IOL-Master revealed corneal power measurements averaging 43.57 ± 1.45 D, with an associated corneal astigmatism of -1.31 ± 0.78 D. Furthermore, this study utilized the IOL Master 700, which was equipped with novel software, to assess both the traditional K and TK, which reflect the refractive power of both the anterior and posterior corneal surfaces. The measurements derived from the K and TK exhibit strong concordance. Comparable results were found in a study by Kommineni [24], emphasizing the reliability of IOLMaster measurements in assessing corneal parameters in myopic eyes.

In clinical situations, it is crucial to comprehend not just the AL but also the individual contributions of each part, which may be determined using ASL and PSL measurements. Advanced biometry instruments enable extensive measurements of the eye's dimensions, therefore enhancing our comprehension of its anatomy. These characteristics provide doctors with a more comprehensive viewpoint for strategizing myopia prevention and refractive procedures, choosing intraocular lenses and handling different ocular disorders. Many effective strategies for preventing and controlling myopia have been developed recently; these include outdoor activities, low-dose atropine eye drops, multifocal spectacle and orthokeratology [25]. The prevention and management of myopia are major concerns for ophthalmologists as well as the general public. Future refractive observations of individuals at risk of myopia should focus more on the ASL and PSL in addition to the AL since the AL has a significant positive correlation with the PSL and a negative correlation with the ASL/PSL ratio. It is essential to identify these characteristics in order to create effective preventative measures and early treatments, which might help to slow down the evolution of myopia and decrease related consequences [26].The results of this study might have implications for tailored therapeutic treatments and the overall comprehension of myopia in Northern China. Refractive calculators currently in use for cataract surgery and phakic intraocular lens implantation typically employ regression or artificial intelligence to forecast the postoperative refractive state based on biometric parameters like the AL, K, ACD, LT, etc. [27]. The calculation might be more accurate if the parameters of the posterior segment of the eyes are taken into consideration. Furthermore, the findings of the study may stimulate additional inquiries into the genetic and environmental determinants that impact the ASL and PSL. Additionally, prior studies have described the characteristics of the PSL in patients with retinal diseases like ROP and CRAO [11,12]. Further investigation is essential to confirm whether the PSL has a distinct manifestation in common diseases like diabetic retinopathy or posterior vitreous detachment. The ASL, PSL and ASL/PSL ratio have potential for an in-depth explanation of the traits of pathological myopia and microphthalmia as well as the tracking of their occurrence processes.

Although the study provides helpful insights, it is crucial to recognize its limitations. This study primarily analyzes the biometric parameters measured by the IOLMaster 700. For a study on a myopic population, it is necessary to present the distribution of myopia diopters. However, due to the papery archiving of refractive results at this ophthalmology center, the large sample size made it difficult to collect and statistically analyze the refractive results. The use of a cross-sectional design hinders our capacity to identify causal linkages. Longitudinal research would provide a more comprehensive and detailed understanding of the development of myopia and its related alterations in the eye. These studies would focus on how these parameters evolve over time and their influence on ocular health and the advancement of diseases. Moreover, the study's emphasis on a particular geographic area might limit the applicability of the results to different populations. Subsequent investigations should strive to incorporate a broader spectrum of individuals from various places in China to account for any disparities in ocular attributes. To gain a greater knowledge of the multifactorial nature of myopia, future research should consider including additional criteria like corneal biomechanics and retinal morphology. Further investigation is required to examine the fundamental processes that contribute to the variations in the ASL and PSL based on age and gender. Furthermore, investigating the genetic and environmental variables that contribute to differences in ocular biometry might improve our comprehension of myopia and other ocular diseases.

In conclusion, this research provides data on the ocular characteristics of the myopic population in Northern China. This study's findings highlight the intricate relationship between ocular biometry parameters and their clinical significance. In this myopic population, male gender and older age were associated with prolonged ASLs and PSLs. The AL strongly correlates positively with the PSL and negatively correlates with the ASL/PSL ratio. The posterior segment's elongation could be the main cause of the eyeball's lengthening. There are no perceptible correlations between axial dimensions and the CCT or SE. The comprehensive ocular biometry provided may guide practitioners in optimizing treatment strategies for myopic individuals with diverse anatomical features. It is essential to identify these characteristics in order to create effective preventative measures and early treatments, which might help to slow down the progression of myopia and minimize related consequences.

Author Contributions: Conceptualization, L.B. and H.Q.; formal analysis, R.Q., Z.S., L.Z., Y.Z., D.L., Y.L. and T.S.; funding acquisition, H.Q.; investigation, R.Q., Z.S., L.Z., Y.Z., D.L., Y.L. and T.S.; methodology, L.B. and W.L.; resources, H.Q.; writing—original draft, L.B.; writing—review and editing, L.B., W.L., R.Q. and Z.S. All authors have read and agreed to the published version of the manuscript.

Funding: The study was supported by National Natural Science Foundation of China (82171022, 81974128, 82371026).

Institutional Review Board Statement: The study was approved by the Ethics Committee of the Peking University Third Hospital (M2023687, approval date 30 November 2023) and was performed in accordance with the tenets of the Declaration of Helsinki.

Informed Consent Statement: Informed consent was obtained from all subjects involved in the study.

Data Availability Statement: The data presented in this study are available on request from the corresponding author.

Conflicts of Interest: The authors declare no conflicts of interest.

References

1. Gao, H.-J.; Zhang, H.-M.; Dang, W.-Y.; Liu, L.; Zhu, Y.; He, Q.; Wang, X.; Chen, Y.-H.; Gao, F.; Wang, Q.-X.; et al. Prevalence and inconformity of refractive errors and ocular biometry of 3573 medical university freshman students for 4 consecutive years. *Int. J. Ophthalmol.* **2022**, *15*, 807–812. [CrossRef]
2. Miao, A.; Tang, Y.; Zhu, X.; Qian, D.; Zheng, T.; Lu, Y. Associations between anterior segment biometry and high axial myopia in 3438 cataractous eyes in the Chinese population. *BMC Ophthalmol.* **2022**, *22*, 71. [CrossRef] [PubMed]
3. Qi, J.; He, W.; Meng, J.; Wei, L.; Qian, D.; Lu, Y.; Zhu, X. Distribution of Ocular Anterior and Posterior Segment Lengths Among a Cataract Surgical Population in Shanghai. *Front. Med.* **2021**, *8*, 688805. [CrossRef] [PubMed]
4. Pakuliene, G.; Zimarinas, K.; Nedzelskiene, I.; Siesky, B.; Kuzmiene, L.; Harris, A.; Januleviciene, I. Anterior segment optical coherence tomography imaging and ocular biometry in cataract patients with open angle glaucoma comorbidity. *BMC Ophthalmol.* **2021**, *21*, 127. [CrossRef] [PubMed]
5. Lei, Q.; Tu, H.; Feng, X.; Ortega-Usobiaga, J.; Cao, D.; Wang, Y. Distribution of ocular biometric parameters and optimal model of anterior chamber depth regression in 28,709 adult cataract patients in China using swept-source optical biometry. *BMC Ophthalmol.* **2021**, *21*, 178. [CrossRef] [PubMed]
6. Shi, Y.; Wang, Y.; Cui, A.; Liu, S.; He, X.; Qiu, H.; Cui, H.; Gao, Y.; Yang, J. Myopia prevalence and ocular biometry: A cross-sectional study among minority versus Han schoolchildren in Xinjiang Uygur autonomous region, China. *Eye Lond. Engl.* **2022**, *36*, 2034–2043. [CrossRef] [PubMed]
7. Pedersen, H.R.; Svarverud, E.; Hagen, L.A.; Gilson, S.J.; Baraas, R.C. Comparing ocular biometry and autorefraction measurements from the Myopia Master with the IOLMaster 700 and the Huvitz HRK-8000A autorefractor. *Ophthalmic Physiol. Opt. J. Br. Coll. Ophthalmic Opt. Optom.* **2023**, *43*, 410–417. [CrossRef] [PubMed]
8. Rozema, J.; Dankert, S.; Iribarren, R.; Lanca, C.; Saw, S.M. Axial Growth and Lens Power Loss at Myopia Onset in Singaporean Children. *Investig. Ophthalmol. Vis. Sci.* **2019**, *60*, 3091–3099. [CrossRef] [PubMed]
9. Paritala, A.; Takkar, B.; Gaur, N.; Soni, D.; Ali, M.H.; Rathi, A. Correlation of vitreous chamber depth with ocular biometry in high axial myopia. *Indian J. Ophthalmol.* **2022**, *70*, 914–920. [CrossRef]
10. Jian, W.; Shen, Y.; Chen, Y.; Tian, M.; Zhou, X. Ocular dimensions of the Chinese adolescents with keratoconus. *BMC Ophthalmol.* **2018**, *18*, 43. [CrossRef]
11. Kent, D.; Pennie, F.; Laws, D.; White, S.; Clark, D. The influence of retinopathy of prematurity on ocular growth. *Eye Lond. Engl.* **2000**, *14*, 23–29. [CrossRef] [PubMed]
12. Moghimi, S.; Mirshahi, A.; Lasheie, A.; Maghsoudipour, M.; Beheshtnejaad, A. Biometric indices evaluation in central retinal vein occlusion using partial coherence laser interferometry. *Eur. J. Ophthalmol.* **2007**, *17*, 383–387. [CrossRef]
13. Wanichwecharungruang, B.; Amornpetchsathaporn, A.; Wongwijitsook, W.; Kongsomboon, K.; Chantra, S. Evaluation of ocular biometry in primary angle-closure disease with two swept source optical coherence tomography devices. *PLoS ONE* **2022**, *17*, e0265844. [CrossRef]
14. Nguyen, P.; Chopra, V. Applications of optical coherence tomography in cataract surgery. *Curr. Opin. Ophthalmol.* **2013**, *24*, 47–52. [CrossRef] [PubMed]
15. Mohamed, A.; Nandyala, S.; Ho, A.; Manns, F.; Parel, J.M.A.; Augusteyn, R.C. Relationship of the cornea and globe dimensions to the changes in adult human crystalline lens diameter, thickness and power with age. *Exp. Eye Res.* **2021**, *209*, 108653. [CrossRef]
16. Bullimore, M.A.; Lee, S.S.-Y.; Schmid, K.L.; Rozema, J.J.; Leveziel, N.; Mallen, E.A.H.; Jacobsen, N.; Iribarren, R.; Verkicharla, P.K.; Polling, J.R.; et al. IMI-Onset and Progression of Myopia in Young Adults. *Investig. Ophthalmol. Vis. Sci.* **2023**, *64*, 2. [CrossRef] [PubMed]
17. Asfuroğlu, Y.; Kan, Ö.; Asfuroğlu, M.; Baser, E. Association Between Dry Eye and Polycystic Ovary Syndrome: Subclinical Inflammation May Be Part of the Process. *Eye Contact Lens.* **2021**, *47*, 27–31. [CrossRef]
18. Flaskó, Z.; Zemova, E.; Eppig, T.; Módis, L.; Langenbucher, A.; Wagenpfeil, S.; Seitz, B.; Szentmáry, N. Hypothyroidism is Not Associated with Keratoconus Disease: Analysis of 626 Subjects. *J. Ophthalmol.* **2019**, *2019*, 3268595. [CrossRef]
19. Seven, E.; Yıldız, S.; Tekin, S.; Altaş, A.S.; Özer, M.D.; Batur, M.; Üçler, R.; Yaşar, T. Effect of Insulin Therapy on Ocular Biometric Parameters in Diabetic Patients. *J. Ocul. Pharmacol. Ther. Off. J. Assoc. Ocul. Pharmacol. Ther.* **2020**, *36*, 102–108. [CrossRef]
20. Buonsanti, D.; Raimundo, M.; Findl, O. Online intraocular lens calculation. *Curr. Opin. Ophthalmol.* **2023**. [CrossRef]
21. Minami, K.; Kataoka, Y.; Matsunaga, J.; Ohtani, S.; Honbou, M.; Miyata, K. Ray-tracing intraocular lens power calculation using anterior segment optical coherence tomography measurements. *J. Cataract. Refract. Surg.* **2012**, *38*, 1758–1763. [CrossRef]

22. Tan, Q.; Lin, D.; Wang, L.; Chen, B.; Tang, Q.; Chen, X.; Chen, M.; Tan, J.; Zhang, J.; Wu, L.; et al. Comparison of IOL Power Calculation Formulas for a Trifocal IOL in Eyes With High Myopia. *J. Refract. Surg.* **2021**, *37*, 538–544. [CrossRef]
23. Ohno-Matsui, K.; Wu, P.-C.; Yamashiro, K.; Vutipongsatorn, K.; Fang, Y.; Cheung, C.M.G.; Lai, T.Y.Y.; Ikuno, Y.; Cohen, S.Y.; Gaudric, A.; et al. IMI Pathologic Myopia. *Investig. Ophthalmol. Vis. Sci.* **2021**, *62*, 5. [CrossRef]
24. Kommineni, U.B.; Mohamed, A.; Vaddavalli, P.K.; Reddy, J.C. Comparison of total keratometry with corneal power measured by optical low-coherence reflectometry and placido-dual Scheimpflug system. *Eur. J. Ophthalmol.* **2022**, *32*, 1496–1503. [CrossRef] [PubMed]
25. Jonas, J.B.; Ang, M.; Cho, P.; Guggenheim, J.A.; He, M.G.; Jong, M.; Logan, N.S.; Liu, M.; Morgan, I.; Ohno-Matsui, K.; et al. IMI Prevention of Myopia and Its Progression. *Investig. Ophthalmol. Vis. Sci.* **2021**, *62*, 6. [CrossRef] [PubMed]
26. Morgan, I.G.; French, A.N.; Ashby, R.S.; Guo, X.; Ding, X.; He, M.; Rose, K.A. The epidemics of myopia: Aetiology and prevention. *Prog. Retin. Eye Res.* **2018**, *62*, 134–149. [CrossRef] [PubMed]
27. Stopyra, W.; Langenbucher, A.; Grzybowski, A. Intraocular Lens Power Calculation Formulas-A Systematic Review. *Ophthalmol. Ther.* **2023**, *12*, 2881–2902. [CrossRef] [PubMed]

Disclaimer/Publisher's Note: The statements, opinions and data contained in all publications are solely those of the individual author(s) and contributor(s) and not of MDPI and/or the editor(s). MDPI and/or the editor(s) disclaim responsibility for any injury to people or property resulting from any ideas, methods, instructions or products referred to in the content.

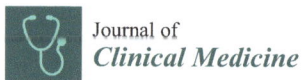

Article

Evaluation of the Diagnostic Capability of Spectralis SD-OCT 8 × 8 Posterior Pole Software with the Grid Tilted at 7 Degrees and Horizontalized in Glaucoma

Aurora Alvarez-Sarrion [1], Jose Javier Garcia-Medina [1,2,3,4,*], Ana Palazon-Cabanes [5], Maria Dolores Pinazo-Duran [3,4,6] and Monica Del-Rio-Vellosillo [7,8]

[1] Department of Ophthalmology and Optometry, University of Murcia, 30120 Murcia, Spain; aurora.alvarezopt@gmail.com
[2] Department of Ophthalmology, General University Hospital Morales Meseguer, 30008 Murcia, Spain
[3] Ophthalmic Research Unit "Santiago Grisolia", 28029 Valencia, Spain; dolores.pinazo@uv.es
[4] Spanish Net of Inflammatory Diseases RICORS, Institute of Health Carlos III, 28029 Madrid, Spain
[5] Department of Ophthalmology, Hospital Virgen del Castillo, Yecla, 30510 Murcia, Spain; a.palazoncabanes@gmail.com
[6] Cellular and Molecular Ophthalmo-Biology Group, Department of Surgery, University of Valencia, 46010 Valencia, Spain
[7] Department of Anesthesiology, General University Hospital Morales Meseguer, 30008 Murcia, Spain; monica.delrio@um.es
[8] Department of Surgery, Obstetrics and Gynecology and Pediatrics, University of Murcia, 30120 Murcia, Spain
* Correspondence: jj.garciamedina@um.es

Abstract: Background: The goal was to evaluate the diagnostic capability of different parameters obtained with the posterior pole (PP) software in Spectralis SD-OCT with the 8 × 8 grid tilted at 7° and horizontalized in glaucomatous eyes. **Methods**: A total of 299 eyes were included, comprising 136 healthy eyes and 163 with primary open-angle glaucoma (POAG). The following segmentations were evaluated: complete retina, retinal nerve fiber layer (RNFL), ganglion cell layer (GCL), GCL and inner plexiform layer (GCLIPL), ganglion cell complex (GCC), outer plexiform layer and outer nuclear layer (OPLONL), inner retinal layer (IRL), and outer retinal layer (ORL). Different patterns of macular damage were represented using heatmaps for each studied layer, where the areas under the curve (AUROC) values and a retinal thickness cutoff point were defined to discriminate POAG patients. **Results**: There was not any difference in the diagnostic capability for detecting glaucoma between the grid tilted at 7° and horizontalized. The macular segmentations that offer the highest diagnostic ability in glaucoma discrimination were, in the following order, RNFL (AUROC = 0.796), GCC (AUROC = 0.785), GCL (AUROC = 0.784), GCLIPL (AUROC = 0.770), IRL (AUROC = 0.755), and the complete retina (AUROC = 0.752). In contrast, ORL and OPLONL do not appear to be helpful for discriminating POAG. **Conclusions**: Some results of PP software may be useful for discriminating POAG.

Keywords: glaucoma; posterior pole; macula; thickness; layer; segmentation; map; 8 × 8; sensitivity; specificity

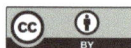

1. Introduction

Primary open-angle glaucoma (POAG), in most cases, begins as a disease of the anterior segment of the eye, where there is increased resistance to the drainage of aqueous humor, resulting in elevated intraocular pressure (IOP), or pressure that is too high for the patient's eye [1]. This condition causes a progressive and chronic optic neuropathy [2,3] characterized by optic nerve (ON) atrophy, papillary excavation, increased IOP, and a decrease in intraretinal thickness [4–6]. It has been classified as one of the leading causes of blindness worldwide [3,7,8].

An emerging method for diagnosing POAG and monitoring its progression is through the use of ON imaging and measurements of different retinal thicknesses with optical coherence tomography (OCT) [9–11]. Scientific evidence of early and even initial glaucomatous damage in the macula can be found in the literature. The assessment of macular thickness can be a valuable tool in evaluating glaucomatous structural changes [12–16]. To detect this damage with OCT, a macular scan should be obtained [17]. Additionally, understanding sequences of macular damage and specific macular patterns can provide relevant information for monitoring glaucomatous progression [18].

OCT allows for the quantitative evaluation of structural parameters of the retina [19–21]. The posterior pole (PP) software in Spectralis SD-OCT (Heidelberg Engineering, Germany) provides the total value of retinal thickness in an automatically tilted 8 × 8 grid (with 64 macular cells or superpixels) aligned at 7 degrees, which is the more common disc-fovea axis inclination. Other devices and software do not take this inclination into account and present the different grids horizontalized.

Furthermore, Spectralis SD-OCT allows for the segmentation of different retinal layers to obtain the isolated thickness of each layer or the thickness resulting from the combination of different layers. It is unknown which method offers the best results. Therefore, the objective of this study is to evaluate the diagnostic capacity of the PP algorithm in Spectralis SD-OCT with the 8 × 8 grid, tilted at 7° and horizontally aligned in glaucomatous eyes, through the analysis of the area under the curve (AUROC) values of thickness patterns obtained from the segmentation of different retinal layers or sets of layers with both inclinations.

2. Materials and Methods

This is a cross-sectional study that includes a total of 299 eyes, comprising 136 healthy eyes and 163 eyes with POAG. The Spectralis SD-OCT PP 8 × 8 software was employed for the study. This algorithm is made up of 64 cells or superpixels. The following segmentations were evaluated: complete retina, retinal nerve fiber layer (RNFL), ganglion cell layer (GCL), GCL and inner plexiform layer (GCLIPL), ganglion cell complex (RNFL+ GCLIPL), combination of outer plexiform layer and outer nuclear layer (OPLONL), inner retinal layers (IRL), and outer retinal layers (ORL) (Figure 1).

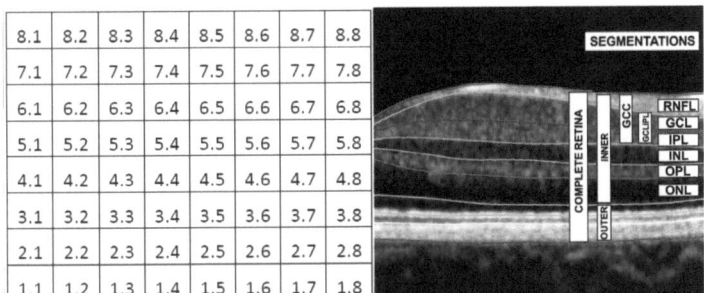

Figure 1. Denomination of cells or superpixels in the 8 × 8 posterior pole algorithm. The cells are named 1.1 at the lower temporal corner, 1.8 at the lower nasal corner, 8.1 at the upper temporal corner, and 8.8 at the upper nasal corner (**left figure**). Spectralis SD-OCT segmentations are also shown (**right figure**). RNFL = retinal nerve fiber layer, GCL = ganglion cell layer, IPL = inner plexiform layer, INL = inner nuclear layer, OPL = outer plexiform layer, ONL = outer nuclear layer, GCC = ganglion cell complex, GCLIPL = GCL+IPL, INNER = inner retina layer (IRL), OUTER = outer retina layer (ORL).

Inclusion criteria were defined as follows: obtaining PP maps centered on the fovea, correctly segmented OCT scans, patients diagnosed solely with POAG (case group), healthy subjects (control group), and subjects of Caucasian race. Exclusion criteria encompassed decentered PP maps from the fovea, poorly segmented OCT scans or inadequate image quality (signal strength < 20), individuals with ocular pathologies other than POAG or general pathologies that could affect macular thickness determination, best-corrected visual acuity (BCVA) less than 20/60, and individuals with isolated ocular hypertension.

Regarding the data collection method, the research was conducted at the University General Hospital Reina Sofía (Murcia, Spain), with 632 eyes classified as healthy or glaucomatous. The study protocol adhered to the ethical principles of the Declaration of Helsinki and was approved by the Local Ethics Committee at the University General Hospital Reina Sofía in Murcia, Spain (protocol number 02/18). Initially, demographic and ophthalmological characteristics of both groups (gender, age, IOP), optic disc cupping, mean deviation (MD), pattern standard deviation (PSD), and the presence of other pathologies were compiled (results in Table 1). Subsequently, retinal thickness data collection occurred in two phases. First, eyes were identified in Spectralis SD-OCT, and PP maps were selected, automatically tilted by 7 degrees, checked for appropriate segmentation, and thickness values from different segmentations were exported. Then, manual horizontalization of the PP 8 × 8 grid was performed (Figure 2), and thickness values were exported again. Each cell was symmetrically labeled according to whether it was the right or left eye. All eyes were considered and depicted as if they were right eyes in this study.

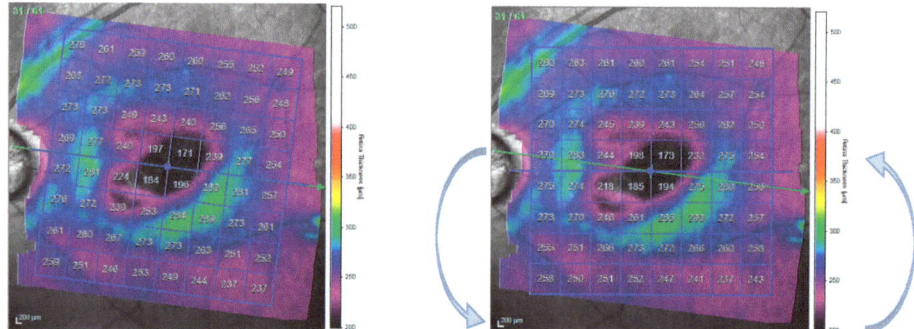

Figure 2. 8 × 8 grid of the posterior pole (PP) from Spectralis SD-OCT automatically tilted 7 degrees by the device (**left**). Horizontalized 8 × 8 grid of PP from Spectralis SD-OCT (**right**).

Table 1. Demographic and ophthalmic clinical analysis of the sample. Best corrected visual acuity (BCVA), Intraocular pressure (IOP), standard deviation (SD).

	Group		Test	p-Value
	Control	Glaucoma		
Eyes according to sex n (%)			$\chi^2 = 0.389$	0.533 (chi-squared test)
Men	61 (44.85)	79 (48.5)		
Women	75 (55.15)	84 (51.5)		
Patients according to sex n (%)			$\chi^2 = 1.097$	0.295 (chi-squared test)
Men	35 (43.2)	53 (51)		
Women	46 (56.8)	51 (49)		
Patients according to age Mean (SD)	66.7 (16.4)	75.5 (12.5)	$t(181) = -4.13$	<0.001 (t test)
Eyes according to age Mean (SD)	65.4 (16.4)	75.8 (12.2)	$t(297) = -6.27$	<0.001 (t test)
Decimal BCVA. Mean (SD)	0.9 (0.2)	0.87 (0.55)	$t(291) = 0.70$	0.485 (t test)
IOP Mean (SD)	17.22 (3.04)	17.13 (3.75)	$t(297) = 0.23$	0.819 (t test)
Vertical optic disc cupping Mean (SD)	0.39 (0.25)	0.57 (0.25)	$t(259) = -5.77$	<0.001 (t test)
Mean deviation. Mean (SD)	−1.13 (1.38)	−6.99 (7.11)	$t(257) = 7.97$	<0.001 (t test)
Pattern standard deviation Mean (SD)	1.84 (0.71)	5.47 (3.69)	$t(257) = -9.51$	<0.001 (t test)

Statistical Analysis

The statistical analysis was conducted using SPSS 27.0 for Windows. Differences were considered statistically significant when $p < 0.05$.

A descriptive analysis of qualitative and quantitative variables was performed, along with a comparison of means for both quantitative and qualitative variables. The diagnostic capability of the thickness of each cell in the 8×8 grid was calculated and represented in heatmaps. Subsequently, two global indices, mean and weighted, were calculated. Global indices were compared between grids and between layers within the same grid. Finally, cutoff points were determined for each layer and diagnostic capability indices.

In the descriptive analysis of qualitative variables, the number of cases in each category and their corresponding percentages were obtained, while for quantitative variables, minimum and maximum values, means, and standard deviation were calculated.

For the comparison of means of quantitative variables between the two groups, the independent samples t-test was employed after verifying the assumptions of normality with the Kolmogorov–Smirnov test. For qualitative variables, comparisons between the groups were performed using the Pearson chi-squared test.

The diagnostic capability of retinal macular thickness was calculated using the area under the curve (AUROC) for each cell in the 8×8 grid in each layer and in both grids. This was represented in heatmaps, where AUROC ≤ 0.5 was shown in blue, between 0.6 and 0.69 in white, and AUROC ≥ 0.70 in red.

To calculate the global indices for each layer or combination of layers studied in both grids, cells with AUROC ≥ 0.70 were selected. Two global indices were calculated—mean and weighted indices—and were compared using a related samples design. The mean index is the average thickness of selected cells, while the weighted index is the average of thickness values multiplied by the AUROC of the selected cells. These indices were compared in each segmentation and in each grid with the DeLong test.

Finally, cutoff points of the mean index in the inclined grid were determined for each layer, establishing the maximum thickness to classify a patient as diseased. Diagnostic validity indices were then calculated with 95% confidence intervals: sensitivity, specificity, positive predictive value (PPV), and negative predictive value (NPV).

3. Results

3.1. Analysis of Demographic and Ophthalmic Data

The final sample of the study consisted of 299 eyes from 185 subjects, with 47.6% being male ($n = 88$) and 52.4% female ($n = 97$). The mean age of the subjects was 71.6 years (Min.–Max.: 20–97, SD = 14.9). The number of eyes and subjects participating in the study were compared between healthy and glaucomatous groups based on gender, age, BCVA, IOP, optic disc excavation, mean deviation (MD), and pattern standard deviation (PSD). Significant differences were found between the two groups in optic disc excavation, MD, PSD, and age, with healthy subjects being younger than diseased subjects (Table 1).

3.2. Analysis of AUROCs

Supplementary Tables S2–S8 present the AUROCs, 95% confidence intervals, and p-values for the layers and layer combinations studied with the 7° inclined and horizontalized PP grids.

The heatmaps of AUROC for each studied layer (RNFL, GCL) and layer combinations (complete retina, IRL, ORL, GCLIPL, OPLONL, and ganglion cell complex) are then presented for each cell in the horizontalized (Figure 3) and 7° inclined (Figure 4) grids. Blue cells indicate lower diagnostic capability. Red cells represent a greater AUROC, and consequently, a higher diagnostic capability and more significant changes in retinal thickness between healthy and glaucomatous subjects.

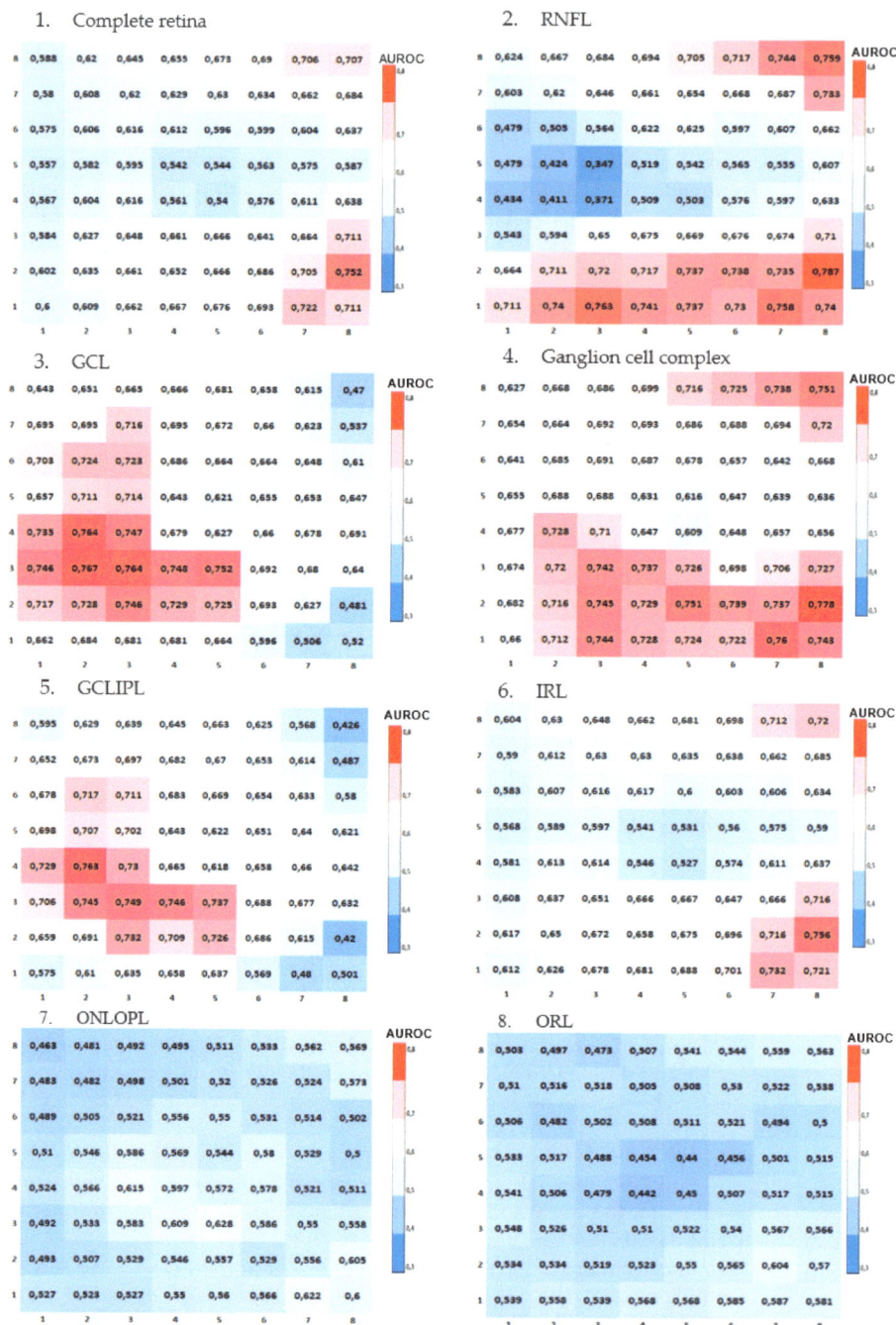

Figure 3. Heatmaps of AUROCs for the studied layers in the horizontalized grid using the 8 × 8 grid of the posterior pole from Spectralis SD-OCT. (**1**) Complete retina. (**2**) Retinal nerve fiber layer (RNFL). (**3**) Ganglion cell layer (GCL). (**4**) Ganglion cell complex. (**5**) Ganglion cell layer + inner plexiform layer (GCLIPL). (**6**) Inner retinal layer (IRL). (**7**) Outer nuclear layer + outer plexiform layer (ONLOPL). (**8**) Outer retinal layer (ORL).

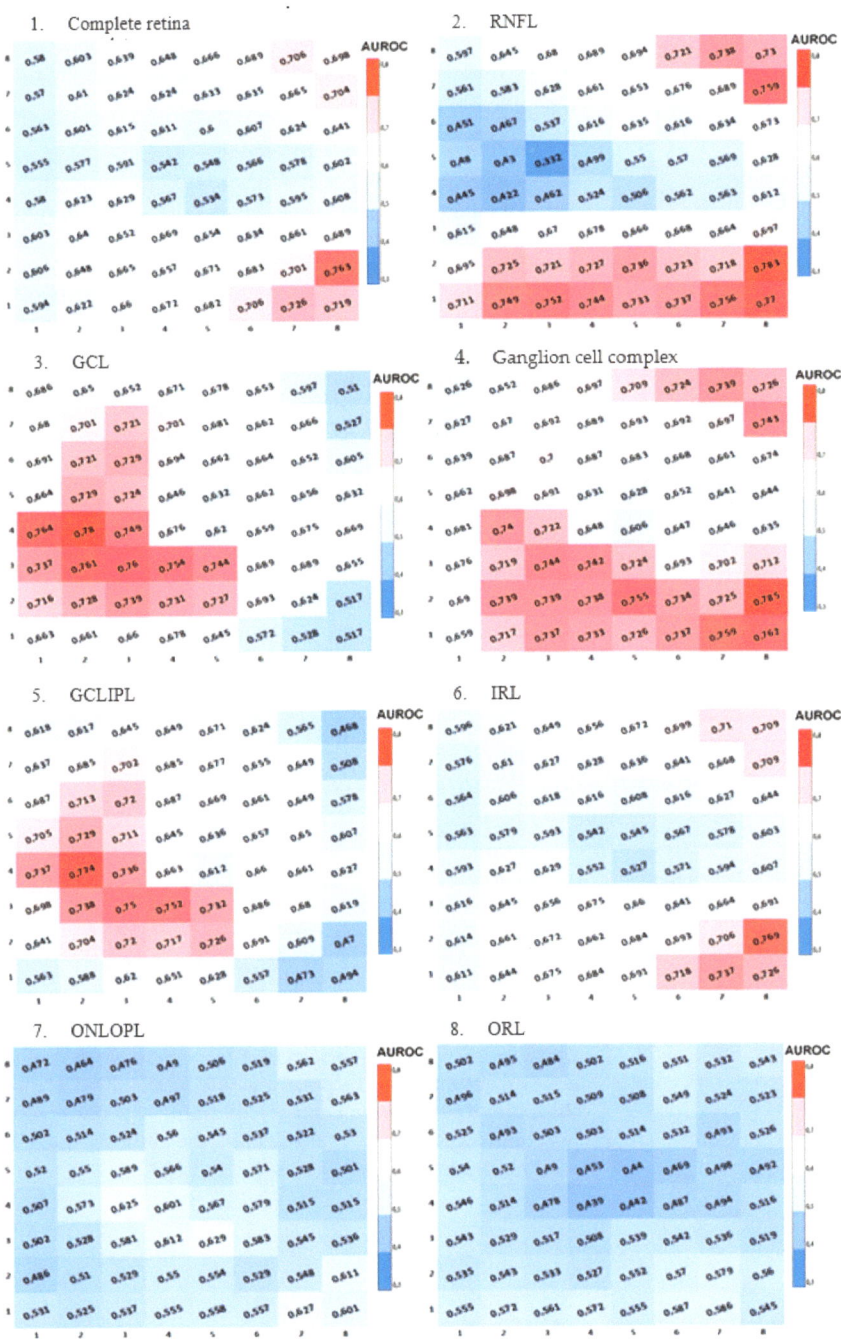

Figure 4. Heatmaps of AUROCs for the studied layers in the inclined grid (disc-fovea axis) using the 8 × 8 grid of the posterior pole from Spectralis SD-OCT. (**1**) Complete retina. (**2**) Retinal nerve fiber layer (RNFL). (**3**) Ganglion cell layer (GCL). (**4**) Ganglion cell complex. (**5**) Ganglion cell layer + inner plexiform layer (GCLIPL). (**6**) Inner retinal layer (IRL). (**7**) Outer nuclear layer + outer plexiform layer (ONLOPL). (**8**) Outer retinal layer (ORL).

Across all the heatmaps, in all studied layers and layer combinations, a very similar pattern is observed between the results obtained with the inclined and horizontalized 8 × 8 grids. The ganglion cell complex is the segmentation that shows the most cells with good diagnostic capability (AUROC $\geq$ 0.7).

3.3. Analysis of Global Indices

Following the calculation of AUROC for each cell in the 8 × 8 PP grid in the studied layers, both in the 7° inclined and horizontal grids, two global indices were calculated: mean index and weighted index. The AUROC obtained for these indices did not show statistically significant differences in any of the layers and grids ($p > 0.05$, DeLong test). Therefore, the mean index was chosen to continue the research, as it is a more straightforward methodology for replication in any future investigation. Supplementary Tables S9–S14 show the AUROC for each layer and comparisons between indices based on the grid position. The AUROC for the global indices of the ONLOPL and ORL were < 0.70, so they were excluded as data of interest in the results.

The results of the comparison of mean indices for the Spectralis SD-OCT PP 8 × 8 grid indicate no statistically significant differences in any of the layers between horizontalized and inclined grids (Table 2). Consequently, the inclined grid, obtained automatically in Spectralis SD-OCT, was selected to continue the research. The layer that offers the highest diagnostic yield is RNFL.

Table 2. Comparison of the mean index between the inclined and horizontal grids of the 8 × 8 grid of the posterior pole in the layers and layer combinations of the studied macular retina: complete retina, retinal nerve fiber layer (RNFL), ganglion cell layer (GCL), ganglion cell complex, combination formed by the ganglion cell layer and the inner plexiform layer (GCLIPL), and inner retinal layers (IRL).

Segmentation	Position of the Grid. AUROC (CI95%)		Comparison	
	Horizontalized	Inclined	Z	p-Value (DeLong Test)
Complete retina	0.743 (0.688–0.798)	0.752 (0.698–0.806)	1.594	0.111
RNFL	0.794 (0.744–0.843)	0.796 (0.746–0.845)	0.821	0.412
GCL	0.781 (0.729–0.834)	0.784 (0.732–0.836)	0.558	0.577
Ganglion cell complex	0.784 (0.733–0.835)	0.785 (0.734–0.835)	0.195	0.845
GCLIPL	0.769 (0.715–0.823)	0.770 (0.717–0.824)	0.405	0.685
IRL	0.751 (0.697–0.806)	0.755 (0.701–0.809)	0.886	0.376

3.4. Analysis of Cutoff Points for the Mean Indices

After determining the AUROC for each layer, the thickness value (cutoff point) of the mean index was chosen to classify a patient, such that if their thickness was below the selected cutoff point, the patient would be classified as diseased. The criterion for selecting this point was based on choosing the value at which sensitivity and specificity are as equal and high as possible. After selecting the value for each layer, diagnostic validity indices were calculated. Table 3 shows these results.

Table 3. Cutoff points of the mean index (in microns) for classifying a patient as healthy (if the thickness is above the cutoff point) or as glaucomatous (if the thickness is below the cutoff point), and diagnostic capability indices for different retinal layers and layer combinations. Retinal nerve fiber layer (RNFL), ganglion cell layer (GCL), ganglion cell complex, combination formed by the ganglion cell layer and the inner plexiform layer (GCLIPL), and inner retinal layers (IRL).

Segmentation	Cuttof Point (Microns)	Specificity % (CI95%)	Sensitivity % (CI95%)	PPV % (CI95%)	NPV % (CI95%)
Complete retina	286.00	64.42 (56.76–72.07)	74.26 (66.55–81.98)	75 (67.47–82.53)	63.52 (55.73–71.32)
RNFL	52.24	71.17 (63.9–78.43)	72.79 (64.95–80.64)	75.82 (68.71–82.93)	67.81 (59.89–75.73)
GCL	32.40	71.17 (63.9–78.43)	72.79 (64.95–80.64)	75.82 (68.71–82.93)	67.81 (59.89–75.73)
Ganglion cell complex	96.21	66.26 (58.69–73.82)	74.26 (66.55–81.98)	75.52 (68.13–82.92)	64.74 (56.93–72.56)
GCLIPL	62.85	72.39 (65.22–79.56)	72.79 (64.95–80.64)	76.13 (69.1–83.16)	68.75 (60.83–76.67)
IRL	210.50	65.03 (57.4–72.66)	72.06 (64.15–79.97)	73.61 (66.07–81.16)	63.23 (55.31–71.14)

4. Discussion

In this research, the diagnostic ability of the Spectralis SD-OCT PP software with the 8 × 8 grid automatically tilted along the disc-fovea axis at 7° and the grid horizontalized was studied in the thickness of RNFL, GCL, IRL, ORL, complete retina, the ganglion cell complex (RNFL + GCL + IPL), the complex formed by OPLONL, and the complex formed by GCLIPL in the macular area of healthy and glaucomatous subjects. The topographical evaluation of the effect of different states on the thickness of various intraretinal layers was conducted to identify the diagnostic capacity of different changes. Clinical consideration was given to whether it is more effective to use the horizontalized or inclined grid based on the disc-fovea axis. Additionally, a global index was determined for each studied layer, both with the inclined and horizontalized grids, identifying the layer with the highest diagnostic capability. Diagnostic capacities of different topographic patterns were calculated using ROC curves (receiver operating characteristic curve) results. Finally, the diagnostic capability of each studied layer and layer combination was determined after selecting a cutoff point based on sensitivity and specificity to correctly detect the presence of glaucoma.

In an extensive literature search, no other study following a similar methodology to this research was found, except for the study conducted by Del-Rio-Vellosillo et al. [22], performed by the present research group, where we compared the diagnostic capability of the ganglion cell complex thickness with the 8 × 8 grid of the 7-degree inclined and horizontalized PP algorithm to distinguish between healthy and glaucomatous eyes.

Numerous authors have studied the influence of the disc-fovea axis on retinal thickness in glaucoma diagnosis. Some authors [23], similarly to this study, found no statistically significant differences in retinal thickness when modifying the disc-fovea axis. In contrast, many other authors did find small differences between both axes, although, like in this research, compensating for the inclination of the disc-fovea axis did not seem to offer clear clinical advantages [24–32].

Nouri-Mahdavi et al. [20] compared macular GCLIPL with peripapillary RNFL and confirmed similar results. In the present study, when comparing macular GCLIPL, similar results were obtained with mRNFL and the macular ganglion cell complex. Budenz et al. and Martínez de la Casa et al., similarly to this study, indicated that RNFL has a higher discrimination capability for subjects with glaucoma than other layers [2,33]. However, Rao et al. [34] claimed that IRL parameters are as valid as RNFL. It is noteworthy that the subjects in their study were of Hindu race.

Like some authors [35–39], the present research group found that the thickness of the inner layers of the macula has a higher diagnostic capability than total retinal thickness. Other researchers [29,40–44] have indicated, as it has been observed in the present piece of investigation, that macular thickness and RNFL have high diagnostic sensitivity and specificity to discriminate between healthy and glaucomatous eyes.

Khanal et al. [43] suggested that overall macular thickness could lead to lower sensitivity than segmenting thickness in different layers or layer combinations, in accordance with the results of the present study, as the macula contains regions that are not sensitive to glaucomatous changes. Pazos et al. [42] achieved a high diagnostic capability in the macular ganglion cell complex, although it did not surpass macular RNFL.

Among the different types of existing macular glaucoma diagnostic methods in the literature, there are two that are especially remarkable: the schematic model of glaucomatous damage by Hood et al. [14] and the reduction of intraretinal thickness. Hood et al. created a schematic model of visual field defects in the macula by overlaying OCT-obtained maps onto visual fields. The schematic model predicts the arched defects of initial macular damage and the relatively preserved "central island" in the macula in patients with advanced glaucoma. Numerous authors indicate that to improve sensitivity and specificity, topographic information from visual fields should be combined with OCT images [45,46], analyzing the thickness of pRNFL, macular GCC, and GCL from both optic disc and macular scanning cubes [47,48]. In Figure 5, it can be observed how cells with higher diagnostic capability (cells in red) obtained in this study coincide with the prediction of macular glaucomatous damage defects found by Hood et al. [14].

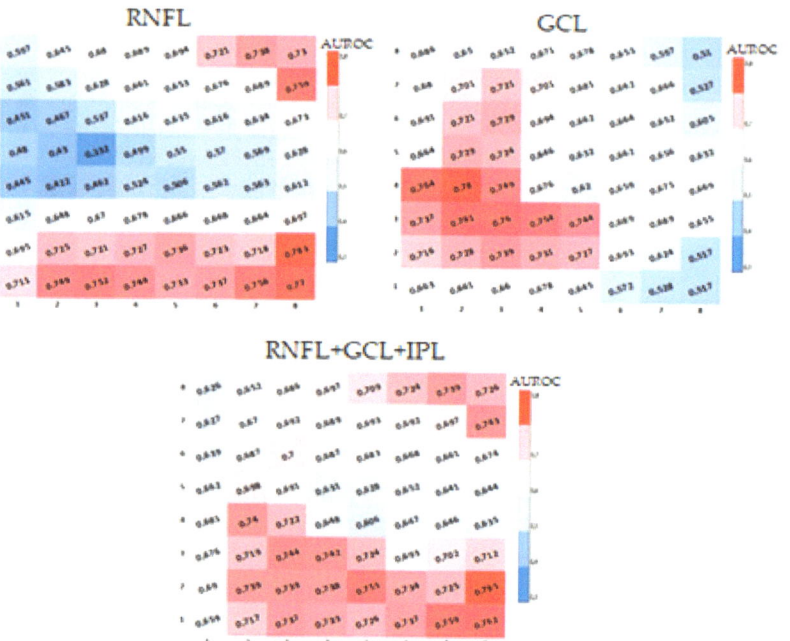

Figure 5. Heatmaps of AUROCs for RNFL, GCL, and the macular ganglion cell complex obtained in this study with the 8 × 8 grid of the Spectralis SD-OCT posterior pole, tilted at 7°, similar to the model described by Hood et al. [14]. Retinal nerve fiber layer (RNFL); ganglion cell layer (GCL); inner plexiform layer (IPL).

The progression of POAG involves a decrease in intraretinal thickness, and numerous researchers have studied it using various methods. Many authors [49–53] have focused on individual studies of macular RNFL and GCL thickness, while others [12,54], in addition to these studies, have included the photoreceptor layer and the retinal pigment epithelium in their studies. Some authors, however, have focused their work on GCL [4,12,35,36,42,55–58].

Regarding the method of retinal study, Bambo et al. [58] used the ETDRS grid for the analysis of retinal thickness. They indicated that the inner layers of the macula, especially the temporal sector of GCL, provided a good diagnostic capacity for glaucoma. Although the data obtained in this research have coincided, the AUROC analysis results of these authors show greater AUROC values than those found in the present work. However, in another study focusing on the study of RNFL, GCL, and IPL, Garcia-Medina et al. [6] concluded that the PP 8×8 asymmetry protocol is superior to the ETDRS protocol in assessing the diagnostic capacity to differentiate between ocular hypertension and POAG, which is why we decided to investigate with the 8×8 grid.

The thickness of the macula in all its regions, as it has been observed in this study, is asymmetric. Ooto et al. [59] also concluded, similarly to the present study, that GCL thickness was significantly lower in the temporal region compared to the nasal region of the macula in glaucoma. Moreover, they created thickness maps that showed vertical asymmetry for all layers, including the inner layers of the retina.

The results of this research coincide with numerous studies indicating that segmented macular IRL thickness has a greater diagnostic yield than total macular thickness and is similar (though not better) than pRNFL thickness in glaucoma diagnosis [55,60,61]. Most OCT studies that independently or through combinations evaluate the inner layers of the retina in the macula have demonstrated diagnostic accuracy similar to pRNFL thickness. Nevertheless, to date, it is still unknown how the isolated analysis of GCL improves glaucomatous diagnostic capacity [35,36,42,50,55–58]. In this study, after performing an isolated GCL analysis, it was verified that its diagnostic capacity is not superior to that of other retinal layers, using the 8×8 macular grid in Spectralis SD-OCT as the evaluation method.

One may argue that the difference in mean age between healthy and glaucoma patients in this study (Table 1) could affect its results, but it has been shown that a 10-year age difference does not significantly influence either the sensitivity of automated perimetry [62] or retinal thickness measured by OCT [19]. It also was found that there is no difference in IOP between the groups. This result may be attributed to the fact that all participants in the POAG group were under hypotensive topical treatment.

This study has several limitations to consider: predictive values and overall diagnostic accuracy cannot be easily generalized beyond the study population in which they were estimated [63]. Plus, the groups of subjects, both healthy and glaucomatous, consisted of Caucasian patients with POAG, so the results cannot be extrapolated to other ethnicities. In addition, this research is a cross-sectional study, so, due to its nature, it does not allow the study of progressive changes in POAG. Finally, in this study, the degree of glaucoma is not differentiated, which may affect the overall values obtained. To reduce bias and increase diagnostic accuracy, future research should focus on segregating different severity levels. This way, the affected zones and layers could be determined based on the progression and classification of the disease.

5. Conclusions

The original findings obtained in this study include the identification of different patterns of macular damage based on the studied layers using a new methodology, a global index indicating the diagnostic capacity of each layer studied in two grids (tilted at 7° and horizontal), and evidence that modifying the orientation of the macular grid does not seem profitable. The retinal layers with the highest diagnostic yield were identified using an objective methodology, along with a cutoff point for retinal thickness in each studied layer facilitating the discrimination of patients with POAG.

Both the heatmap patterns and the results of global index comparisons indicate that the diagnostic capacity of the studied segmentations is similar when considering the 8×8 macular grid tilted at 7° or horizontalized. The macular segmentations that offer the highest diagnostic yield in glaucoma discrimination are, in the following order, RNFL, the ganglion cell complex, GCL, GCLIPL, IRL, and the complete retina. In contrast, the thickness of the ORL and OPLONL does not seem useful for discriminating between healthy individuals and those with glaucoma.

To sum up, the 8×8 macular grid from the PP software in Spectralis SD-OCT provides a good diagnostic capacity in different layers and combinations of inner retina layers as a complementary method that may be useful for diagnosing POAG.

Supplementary Materials: The following supporting information can be downloaded at: https://www.mdpi.com/article/10.3390/jcm13041016/s1. Table S1. Area Under the Curve (AUROC) value, 95% Confidence Interval (CI) and p-value for each cell of the 8×8 macular grid of the macular Retinal Nerve Fiber Layer (RNFL) with the grid tilted at 7° and with the grid horizontalized. Table S2. Area Under the Receiver Operating Characteristic Curve (AUROC) value, 95% Confidence Interval (CI) and p-value for each cell of the 8×8 macular grid of the Ganglion Cell Layer (GCL) with the grid tilted at 7° and with the grid horizontalized. Table S3. Area Under the Receiver Operating Characteristic Curve (AUROC) value, 95% Confidence Interval (CI) and p-value for each cell of the 8×8 macular grid of the entire retina with the grid tilted at 7° and with the grid horizontalized. Table S4. Area Under the Receiver Operating Characteristic Curve (AUROC) value, 95% Confidence Interval (CI) and p-value for each cell of the 8×8 macular grid of the ganglion cell complex (RNFL+GCL+IPL) with the grid tilted at 7° and with the grid horizontalized. Table S5. Area Under the Receiver Operating Characteristic Curve (AUROC) value, 95% Confidence Interval (CI) and p-value for each cell of the 8×8 macular grid of the ganglion cell layer+inner plexiform layer (GCLIPL) with the grid tilted at 7° and with the grid horizontalized. Table S6. Area Under the Receiver Operating Characteristic Curve (AUROC) value, 95% Confidence Interval (CI) and p-value for each cell of the 8×8 macular grid of the outer plexiform layer+outer nuclear layer (OPLONL) with the grid tilted at 7° and with the grid horizontalized. Table S7. Area Under the Receiver Operating Characteristic Curve (AUROC) value, 95% Confidence Interval (CI) and p-value for each cell of the 8×8 macular grid of the inner retinal layers (INL) with the grid tilted at 7° and with the grid horizontalized. Table S8. Area Under the Receiver Operating Characteristic Curve (AUROC) value, 95% Confidence Interval (CI) and p-value for each cell of the 8×8 macular grid of the outer retinal layer (ORL) with the grid tilted at 7° and with the grid horizontalized. Table S9. AUROC and comparison of mean and weighted indices for the 8×8 grid of the Posterior Pole (PP) using Spectralis SD-OCT in the thickness of the complete retina. Table S10. AUROC and comparison of mean and weighted indices for the 8×8 grid of the Posterior Pole (PP) using Spectralis SD-OCT in the thickness of the RNFL. Table S11. AUROC and comparison of mean and weighted indices for the 8×8 grid of the Posterior Pole (PP) using Spectralis SD-OCT in the thickness of the GCL. Table S12. AUROC and comparison of mean and weighted indices for the 8×8 grid of the Posterior Pole (PP) using Spectralis SD-OCT in the thickness of the ganglion cell complex. Table S13. AUROC and comparison of mean and weighted indices for the 8×8 grid of the Posterior Pole (PP) using Spectralis SD-OCT in the thickness of GCLIPL. Table S14. AUROC and comparison of mean and weighted indices for the 8×8 grid of the Posterior Pole (PP) using Spectralis SD-OCT in the thickness of the IRL.

Author Contributions: Conceptualization and methodology, writing original draft preparation: all authors; validation, formal analysis, and investigation: all authors; data curation: A.A.-S.; critically reviewed the last draft of the paper: all authors; supervision: J.J.G.-M. All authors have read and agreed to the published version of the manuscript.

Funding: Partly financed by the members (J.J.G.-M. and M.D.P.-D.) of the Spanish Research Net REI-RICORS (RD21/0002/0032), Institute of Health Carlos III, Madrid, Spain and the NextGenerationEU FIS/FEDER fundus.

Institutional Review Board Statement: The study was conducted in accordance with the Declaration of Helsinki, and approved by the Institutional Review Board (or Ethics Committee) of the University General Hospital Reina Sofía in Murcia, Spain (protocol number 02/18).

Informed Consent Statement: Informed consent was obtained from all subjects involved in the study.

Data Availability Statement: The data presented in this study are available on reasonable request from the corresponding author.

Acknowledgments: We would like to thank José Manuel Tamarit (Heidelberg Engineering, Heidelberg, Germany) for his technical support with the Spectralis SD-OCT device. Some preliminary results of this study were presented during the Association for Research in Vision and Ophthalmology (ARVO) Annual Meeting, originally scheduled for 2–6 May in San Francisco, CA, USA, 2021, but finally presented as a Virtual Meeting. The content of this manuscript is included in a doctoral thesis entitled "Evaluation of the diagnostic ability of Spectralis SD-OCT posterior pole software with the 8 × 8 grid tilted at 7° and horizontalized in glaucomatous eyes", presented by Aurora Alvarez-Sarrion on 19 October 2023 at the University of Murcia, Spain. This thesis was directed by Jose Javier Garcia-Medina.

Conflicts of Interest: The authors declare no conflicts of interest.

References

1. Pastor-Jimeno, J.C.; Maldonado-López, M.J. *Guiones de Oftalmología*, 2nd ed.; McGraw-Hill Interamericana de España S.L.: Madrid, Spain, 2011.
2. Budenz, D.L.; Michael, A.; Chang, R.T.; McSoley, J.; Katz, J. Sensitivity and specificity of the StratusOCT for perimetric glaucoma. *Ophthalmology* **2005**, *112*, 3–9. [CrossRef] [PubMed]
3. Weinreb, R.N.; Aung, T.; Medeiros, F.A. The pathophysiology and treatment of glaucoma: A review. *JAMA* **2014**, *311*, 1901–1911. [CrossRef]
4. Chen, M.J.; Yang, H.Y.; Chang, Y.F.; Hsu, C.C.; Ko, Y.C.; Liu, C.J. Diagnostic ability of macular ganglion cell asymmetry in Preperimetric Glaucoma. *BMC Ophthalmol.* **2019**, *19*, 12. [CrossRef] [PubMed]
5. Kwon, J.W.; Bae, J.M.; Kim, J.S.; Jee, D.; Choi, J.A. Asymmetry of the macular structure is associated with ocular dominance. *Can. J. Ophthalmol.* **2019**, *54*, 237–241. [CrossRef] [PubMed]
6. Garcia-Medina, J.J.; Del-Rio-Vellosillo, M.; Palazon-Cabanes, A.; Alvarez-Sarrión, A.; Martinez-Campillo, L.; Zanon-Moreno, V.; Pinazo-Duran, M.D.; Villegas-Perez, M.P. Diagnostic ability of the thickness of the macular inner retinal layers as measured by 8 × 8 posterior pole and ETDRS protocols to differentiate between ocular hypertension and early primary-open angle glaucoma. *Investig. Ophthalmol. Vis. Sci.* **2020**, *61*, 3901.
7. Castañeda, R.; Jiménez, J.; Iriarte, M.J. Concepto de sospecha de glaucoma de ángulo abierto: Definición, diagnóstico y tratamiento. *Rev. Mex Oftalmol.* **2014**, *88*, 153–160. [CrossRef]
8. Mwanza, J.C.; Budenz, D.L. Glaucoma at the Center of the Earth. *Adv. Ophthalmol. Optom.* **2019**, *4*, 211–222. [CrossRef]
9. Mantravadi, A.V.; Vadhar, N. Glaucoma. *Prim. Care* **2015**, *42*, 437–449. [CrossRef]
10. Perucho, M.S.; Toledano, F.N. *Actualización e Interpretación de las Técnicas Diagnósticas en Oftalmolígia*; ENE: Spain, 2008.
11. Kim, Y.K.; Jeoung, J.W.; Park, K.H. Inferior Macular Damage in Glaucoma: Its Relationship to Retinal Nerve Fiber Layer Defect in Macular Vulnerability Zone. *J. Glaucoma* **2017**, *26*, 126–132. [CrossRef]
12. Chen, Q.; Huang, S.; Ma, Q.; Lin, H.; Pan, M.; Liu, X.; Lu, F.; Shen, M. Ultra-high resolution profiles of macular intra-retinal layer thicknesses and associations with visual field defects in primary open angle glaucoma. *Sci. Rep.* **2017**, *7*, 41100. [CrossRef]
13. Sung, K.R.; Kim, J.S.; Wollstein, G.; Folio, L.; Kook, M.S.; Schuman, J.S. Imaging of the retinal nerve fibre layer with spectral domain optical coherence tomography for glaucoma diagnosis. *Br. J. Ophthalmol.* **2011**, *95*, 909–914. [CrossRef]
14. Hood, D.C.; Raza, A.S.; de Moraes, C.G.; Liebmann, J.M.; Ritch, R. Glaucomatous damage of the macula. *Prog. Retin. Eye Res.* **2013**, *32*, 1–21. [CrossRef]
15. Kim, Y.K.; Ha, A.; Na, K.I.; Kim, H.J.; Jeoung, J.W.; Park, K.H. Temporal Relation between Macular Ganglion Cell-Inner Plexiform Layer Loss and Peripapillary Retinal Nerve Fiber Layer Loss in Glaucoma. *Ophthalmology* **2017**, *124*, 1056–1064. [CrossRef]
16. Hood, D.C.; De Moraes, C.G. Four Questions for Every Clinician Diagnosing and Monitoring Glaucoma. *J. Glaucoma* **2018**, *27*, 657–664. [CrossRef] [PubMed]
17. Hood, D.C.; De Cuir, N.; Blumberg, D.M.; Liebmann, J.M.; Jarukasetphon, R.; Ritch, R.; De Moraes, C.G. A Single Wide-Field OCT Protocol Can Provide Compelling Information for the Diagnosis of Early Glaucoma. *Transl. Vis. Sci. Technol.* **2016**, *5*, 4. [CrossRef] [PubMed]
18. Shin, J.W.; Sung, K.R.; Park, S.W. Patterns of Progressive Ganglion Cell-Inner Plexiform Layer Thinning in Glaucoma Detected by OCT. *Ophthalmology* **2018**, *125*, 1515–1525. [CrossRef] [PubMed]
19. Mwanza, J.C.; Durbin, M.K.; Budenz, D.L.; Sayyad, F.E.; Chang, R.T.; Neelakantan, A.; Godfrey, D.G.; Carter, R.; Crandall, A.S. Glaucoma diagnostic accuracy of ganglion cell-inner plexiform layer thickness: Comparison with nerve fiber layer and optic nerve head. *Ophthalmology* **2012**, *119*, 1151–1158. [CrossRef] [PubMed]
20. Nouri-Mahdavi, K.; Nowroozizadeh, S.; Nassiri, N.; Cirineo, N.; Knipping, S.; Giaconi, J.; Caprioli, J. Macular ganglion cell/inner plexiform layer measurements by spectral domain optical coherence tomography for detection of early glaucoma and comparison to retinal nerve fiber layer measurements. *Am. J. Ophthalmol.* **2013**, *156*, 1297–1307.e2. [CrossRef] [PubMed]

21. Hu, H.; Li, P.; Yu, X.; Wei, W.; He, H.; Zhang, X. Associations of Ganglion Cell-Inner Plexiform Layer and Optic Nerve Head Parameters with Visual Field Sensitivity in Advanced Glaucoma. *Ophthalmic Res.* **2021**, *64*, 310–320. [CrossRef] [PubMed]
22. Del-Rio-Vellosillo, M.; Álvarez-Sarrión, A.; Lopez-Bernal, M.D.; Rubio-Velazquez, E.; Pinazo-Duran, M.D.; Garcia-Medina, J.J. Comparison of diagnosis accuracy of the ganglion cell complex thickness in the 7-degree inclined versus horizontalized 8 × 8 grid of the posterior pole algorithm to distinguish between healthy and glaucomatous eyes. *Investig. Ophthalmol. Vis. Sci.* **2021**, *62*, 2462.
23. Choi, J.A.; Kim, J.S.; Park, H.Y.; Park, H.; Park, C.K. The foveal position relative to the optic disc and the retinal nerve fiber layer thickness profile in myopia. *Investig. Ophthalmol. Vis. Sci.* **2014**, *55*, 1419–1426. [CrossRef]
24. Valverde-Megías, A.; Martinez-de-la-Casa, J.M.; Serrador-García, M.; Larrosa, J.M.; García-Feijoó, J. Clinical relevance of foveal location on retinal nerve fiber layer thickness using the new FoDi software in spectralis optical coherence tomography. *Investig. Ophthalmol. Vis. Sci.* **2013**, *54*, 5771–5776. [CrossRef]
25. Amini, N.; Nowroozizadeh, S.; Cirineo, N.; Henry, S.; Chang, T.; Chou, T.; Coleman, A.L.; Caprioli, J.; Nouri-Mahdavi, K. Influence of the disc-fovea angle on limits of RNFL variability and glaucoma discrimination. *Investig. Ophthalmol. Vis. Sci.* **2014**, *55*, 7332–7342. [CrossRef]
26. He, L.; Ren, R.; Yang, H.; Hardin, C.; Reyes, L.; Reynaud, J.; Gardiner, S.K.; Fortune, B.; Demirel, S.; Burgoyne, C.F. Anatomic vs. acquired image frame discordance in spectral domain optical coherence tomography minimum rim measurements. *PLoS ONE* **2014**, *9*, e92225. [CrossRef] [PubMed]
27. Resch, H.; Pereira, I.; Hienert, J.; Weber, S.; Holzer, S.; Kiss, B.; Fischer, G.; Vass, C. Influence of disc-fovea angle and retinal blood vessels on interindividual variability of circumpapillary retinal nerve fibre layer. *Br. J. Ophthalmol.* **2016**, *100*, 531–536. [CrossRef]
28. Jonas, R.A.; Wang, Y.X.; Yang, H.; Li, J.J.; Xu, L.; Panda-Jonas, S.; Jonas, J.B. Optic Disc—Fovea Angle: The Beijing Eye Study 2011. *PLoS ONE* **2015**, *10*, e0141771. [CrossRef]
29. Mayama, C.; Saito, H.; Hirasawa, H.; Tomidokoro, A.; Araie, M.; Iwase, A.; Ohkubo, S.; Sugiyama, K.; Hangai, M.; Yoshimura, N. Diagnosis of Early-Stage Glaucoma by Grid-Wise Macular Inner Retinal Layer Thickness Measurement and Effect of Compensation of Disc-Fovea Inclination. *Investig. Ophthalmol. Vis. Sci.* **2015**, *56*, 5681–5690. [CrossRef]
30. Mwanza, J.C.; Lee, G.; Budenz, D.L. Effect of Adjusting Retinal Nerve Fiber Layer Profile to Fovea-Disc Angle Axis on the Thickness and Glaucoma Diagnostic Performance. *Am. J. Ophthalmol.* **2016**, *161*, 12–21.e212. [CrossRef]
31. Tuncer, Z.; Altuğ, M. Does Foveal Position Relative to the Optic Disc Affect Optical Coherence Tomography Measurements in Glaucoma? *Turk. J. Ophthalmol.* **2018**, *48*, 178–184. [CrossRef] [PubMed]
32. Alluwimi, M.S.; Swanson, W.H.; King, B.J. Identifying Glaucomatous Damage to the Macula. *Optom. Vis. Sci. Off. Publ. Am. Acad. Optom.* **2018**, *95*, 96–105. [CrossRef] [PubMed]
33. Martínez-de-la-Casa, J.M.; Cifuentes-Canorea, P.; Berrozpe, C.; Sastre, M.; Polo, V.; Moreno-Montañes, J.; Garcia-Feijoo, J. Diagnostic ability of macular nerve fiber layer thickness using new segmentation software in glaucoma suspects. *Investig. Ophthalmol. Vis. Sci.* **2014**, *55*, 8343–8348. [CrossRef]
34. Rao, H.L.; Babu, J.G.; Addepalli, U.K.; Senthil, S.; Garudadri, C.S. Retinal nerve fiber layer and macular inner retina measurements by spectral domain optical coherence tomograph in Indian eyes with early glaucoma. *Eye* **2012**, *26*, 133–139. [CrossRef]
35. Tan, O.; Chopra, V.; Lu, A.T.; Schuman, J.S.; Ishikawa, H.; Wollstein, G.; Varma, R.; Huang, D. Detection of macular ganglion cell loss in glaucoma by Fourier-domain optical coherence tomography. *Ophthalmology* **2009**, *116*, 2305–2314.e142. [CrossRef] [PubMed]
36. Nakatani, Y.; Higashide, T.; Ohkubo, S.; Takeda, H.; Sugiyama, K. Evaluation of macular thickness and peripapillary retinal nerve fiber layer thickness for detection of early glaucoma using spectral domain optical coherence tomography. *J. Glaucoma* **2011**, *20*, 252–259. [CrossRef] [PubMed]
37. Tan, O.; Li, G.; Lu, A.T.; Varma, R.; Huang, D. Advanced Imaging for Glaucoma Study Group Mapping of macular substructures with optical coherence tomography for glaucoma diagnosis. *Ophthalmology* **2008**, *115*, 949–956. [CrossRef]
38. Sakamoto, A.; Hangai, M.; Nukada, M.; Nakanishi, H.; Mori, S.; Kotera, Y.; Inoue, R.; Yoshimura, N. Three-dimensional imaging of the macular retinal nerve fiber layer in glaucoma with spectral-domain optical coherence tomography. *Investig. Ophthalmol. Vis. Sci.* **2010**, *51*, 5062–5070. [CrossRef] [PubMed]
39. Mwanza, J.C.; Budenz, D.L.; Godfrey, D.G.; Neelakantan, A.; Sayyad, F.E.; Chang, R.T.; Lee, R.K. Diagnostic performance of optical coherence tomography ganglion cell–inner plexiform layer thickness measurements in early glaucoma. *Ophthalmology* **2014**, *121*, 849–854. [CrossRef]
40. Bussel, I.I.; Wollstein, G.; Schuman, J.S. OCT for glaucoma diagnosis, screening and detection of glaucoma progression. *Br. J. Ophthalmol.* **2014**, *98* (Suppl. 2), ii15–ii19. [CrossRef] [PubMed]
41. Rolle, T.; Manerba, L.; Lanzafame, P.; Grignolo, F.M. Diagnostic Power of Macular Retinal Thickness Analysis and Structure-Function Relationship in Glaucoma Diagnosis Using SPECTRALIS OCT. *Curr. Eye Res.* **2016**, *41*, 667–675. [CrossRef]
42. Pazos, M.; Dyrda, A.A.; Biarnés, M.; Gómez, A.; Martín, C.; Mora, C.; Fatti, G.; Antón, A. Diagnostic Accuracy of Spectralis SD OCT Automated Macular Layers Segmentation to Discriminate Normal from Early Glaucomatous Eyes. *Ophthalmology* **2017**, *124*, 1218–1228. [CrossRef]
43. Khanal, S.; Davey, P.G.; Racette, L.; Thapa, M. Intraeye retinal nerve fiber layer and macular thickness asymmetry measurements for the discrimination of primary open-angle glaucoma and normal tension glaucoma. *J. Optom.* **2016**, *9*, 118–125. [CrossRef]

44. Lee, W.J.; Kim, Y.K.; Park, K.H.; Jeoung, J.W. Trend-based Analysis of Ganglion Cell-Inner Plexiform Layer Thickness Changes on Optical Coherence Tomography in Glaucoma Progression. *Ophthalmology* **2017**, *124*, 1383–1391. [CrossRef] [PubMed]
45. Hood, D.C.; Wang, D.L.; Raza, A.S.; de Moraes, C.G.; Liebmann, J.M.; Ritch, R. The locations of circumpapillary glaucomatous defects seen on frequency-domain OCT scans. *Investig. Ophthalmol. Vis. Sci.* **2013**, *54*, 7338–7343. [CrossRef] [PubMed]
46. Hood, D.C.; Raza, A.S. On improving the use of OCT imaging for detecting glaucomatous damage. *Br. J. Ophthalmol.* **2014**, *98* (Suppl. 2), ii1–ii9. [CrossRef]
47. Hood, D.C.; Fortune, B.; Mavrommatis, M.A.; Reynaud, J.; Ramachandran, R.; Ritch, R.; Rosen, R.B.; Muhammad, H.; Dubra, A.; Chui, T.Y. Details of 175 Glaucomatous Damage Are Better Seen on OCT En Face Images Than on OCT Retinal Nerve Fiber Layer Thickness Maps. *Investig. Ophthalmol. Vis. Sci.* **2015**, *56*, 6208–6216. [CrossRef]
48. Hood, D.C. Improving our understanding, and detection, of glaucomatous damage: An approach based upon optical coherence tomography (OCT). *Prog. Retin. Eye Res.* **2017**, *57*, 46–75. [CrossRef] [PubMed]
49. Guedes, V.; Schuman, J.S.; Hertzmark, E.; Wollstein, G.; Correnti, A.; Mancini, R.; Lederer, D.; Voskanian, S.; Velazquez, L.; Pakter, H.M.; et al. Optical coherence tomography measurement of macular and nerve fiber layer thickness in normal and glaucomatous human eyes. *Ophthalmology* **2003**, *110*, 177–189. [CrossRef]
50. Ishikawa, H.; Stein, D.M.; Wollstein, G.; Beaton, S.; Fujimoto, J.G.; Schuman, J.S. Macular segmentation with optical coherence tomography. *Investig. Ophthalmol. Vis. Sci.* **2005**, *46*, 2012–2017. [CrossRef]
51. Wang, M.; Hood, D.C.; Cho, J.S.; Ghadiali, Q.; De Moraes, C.G.; Zhang, X.; Ritch, R.; Liebmann, J.M. Measurement of local retinal ganglion cell layer thickness in patients with glaucoma using frequency-domain optical coherence tomography. *Arch. Ophthalmol.* **2009**, *127*, 875–881. [CrossRef]
52. Barua, N.; Sitaraman, C.; Goel, S.; Chakraborti, C.; Mukherjee, S.; Parashar, H. Comparison of diagnostic capability of macular ganglion cell complex and retinal nerve fiber layer among primary open angle glaucoma, ocular hypertension, and normal population using Fourier-domain optical coherence tomography and determining their functional correlation in Indian population. *Indian J. Ophthalmol.* **2016**, *64*, 296–302. [CrossRef]
53. Kim, H.J.; Lee, S.Y.; Park, K.H.; Kim, D.M.; Jeoung, J.W. Glaucoma Diagnostic Ability of Layer-by-Layer Segmented Ganglion Cell Complex by Spectral-Domain Optical Coherence Tomography. *Investig. Ophthalmol. Vis. Sci.* **2016**, *57*, 4799–4805. [CrossRef] [PubMed]
54. Fan, N.; Huang, N.; Lam, D.S.; Leung, C.K. Measurement of photoreceptor layer in glaucoma: A spectral-domain optical coherence tomography study. *J. Ophthalmol.* **2011**, *2011*, 264803. [CrossRef] [PubMed]
55. Leung, C.K.; Chan, W.M.; Yung, W.H.; Ng, A.C.; Woo, J.; Tsang, M.K.; Tse, R.K. Comparison of macular and peripapillary measurements for the detection of glaucoma: An optical coherence tomography study. *Ophthalmology* **2005**, *112*, 391–400. [CrossRef] [PubMed]
56. Seong, M.; Sung, K.R.; Choi, E.H.; Kang, S.Y.; Cho, J.W.; Um, T.W.; Kim, Y.J.; Park, S.B.; Hong, H.E.; Kook, M.S. Macular and peripapillary retinal nerve fiber layer measurements by spectral domain optical coherence tomography in normal-tension glaucoma. *Investig. Ophthalmol. Vis. Sci.* **2010**, *51*, 1446–1452. [CrossRef] [PubMed]
57. Francoz, M.; Fenolland, J.R.; Giraud, J.M.; El Chehab, H.; Sendon, D.; May, F.; Renard, J.P. Reproducibility of macular ganglion cell-inner plexiform layer thickness measurement with cirrus HD-OCT in normal, hypertensive and glaucomatous eyes. *Br. J. Ophthalmol.* **2014**, *98*, 322–328. [CrossRef] [PubMed]
58. Bambo, M.P.; Cameo, B.; Hernandez, R.; Fuentemilla, E.; Güerri, N.; Ferrandez, B.; Polo, V.; Larrosa, J.M.; Pablo, L.E.; Garcia-Martin, E. Diagnostic ability of inner macular layers to discriminate early glaucomatous eyes using vertical and horizontal B-scan posterior pole protocols. *PLoS ONE* **2018**, *13*, e0198397. [CrossRef] [PubMed]
59. Ooto, S.; Hangai, M.; Tomidokoro, A.; Saito, H.; Araie, M.; Otani, T.; Kishi, S.; Matsushita, K.; Maeda, N.; Shirakashi, M.; et al. Effects of age, sex, and axial length on the three-dimensional profile of normal macular layer structures. *Investig. Ophthalmol. Vis. Sci.* **2011**, *52*, 8769–8779. [CrossRef]
60. Medeiros, F.A.; Zangwill, L.M.; Bowd, C.; Vessani, R.M.; Susanna, R., Jr.; Weinreb, R.N. Evaluation of retinal nerve fiber layer, optic nerve head, and macular thickness measurements for glaucoma detection using optical coherence tomography. *Am. J. Ophthalmol.* **2005**, *139*, 44–55. [CrossRef]
61. Sung, K.R.; Wollstein, G.; Kim, N.R.; Na, J.H.; Nevins, J.E.; Kim, C.Y.; Schuman, J.S. Macular assessment using optical coherence tomography for glaucoma diagnosis. *Br. J. Ophthalmol.* **2012**, *96*, 1452–1455. [CrossRef]
62. Brenton, R.S.; Phelps, C.D. The normal visual field on the Humphrey field analyzer. Ophthalmologica. Journal international d'ophtalmologie. *Int. J. Ophthalmol. Z. Augenheilkd.* **1986**, *193*, 56–74. [CrossRef]
63. Vetter, T.R.; Schober, P.; Mascha, E.J. Diagnostic Testing and DecisionMaking: Beauty Is Not Just in the Eye of the Beholder. *Anesth. Analg.* **2018**, *127*, 1085–1091. [CrossRef] [PubMed]

Disclaimer/Publisher's Note: The statements, opinions and data contained in all publications are solely those of the individual author(s) and contributor(s) and not of MDPI and/or the editor(s). MDPI and/or the editor(s) disclaim responsibility for any injury to people or property resulting from any ideas, methods, instructions or products referred to in the content.

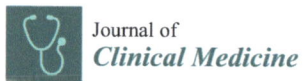

Article

Evaluation of Anatomical and Tomographic Biomarkers as Predictive Visual Acuity Factors in Eyes with Retinal Vein Occlusion Treated with Dexamethasone Implant

Giuseppe Covello [1,*], Maria Novella Maglionico [1], Michele Figus [1,2], Chiara Busoni [1], Maria Sole Sartini [2], Marco Lupidi [3,4] and Chiara Posarelli [1,2]

1. Department of Surgical, Medical, Molecular Pathology and Critical Care Medicine, University of Pisa, 56126 Pisa, Italy; m.novella.maglionico@gmail.com (M.N.M.); michele.figus@unipi.it (M.F.); chiarabuso@gmail.com (C.B.); chiara.posarelli@med.unipi.it (C.P.)
2. Ophthalmology, Department of Medical and Surgical Specialties, Azienda Ospedaliero Universitaria Pisana, 56124 Pisa, Italy; mssartini5@gmail.com
3. Eye Clinic, Department of Experimental and Clinical Medicine, Polytechnic University of Marche, 60131 Ancona, Italy; marcomed2@gmail.com
4. Fondazione per la Macula Onlus, Dipartimento di Neuroscienze, Riabilitazione, Oftalmologia, Genetica e Scienze Materno-Infantili (DINOGMI), University Eye Clinic, 16132 Genova, Italy
* Correspondence: giucovello@gmail.com; Tel.: +39-3880582241

Abstract: Background: This prospective study evaluated the impact of anatomical and tomographic biomarkers on clinical outcomes of intravitreal dexamethasone implants in patients with macular edema secondary to retinal vein occlusion (RVO). **Methods**: The study included 46 patients (28 with branch RVO (BRVO) and 18 with central RVO (CRVO)). Best corrected visual acuity (BCVA) significantly improved from a mean baseline of 0.817 ± 0.220 logMAR to 0.663 ± 0.267 logMAR at six months and 0.639 ± 0.321 logMAR at twelve months ($p < 0.05$). Central retinal thickness (CRT) showed a significant reduction from 666.2 ± 212.2 μm to 471.1 ± 215.6 μm at six months and 467 ± 175.7 μm at twelve months ($p < 0.05$). No significant differences were found in OCT biomarkers between baseline and follow-ups. **Results**: The study analysed improvements in visual acuity relative to baseline biomarkers. At six months, ellipsoid zone disruption (EZD) was significant for all subgroups. Disorganization of retinal inner layers (DRIL), external limiting membrane (ELM) disruption, macular ischemia (MI), CRT, and BRVO showed significance for any improvement, while DRIL and ELM were significant for changes greater than 0.3 logMAR ($p < 0.05$). At twelve months, EZD remained significant for all subgroups. ELM, MI, CRT, and BRVO were significant for any improvement, while MI and BRVO were significant for changes greater than 0.3 logMAR ($p < 0.05$). Hyperreflective foci were not statistically significant at either time point ($p > 0.05$). **Conclusions**: The regression model suggested that MI and CRVO could be negative predictive factors for visual outcomes, while ELM and EZD were associated with BCVA improvement one-year post-treatment.

Keywords: retinal vein occlusion; macular edema; OCT; EZD; ELM; DRIL; MI

1. Introduction

Retinal vein occlusion (RVO) is the second most common retinal vascular disease in the world affecting approximately 0.5% of people aged from 31 to 101 years [1,2]. According to anatomic location of occlusion, RVO can be divided into two main types: branch retinal vein occlusion (BRVO) and central retinal vein occlusion (CRVO). Visual loss is due to the development of macular edema (ME) and/or macular ischemia (MI). Blocked venous drainage induces the upregulation of vascular endothelial growth factor (VEGF) and inflammatory mediators, thereby increasing the permeability of vessels and causing a breakdown of the blood–retinal barrier. Treatment of macular edema is based on anti-VEGF intravitreal injections and steroid intravitreal implants. In addition to inhibiting the VEGF pathway, corticosteroids can also reduce the activity of other proinflammatory mediators [3]. The sustained-release intravitreal dexamethasone (DEX) implant, known as Ozurdex® and manufactured by Allergan, Inc. in Irvine, CA, USA, was introduced as a treatment choice for patients with RVO-ME. The GENEVA study reported notably improved functional and anatomical outcomes in the eyes of RVO-ME patients following the administration of DEX [4,5]. The criteria to determine the appropriate intravitreal treatment are visual acuity (VA) and optical coherence tomography (OCT) parameters, such as type of edema (intraretinal, subretinal, cystoid) or central macular thickness. However, many studies have demonstrated a large variability in response to treatment protocols. After 1 year of anti-VEGF injections, although 47% to 70.7% of patients gain at least three VA lines, between 28.1% and 49.2% remain within three lines, and 1% to 5.9% lose at least three lines [6–8]. Beyond visual acuity, even OCT could show a reduction, a persistence, or an improvement in macular edema. Moreover, a correlation between VA and OCT parameters is not always present [9]. Despite resolution of macular edema, visual acuity does not always improve [10]. It is currently unclear how OCT imaging features relate to visual acuity in RVO-ME. Prior studies have investigated correlations between VA and some OCT parameters that have associations with biomarkers such as intraretinal hyperreflective foci (HRF); disorganization of the retinal inner layers (DRIL); the photoreceptor's layers' disruption such as external limiting membrane (ELM) and ellipsoid zone disruption (EZD); and retinal and choroidal thickness [11–16]. However, reaching definite conclusions is difficult because of the study design and sample size limitations, non-standardized treatment protocols, and failure to address other confounding variables (i.e., inner retinal changes, cysts, and cone outer segment tip visibility) [10,17,18]. For example, DRIL is an OCT feature represented by a disruption of any of the two boundaries between the ganglion cell inner plexiform layer, inner nuclear layer, and outer plexiform layer. In diabetic ME, reduced recovery of DRIL over 4 months after anti-VEGF treatment predicted VA worsening over 8 months, supporting a prognostic role for this marker [19,20]. Because ischemia in RVO impacts the inner retina, DRIL therefore may be a similarly useful biomarker [15]. The identification of OCT imaging characteristics that can predict clinical outcomes is essential for guiding the most effective treatment strategy. To establish correlations between anatomical and tomographic biomarkers and treatment results, the present study examined these parameters in a group of patients with RVO-ME who received DEX implant therapy.

2. Materials and Methods

This is a prospective, cohort study involving a population affected by RVO complicated by macular edema and treated with DEX implant between June 2022 and January 2023. This study was performed according to the tenets of the Declaration of Helsinki and approved by the Area Vasta Nord Ovest Ethical Committee (CEAVNO) with code number 22338. A written informed consent was signed by all the patients included in the study. Inclusion criteria comprised an angiographic diagnosis of RVO, both central or branch, after ophthalmoscopic evaluation, and the presence of RVO–ME, defined by a loss of the foveal pit and a central retinal thickness (CRT) > 250 micron on spectral domain optical coherence tomography (SD-OCT) [21]. Patients previously treated for RVO-ME or macular edema secondary to other any condition different to RVO (i.e., diabetes, uveitis, etc.), any intercurrent disease, either ophthalmic or systemic, that could prevent visual acuity recovery, or uncontrolled glaucoma (defined as a medically treated intraocular pressure > 24 mmHg) were excluded from the study. Moreover, images with poor quality due to eye movement, media opacities caused by corneal diseases and/or cataract, and thick retinal haemorrhages were excluded.

The OCT biomarkers were CRT, as explained above; DRIL; ELM; HRF; and EZD. All SD-OCT scans images were obtained using the Spectralis HRA + OCT2 platform (Heidelberg Engineering, Heidelberg, Germany) and conducted using a macular volumetric raster with dimensions of 30 × 25 degrees and 25-line scans spaced at 241 μm in high-speed

(HS) mode with >12 automatic real-time tracking (ART). All biomarkers were evaluated in OCT scans passing through the fovea. CRT (μm) was calculated as the thickness of the central 1 mm circle in the ETDRS Grid. OCT biomarkers were measured by a single experienced ophthalmologist (G.C.). Particularly, DRIL, EZD, ELM and HRF were highlighted as binomial variables (present/absent).

The anatomical biomarkers were the type of RVO and the presence of macular ischemia using fluorescein angiography (FA) [21]. For FA evaluation, the ETDRS study grid was utilized, defining a non-perfusion area within the central 1 mm circle, with or without involvement of the inner and outer regions, as indicative of macular ischemia [22].

Patients were followed prospectively for 12 months and managed as in real life clinical practice in our institution. For each patient we collected data regarding best corrected visual acuity (BCVA) measured as logMAR; intraocular pressure (IOP) expressed as mmHg; the above-mentioned OCT and FA parameters; the number of injections; the number of visits and diagnostic procedures performed; and all the adverse events and the procedure related to them. Follow-up visits at six months and twelve months after the DEX injection were documented.

A 0.7 mg DEX implant (Ozurdex; Allergan, Inc.) was administered via intravitreal injection under aseptic conditions in an operating room. Two minutes before the injection, the patient's study eye received an initial drop of oxibuprocaine (4 mg/mL), followed by a 5% povidone-iodine solution. The eyelid margins, eyelids, and periocular skin were cleansed with povidone-iodine. The eye was then draped in a sterile manner, and the surgeon inserted a sterile lid speculum. The implant was injected into the vitreous cavity using a 22-gauge needle. Patients were prescribed topical antibiotics, such as moxifloxacin, for seven days following the procedure.

In case of recurrent ME, a second DEX implant was injected after the six-month follow-up visit, adhering to the strict treatment regimen imposed by our region (Tuscany), which prohibits a second DEX implant within six months. Therefore, we scheduled follow-up visits at exactly six months to evaluate the necessity of additional treatment.

2.1. Outcomes

The primary endpoint was the mean change in BCVA from baseline to six- and twelve-month visits after treatment.

Secondary outcomes included the impact of the different OCT biomarkers on functional outcomes, expressed as BCVA at the two time points, and the impact of treatment on the different OCT biomarkers, reflected in their changes after the DEX implant at the two time points.

2.2. Statistical Analysis

SPSS IBM Corp. Released 2019 (IBM SPSS Statistics for Windows, Version 26.0. Armonk, NY, USA: IBM Corp) was used to perform the statistical analysis. Sample size was calculated a priori and indicated that 40 subjects were required, with a confidence level of 95% and a significance level of 5%, based on prior published studies [17,18,22]. Moreover, we performed a post hoc analysis to confirm the adequacy of the sample size [23]. The post hoc power analysis was conducted using an alpha level of 0.05, a power of 0.80, an effect size of 0.5 and the study sample size. After checking if any variable was normally distributed using the Shapiro–Wilk test, descriptive analyses were performed. Categorical variables were reported as counts and percentages and were compared with the chi-square test and Fisher's exact test, as needed. To compare non-parametric values the Mann–Whitney U, Wilcoxon and McNemar tests were employed, as appropriate. A p value of less than 0.05 was considered significant. The ordinary least squares regression was used to understand the OCT biomarkers' predictive value for visual acuity.

3. Results

Forty-six patients were enrolled after the evaluation of inclusion and exclusion criteria. Of those, 44 completed the 6-month follow-up visit and 40 patients completed the full study one year after the first DEX implant. Twenty-eight patients received a second implant due to the persistence of macular edema. Table 1 summarises the main demographic and clinical characteristics of the studied patients. Demographic characteristics showed that 24 (52.2%) patients were female and 22 (47.8%) were male. The mean age was 74.69 ± 12.49. Out of all the participants, 22 (47.8%) had undergone cataract surgery at the time of enrolment, and none of the patients developed a cataract severe enough to require surgical intervention.

Table 1. Demographic and clinical data of patients.

	Baseline (n = 46)
Age (years) mean ± SD 95% CI	74.69 ± 12.49 68.92 to 77.28
Gender, female n (%)	24 (52.2%)
Gender, male n (%)	22 (47.8%)
Right eye n (%)	22 (47.8%)
Left eye n (%)	24 (52.2%)
Type-BRVO n (%)	28 (60.8%)
Type-CRVO n (%)	18 (39.2%)
Macular ischemia, n (%)	28 (60.8%)
Pseudophakia, n (%)	22 (47.8%)
Second implant, n (%)	28 (60.8%)
IOP, mmHg ± SD, 95% CI	16.4 ± 1.4 15.9 to 16.8
BCVA, mean ± SD, 95% CI	0.817 ± 0.220 0.4 to 1
CRT, μm ± SD, 95% CI	666.2 ± 212.2 596.1 to 735.7

N: number; SD: standard deviation; CI: confidence interval: BRVO: branch retinal vein occlusion; CRVO: central retinal vein occlusion, IOP: intraocular pressure.

As shown in Table 2, we observed a progressive, statistically significant improvement in visual acuity from a mean baseline value of 0.817 ± 0.220 logMAR to 0.663 ± 0.267 logMAR at six months and 0.639 ± 0.321 logMAR at twelve months ($p < 0.05$). There has been a statistically significant decrease in CRT at both follow-up visits, with the mean value declining from 666.17 ± 212.21 μm at the baseline visit to 471.15 ± 215.63 μm after six months and further to 467 ± 175.67 μm at the twelve-month visit. Any statistically significant differences emerged between baseline and follow-up visits regarding OCT biomarkers.

Functional outcomes were categorized into two subgroups: those showing any improvement in BCVA and those with a ≤ 0.3 logMAR improvement. This division aimed to provide a more detailed analysis of the variables and to gain insights into how biomarkers affect visual acuity over time. In Table 3, comparisons between improvements in visual acuity and OCT biomarkers were presented, complete with 95% confidence intervals (CIs) and odds ratios (ORs) for significant values. In this analysis, anatomical biomarkers were considered, with macular ischemia classified as absent, and the anatomical variant of BRVO selected for evaluation. At the six-month visit, EZD exhibited significance for all subgroups. Furthermore, DRIL, ELM, macular ischemia, CRT, and BRVO showed significance for any improvement, while for changes of more than 0.3 logMAR, statistical significance was observed for DRIL and ELM only ($p < 0.05$).

Table 2. Functional and tomographic parameters at each follow-up visit.

	Baseline (n = 46)	6 Months (n = 44)		12 Months (n = 40)	
BCVA, mean ± SD, 95% CI	0.817 ± 0.220 0.4 to 1	0.663 ± 0.267 0.3 to 1	**p < 0.05** [a]	0.639 ± 0.321 0.2 to 1	**p < 0.05** [a]
CRT, μm ± SD 95% CI	666.2 ± 212.2 596.1 to 735.7	471.1 ± 215.6 399.8 to 542.5	**p < 0.05** [a]	467 ± 175.7 409.9 to 525.4	**p < 0.05** [a]
DRIL (yes %)	65.2%	60.9%	$p = 0.5$ [b]	56.5%	$p = 0.3$ [b]
ELM (yes %)	47.8%	47.8%	$p > 0.9$ [b]	43.5%	$p = 0.7$ [b]
HRF (yes %)	69.6%	78.3%	$p = 0.3$ [b]	56.5%	$p = 0.1$ [b]
EZD (yes %)	52.2%	47.8%	$p = 0.7$ [b]	47.8%	$p = 0.7$ [b]

N: number; BCVA: best corrected visual acuity; CRT: central retinal thickness; DRIL: disorganization of retinal inner layers; ELM: external limiting membrane disruption; HRF: hyperreflective foci; EZD: ellipsoid zone disruption; [a]: Wilcoxon test; [b]: McNemar test. Bold character is for statistically significant values.

Table 3. Comparisons between baseline biomarkers and BCVA at 6 and 12 months using chi-squared test ($p < 0.05$ was considered for significance).

Baseline Anatomic and OCT Biomarkers	p for Any BCVA Improvement at 6 Months	p for Improved BCVA ≤ 0.3 at 6 Months	p for Any BCVA Improvement at 12 Months	p for Improved BCVA ≤ 0.3 at 12 Months
DRIL OR, 95% CI	**0.021** 0.14, 0.03 to 0.76	**0.008** 0.13, 0.03 to 0.59	0.143	0.127
ELM OR, 95% CI	**<0.001** 0.04, 0.01 to 0.02	**0.032** 0.17, 0.06 to 0.80	**<0.001** 0.32, 0.01 to 0.2	0.101
HRF OR, 95% CI	0.506	0.739	0.698	0.684
EZD OR, 95% CI	**<0.001** 0.05, 0.01 to 0.3	**0.012** 0.07, 0.03 to 0.64	**<0.001** 0.05, 0.01 to 0.31	**0.042** 0.2, 0.5 to 0.84
MI OR, 95% CI	**0.005** 0.1, 0.02 to 0.56	**0.027** 0.22, 0.06 to 0.79	**0.002** 0.07, 0.11 to 0.41	**0.002** 0.07, 0.11 to 0.41
CRT	**0.006** [a]	0.854 [a]	**0.012** [a]	0.191 [a]
BRVO OR, 95% CI	0.054	0.210	**0.008** 0.13, 0.03 to 0.59	**<0.001** 0.42, 0.26 to 0.67

[a]: Mann–Whitney U test; OCT: optical coherence tomography; BCVA: best corrected visual acuity; CRT: central retinal thickness; DRIL: disorganization of retinal inner layers; ELM: external limiting membrane disruption; HRF: hyperreflective foci; EZD: ellipsoid zone disruption; MI: macular ischemia; BRVO: branch retinal vein occlusion; OR: odds ratio. Bold character is for statistically significant values.

However, at twelve months, EZD remained significant for all subgroups. ELM, macular ischemia, CRT, and BRVO displayed significance for any improvement, while for changes of more than 0.3 logMAR, statistical significance was observed for MI and BRVO ($p < 0.05$). Notably, HRF did not exhibit statistical significance at either time point ($p > 0.05$).

Disruptions of photoreceptors' layers showed a significant association with visual outcome as well as the absence of macular ischemia at baseline and the branch type of RVO at twelve months ($p < 0.05$). Figure 1 shows a case of CRVO at baseline and at six months after treatment.

3.1. Role of Macular Ischemia

As indicated by the prior analysis, macular ischemia emerges as a potential negative predictive factor for visual recovery.

To delve deeper into the role of OCT biomarkers in predicting visual outcomes in patients with baseline macular ischemia, we focused on patients presenting with MI (n = 28). We then conducted a comparative analysis of their baseline biomarkers in relation to BCVA at 6 and 12 months, using the chi-squared test. The findings, detailed in Table 4, revealed that the OCT biomarkers, specifically ELM and EZD, exhibited statistical significance concerning visual recovery both at the 6- and 12-month visits ($p < 0.05$ for both). Additionally, it is worth noting that BRVO appeared to be a prospective positive predictive factor at both time points, especially regarding improvements exceeding 0.3 logMAR.

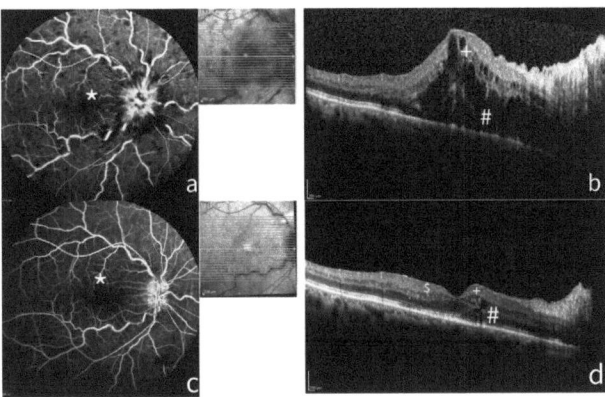

Figure 1. A case of CRVO at baseline and six months after treatment. FA and SD-OCT of a patient before and after treatment. (**a**) FA shows a non-ischemic (*) central retinal vein occlusion (CRVO) with marked delay in arteriovenous transit time, masked by retinal haemorrhages, and vessel wall staining. (**b**) The SD-OCT shows ME with considerable central thickness, absence of DRIL (+), and incomplete disruption of ELM and EZ. (**c**) After six months of treatment, FA shows resolution of the RVO with late staining of optic disc. (**d**) The SD-OCT highlights the reduction in retinal thickness, the presence of HRF ($), resolution of photoreceptor layers (#), and absence of DRIL (+). FA: Fluorescein angiograms; SD-OCT: spectral domain–optical coherence tomography; ME: macula edema; DRIL: disorganization of retinal inner layers; ELM: external limiting membrane disruption; HRF: hyperreflective foci; EZD: ellipsoid zone disruption.

Table 4. Comparisons between biomarkers and visual improvement in 28 patients with macular ischemia.

Baseline Anatomic and OCT Biomarkers	p Value for Any BCVA Improvement at 6 Months	p Value for Improved BCVA ≤ 0.3 at 6 Months	p Value for Any BCVA Improvement at 12 Months	p Value for Improved BCVA ≤ 0.3 at 12 Months
DRIL OR, 95% CI	0.492	>0.99	0.492	>0.99
ELM OR, 95% CI	**<0.001** 0.03, 0.003 to 0.24	0.354	**<0.001** 0.2, 0.03 to 0.2	0.354
HRF OR, 95% CI	0.673	0.289	0.673	0.289
EZD OR, 95% CI	**0.005** 0.07, 0.01 to 0.48	0.147	**0.005** 0.07, 0.01 to 0.48	0.147
BRVO OR, 95% CI	**0.023** 0.12, 0.02 to 0.74	**0.024** 0.62, 0.43 to 0.91	**0.023** 0.12, 0.19 to 0.74	**0.024** 0.62, 0.4 to 0.9

OCT: optical coherence tomography; BCVA: best corrected visual acuity; DRIL: disorganization of retinal inner layers; ELM: external limiting membrane disruption; HRF: hyperreflective foci; EZD: ellipsoid zone disruption; BRVO: branch retinal vein occlusion; OR: odds ratio. Bold character is for statistically significant values.

3.2. Predictive Factors of Visual Acuity

To identify potential predictors of improved visual acuity at 6 and 12 months, we ran the ordinary least squares regression (R-squared: 0.697; coeff.: 0.4446; std err.: 0.207; t:

2.147; P > |t|:0.040; CI: 0.022 to 0.867). All the baseline biomarkers, both anatomical and tomographic, were considered as variables. At 6 months, none of the variables showed a statistical significance ($p > 0.05$). At the final visit, baseline macular ischemia (coeff.: -0.2733; p: 0.009; CI: -0.472 to -0.075) and the branch type of RVO (coeff.: 0.3506; p: 0.005; CI: 0.111 to 0.590) were retained as predictive factors for final BCVA.

Twenty-eight patients (60.8%) required rescue therapy. Ten patients were affected by CRVO and eighteen by BRVO, without statistical differences (p: 0.76; OR: 0.69, 95% CI: 0.21 to 2.33).

Safety analysis revealed no major complications such as endophthalmitis or insert dislocation to the anterior chamber. No patient showed signs of glaucoma before the DEX implant. Moreover, no patient experienced a significant increase (≥ 5 mmHg) in IOP or other adverse events.

4. Discussion

The results of this study confirmed the DEX implant's effectiveness in significantly improving visual acuity in patients affected by RVO-ME. BCVA improved from a baseline mean value of 0.817 ± 0.220 logMAR to 0.663 ± 0.267 logMAR at six months and 0.639 ± 0.321 logMAR at twelve months. Meanwhile, the DEX implant significantly reduced CRT from a mean baseline value of 666.17 ± 212.21 µm to 471.15 ± 215.63 µm and 467 ± 175.67 µm.

The functional and anatomical improvements observed in our study were consistent with existing scientific evidence [16,24,25]. Furthermore, the DEX implant appeared to contribute to the restoration of retinal status (DRIL, ELM, EZD, HRF), albeit without reaching statistical significance. This finding aligns with a prior study conducted by Castro-Navarro et al. [16], which reported that the DEX implant significantly improved ELM integrity in patients with macular edema secondary to retinal vascular disease, although a subsequent study failed to replicate these findings [22]. The authors attributed this inconsistency to differences in the patient sample, with the first study encompassing both diabetic and RVO patients. Additionally, the evaluation of ELM changes in the first study was quantitative, while the second employed a qualitative approach. Our study shared the same limitation: OCT biomarkers were considered as binomial variables (absent/present). However, some OCT biomarkers such as ELM, EZD, and CRT have shown a statistical association with visual improvement at either 6 or 12 months, whereas DRIL only at six months. No significant associations were observed in DRIL at 12 months and HRF. Despite these associations, the ordinary least squares regression results did not observe any relationship between all baseline OCT biomarkers and the clinical outcomes. These results are consistent with previous evidence in the literature, which also emphasized the lack of uniform findings among different studies [15,22,26]. It is possible that a quantitative analysis may have yielded more informative results on these biomarkers. For instance, it has been observed that a higher HRF count at baseline was associated with improved visual outcomes following anti-VEGF injections as a reduction in HRF was correlated with a visual acuity improvement after DEX implant [27,28]. Instead, in our study, HRF did not seem to have any relationship with visual outcomes. Moreover, the definition of HRF in RVO remains controversial. Notably, two distinct HRF populations were identified: fine scattered HRF, likely associated with the leakage of blood constituents, and confluent HRF, mainly found in unaffected areas spared by the retinal occlusion [12,29]. Confluent HRF are believed to be linked to the absorption of water and other molecules. While fine scattered HRF are not visible on fundus photographic images, confluent HRF are thought to represent retinal exudates. In RVO, HRF are distributed topographically along the outer plexiform layer and the ELM. Like other retinal diseases, the presence of HRF at baseline is associated with poor visual outcomes following anti-VEGF treatment. Additionally, DEX implants might be preferred for eyes with numerous HRF and long-standing macular edema secondary to RVO, due to the inflammatory component [29]. However, likely due to the limited sample size, we did not find significant associations between changes in BCVA and HRF. Therefore, further studies are needed to understand the exact definition and role of HRF to establish their diagnostic significance.

Fluorescein angiography remains the gold standard of care imaging modality in determining the risk of neovascularization and areas of retinal non-perfusion after RVOs. The detection of non-perfused retinal areas by standard FA is the basis for the classification of RVOs as "ischemic" or "non-ischemic" [30]. In case of absence of neovascularization, vitreous haemorrhage, tractional retinal detachment or neovascular glaucoma, visual loss is related to macular edema or macular ischemia. Macular edema is well diagnosed and quantified by OCT and treated with anti-VEGF injections or corticosteroids. Nonetheless, the visual prognosis following treatment often hinges on the existence and extent of macular ischemia, along with photoreceptor loss or atrophy. Macular ischemia can be confirmed with FA and OCT angiography (OCTA) [21]. In OCTA, this is seen as an enlarged, irregular foveal avascular zone (FAZ). Some studies have found significant correlations between visual acuity and OCTA parameters such as FAZ, suggesting that OCTA metrics can be useful biomarkers for identifying and monitoring macular ischemia, and can be informative for visual prognoses in RVOs [31,32]. However, in this study, macular ischemia was investigated with fluorescein angiography. This approach was chosen for its effectiveness in both eliminating potential differential diagnoses and assessing the presence of macular ischemia as well as large areas of non-perfusion [33].

Our results have confirmed a significant association between macular ischemia and visual acuity. Patients without MI exhibited greater visual improvement compared to those with MI. Furthermore, the MI biomarker has emerged as a negative predictive factor for visual acuity. To gain a deeper understanding of MI's role, we analysed patients who presented with MI at baseline and explored the associations between OCT biomarkers and visual outcomes.

In this analysis, we found that the integrity of two specific OCT biomarkers, ELM and EZD, demonstrated statistically significant associations ($p < 0.05$). These results align with previous studies [16,33,34] that established a relationship between photoreceptor's integrity and visual improvement. Etheridge et al. [35] suggested that the early recovery of the EZ may be a crucial driver of visual outcomes in patients with RVO. The prompt improvement in EZ integrity likely signifies the resolution of macular edema, which can disrupt photoreceptors. This leads to the re-approximation and/or organization of this visually essential retinal layer. Liu et al. [36] found that an intact initial ELM predicts better visual outcomes after anti-VEGF treatment in RVO patients.

Taken together, these findings suggest that the presence of macular ischemia may limit the restoration of these retinal layers despite treatment. To date, no consensus exists on the extent or location of macular non-perfusion on FA or OCT angiography that can cause loss of vision [21]. FA can more effectively recognize the extent of capillary non-perfusion (CNP) in both the peripheral retina and macula by visualizing areas of the retina with capillary dropout. However, the true severity of CNP, which correlates with the overall metabolic changes resulting from retinal ischemia and ultimately influencing the anatomical and functional outcomes, cannot be comprehensively evaluated through angiography alone [37]. In fact, the interaction of various biochemical factors may contribute to the final clinical presentation, and many of these factors still escape our complete understanding. Therefore, we should explore approaches beyond angiographic assessment to achieve a more accurate evaluation of CNP severity. In this regard, some promising studies have been published concerning the measurement of oxygen saturation and blood flow in cases of retinal vein occlusions [38,39].

It is worth noting that further research is needed, particularly in the form of histologic investigations, to provide a more comprehensive understanding of these relationships.

Meanwhile, the type of RVO, particularly CRVO, has shown a negative predictive factor for visual acuity. This might be attributed to the continuous involvement of the macular region in CRVO-affected patients, whereas BRVO may only partially affect the macular region. This highlights the crucial role of macular, especially foveal, region integrity in visual prognosis [31,33].

This study presents some strengths and limitations. The strengths are as follows: (i) the bias resulting from the type of agent was controlled; the DEX implant was the single intravitreal agent; (ii) and the prospective nature of this protocol with well-defined inclusion/exclusion criteria, strict treatment regimen and follow-up schedule, and standardized protocols for SD-OCT imaging and visual acuity measurements. This study was limited by a small sample size and the presentation of tomographic biomarkers as binomial variables. Measurements and quantitative representation of data as well as a greater sample could change the analysis and the interpretation of results. The automation of OCT measurements using OCT softwares may offer utility in future treatment approaches and in the assessment of visual acuity, as already seen for diabetic macular edema [40]. Moreover, this study did not incorporate other imaging modalities such as OCT angiography (OCT-A). Future studies employing multimodal imaging may improve the predictive power of SD-OCT biomarkers.

5. Conclusions

The DEX implant was confirmed to be an effective treatment in eyes with RVO-ME, on both visual acuity and CRT. The results of this study suggest that DEX is a good influence when restoring tomographic biomarkers. Macular ischemia and CRVO were negative predictive factors for visual outcomes, whereas external limiting membrane and ellipsoid zone disruptions revealed a statistical association with BCVA improvement one year after treatment. Anatomical and tomographic biomarkers are confirmed to be useful to predict treatment response and monitor disease progression. Emerging OCT technologies have demonstrated innovative imaging biomarkers that hold the potential to refine the stratification of treatment responses and aid in medical management choices. These innovative markers complement traditional diagnostic methods like fluorescein angiography, which continue to play a pivotal role in confirming diagnoses and guiding medical decisions. Further studies are needed to better elucidate the impact and predictivity of these and other potential biomarkers.

Author Contributions: Conceptualization, G.C.; methodology, G.C. and C.P.; software, G.C.; validation, G.C., M.S.S. and M.F.; formal analysis, G.C. and C.B.; investigation, G.C and M.S.S.; resources, G.C. and M.S.S.; data curation, G.C., M.S.S. and M.N.M.; writing—original draft preparation, G.C.; writing—review and editing, G.C. and C.P.; visualization, G.C., C.B.; supervision, G.C., C.P. and M.L. All authors have read and agreed to the published version of the manuscript.

Funding: This research received no external funding.

Institutional Review Board Statement: This study was conducted in accordance with the Declaration of Helsinki and was approved by the Area Vasta Nord Ovest Ethical Committee (CEAVNO) with code number 22338 on 9 June 2022.

Informed Consent Statement: Informed consent was obtained from all subjects involved in the study.

Data Availability Statement: Data are fully available upon specific and motivated request to the authors.

Conflicts of Interest: The authors declare no conflicts of interest.

References

1. Wong, T.Y.; Scott, I.U. Retinal-Vein Occlusion. *N. Engl. J. Med.* **2010**, *363*, 2135–2144. [CrossRef] [PubMed]
2. Rogers, S.; McIntosh, R.L.; Cheung, N.; Lim, L.; Wang, J.J.; Mitchell, P.; Kowalski, J.W.; Nguyen, H.; Wong, T.Y. The Prevalence of Retinal Vein Occlusion: Pooled Data from Population Studies from the United States, Europe, Asia, and Australia. *Ophthalmology* **2010**, *117*, 313–319.e1. [CrossRef] [PubMed]
3. Sohn, H.J.; Han, D.H.; Kim, I.T.; Oh, I.K.; Kim, K.H.; Lee, D.Y.; Nam, D.H. Changes in Aqueous Concentrations of Various Cytokines After Intravitreal Triamcinolone Versus Bevacizumab for Diabetic Macular Edema. *Arch. Ophthalmol.* **2011**, *152*, 686–694. [CrossRef] [PubMed]

4. Haller, J.A.; Bandello, F.; Belfort, R.; Blumenkranz, M.S.; Gillies, M.; Heier, J.; Loewenstein, A.; Yoon, Y.-H.; Jacques, M.-L.; Jiao, J.; et al. Randomized, Sham-Controlled Trial of Dexamethasone Intravitreal Implant in Patients with Macular Edema Due to Retinal Vein Occlusion. *Ophthalmology* **2010**, *117*, 1134–1146.e3. [CrossRef] [PubMed]
5. Haller, J.A.; Bandello, F.; Belfort, R.; Blumenkranz, M.S.; Gillies, M.; Heier, J.; Loewenstein, A.; Yoon, Y.H.; Jiao, J.; Li, X.-Y.; et al. Dexamethasone Intravitreal Implant in Patients with Macular Edema Related to Branch or Central Retinal Vein Occlusion. *Ophthalmology* **2011**, *118*, 2453–2460. [CrossRef] [PubMed]
6. Korobelnik, J.F.; Holz, F.G.; Roider, J.; Ogura, Y.; Simader, C.; Schmidt-Erfurth, U.; Lorenz, K.; Honda, M.; Vitti, R.; Berliner, A.J.; et al. Intravitreal Aflibercept Injection for Macular Edema Resulting from Central Retinal Vein Occlusion. *Ophthalmology* **2014**, *121*, 202–208. [CrossRef]
7. Brown, D.M.; Heier, J.S.; Clark, W.L.; Boyer, D.S.; Vitti, R.; Berliner, A.J.; Zeitz, O.; Sandbrink, R.; Zhu, X.; Haller, J.A. Intravitreal Aflibercept Injection for Macular Edema Secondary to Central Retinal Vein Occlusion: 1-Year Results From the Phase 3 COPERNICUS Study. *Arch. Ophthalmol.* **2013**, *155*, 429–437.e7. [CrossRef] [PubMed]
8. Larsen, M.; Waldstein, S.M.; Boscia, F.; Gerding, H.; Monés, J.; Tadayoni, R.; Priglinger, S.; Wenzel, A.; Barnes, E.; Pilz, S.; et al. Individualized Ranibizumab Regimen Driven by Stabilization Criteria for Central Retinal Vein Occlusion. *Ophthalmology* **2016**, *123*, 1101–1111. [CrossRef] [PubMed]
9. Ota, M.; Tsujikawa, A.; Kita, M.; Miyamoto, K.; Sakamoto, A.; Yamaike, N.; Kotera, Y.; Yoshimura, N. Integrity of Foveal Photoreceptor Layer in Central Retinal Vein Occlusion. *Retina* **2008**, *28*, 1502–1508. [CrossRef] [PubMed]
10. Ko, J.; Kwon, O.W.; Byeon, S.H. Optical Coherence Tomography Predicts Visual Outcome in Acute Central Retinal Vein Occlusion. *Retina* **2014**, *34*, 1132–1141. [CrossRef] [PubMed]
11. Jonas, J.B.; Monés, J.; Glacet-Bernard, A.; Coscas, G. Retinal Vein Occlusions. *Macular Edema* **2017**, *58*, 139–167.
12. Bin, M.; Hai-Ying, Z.; Xuan, J.; Feng, Z. Evaluation of hyperreflective foci as a prognostic factor of visual outcome in retinal vein occlusion. *Int. J. Ophthalmol.* **2017**, *10*, 605.
13. Moon, B.G.; Cho, A.R.; Kim, Y.N.; Kim, J.G. Predictors of Refractory Macular Edema After Branch Retinal Vein Occlusion Following Intravitreal Bevacizumab. *Retina* **2018**, *38*, 1166–1174. [CrossRef] [PubMed]
14. Banaee, T.; Singh, R.P.; Champ, K.; Conti, F.F.; Wai, K.; Bena, J.; Beven, L.; Ehlers, J.P. Ellipsoid Zone Mapping Parameters in Retinal Venous Occlusive Disease with Associated Macular Edema. *Ophthalmol. Retin.* **2018**, *2*, 836–841. [CrossRef] [PubMed]
15. Babiuch, A.S.; Han, M.; Conti, F.F.; Wai, K.; Silva, F.Q.; Singh, R.P. Association of Disorganization of Retinal Inner Layers with Visual Acuity Response to Anti–Vascular Endothelial Growth Factor Therapy for Macular Edema Secondary to Retinal Vein Occlusion. *JAMA Ophthalmol.* **2019**, *137*, 38. [CrossRef] [PubMed]
16. Castro-Navarro, V.; Monferrer-Adsuara, C.; Navarro-Palop, C.; Montero-Hernández, J.; Cervera-Taulet, E. Effect of Dexamethasone Intravitreal Implant on Visual Acuity and Foveal Photoreceptor Integrity in Macular Edema Secondary to Retinal Vascular Disease. *Ophthalmologica* **2021**, *244*, 83–92. [CrossRef] [PubMed]
17. Shin, H.J.; Chung, H.; Kim, H.C. Association between integrity of foveal photoreceptor layer and visual outcome in retinal vein occlusion. *Acta Ophthalmol.* **2011**, *89*, e35–e40. [CrossRef] [PubMed]
18. Mitamura, Y.; Fujihara-Mino, A.; Inomoto, N.; Sano, H.; Akaiwa, K.; Semba, K. Optical coherence tomography parameters predictive of visual outcome after anti-VEGF therapy for retinal vein occlusion. *Clin. Ophthalmol.* **2016**, *10*, 1305–1313. [CrossRef] [PubMed]
19. Radwan, S.H.; Soliman, A.Z.; Tokarev, J.; Zhang, L.; van Kuijk, F.J.; Koozekanani, D.D. Association of Disorganization of Retinal Inner Layers With Vision After Resolution of Center-Involved Diabetic Macular Edema. *JAMA Ophthalmol.* **2015**, *133*, 820–825. [CrossRef] [PubMed]
20. Sun, J.K.; Lin, M.M.; Lammer, J.; Prager, S.; Sarangi, R.; Silva, P.S.; Aiello, L.P. Disorganization of the Retinal Inner Layers as a Predictor of Visual Acuity in Eyes With Center-Involved Diabetic Macular Edema. *JAMA Ophthalmol.* **2014**, *132*, 1309–1316. [CrossRef] [PubMed]
21. Schmidt-Erfurth, U.; Garcia-Arumi, J.; Gerendas, B.S.; Midena, E.; Sivaprasad, S.; Tadayoni, R.; Wolf, S.; Loewenstein, A. Guidelines for the Management of Retinal Vein Occlusion by the European Society of Retina Specialists (EURETINA). *Ophthalmologica* **2019**, *242*, 123–162. [CrossRef] [PubMed]
22. Castro-Navarro, V.; Monferrer-Adsuara, C.; Navarro-Palop, C.; Montero-Hernández, J.; Cervera-Taulet, E. Optical coherence tomography biomarkers in patients with macular edema secondary to retinal vein occlusion treated with dexamethasone implant. *BMC Ophthalmol.* **2022**, *22*, 191. [CrossRef] [PubMed]
23. Phadnis, M.A. Sample size calculation for small sample single-arm trials for time-to-event data: Logrank test with normal approximation or test statistic based on exact chi-square distribution? *Contemp. Clin. Trials Commun.* **2019**, *15*, 100360. [CrossRef] [PubMed]
24. Ji, K.; Zhang, Q.; Tian, M.; Xing, Y. Comparison of dexamethasone intravitreal implant with intravitreal anti-VEGF injections for the treatment of macular edema secondary to branch retinal vein occlusion. *Medicine* **2019**, *98*, e15798. [CrossRef] [PubMed]
25. Li, X.; China Ozurdex in RVO Study Group; Wang, N.; Liang, X.; Xu, G.; Li, X.-Y.; Jiao, J.; Lou, J.; Hashad, Y. Safety and efficacy of dexamethasone intravitreal implant for treatment of macular edema secondary to retinal vein occlusion in Chinese patients: Randomized, sham-controlled, multicenter study. *Graefe's Arch. Clin. Exp. Ophthalmol.* **2018**, *256*, 59–69. [CrossRef] [PubMed]

26. Midena, E.; Torresin, T.; Schiavon, S.; Danieli, L.; Polo, C.; Pilotto, E.; Midena, G.; Frizziero, L. The Disorganization of Retinal Inner Layers Is Correlated to Müller Cells Impairment in Diabetic Macular Edema: An Imaging and Omics Study. *Int. J. Mol. Sci.* **2023**, *24*, 9607. [CrossRef] [PubMed]
27. Luís, M.E.; Sampaio, F.; Costa, J.; Cabral, D.; Teixeira, C.; Ferreira, J.T. Dril Influences Short-term Visual Outcome after Intravitreal Corticosteroid Injection for Refractory Diabetic Macular Edema. *Curr. Eye Res.* **2021**, *46*, 1378–1386. [CrossRef] [PubMed]
28. American Diabetes Association. Diagnosis and Classification of Diabetes Mellitus. *Diabetes Care* **2013**, *36* (Suppl. 1), S67–S74. [CrossRef] [PubMed]
29. Fragiotta, S.; Abdolrahimzadeh, S.; Dolz-Marco, R.; Sakurada, Y.; Gal-Or, O.; Scuderi, G. Significance of Hyperreflective Foci as an Optical Coherence Tomography Biomarker in Retinal Diseases: Characterization and Clinical Implications. *J. Ophthalmol.* **2021**, *2021*, 1–10. [CrossRef] [PubMed]
30. Tan, T.-E.; Ibrahim, F.; Chandrasekaran, P.R.; Teo, K.Y.C. Clinical utility of ultra-widefield fluorescein angiography and optical coherence tomography angiography for retinal vein occlusions. *Front. Med.* **2023**, *10*, 1110166. [CrossRef] [PubMed]
31. Wons, J.; Pfau, M.; Wirth, M.A.; Freiberg, F.J.; Becker, M.D.; Michels, S. Optical Coherence Tomography Angiography of the Foveal Avascular Zone in Retinal Vein Occlusion. *Ophthalmologica* **2016**, *235*, 195–202. [CrossRef] [PubMed]
32. Salles, M.C.; Kvanta, A.; Amrén, U.; Epstein, D. Optical Coherence Tomography Angiography in Central Retinal Vein Occlusion: Correlation Between the Foveal Avascular Zone and Visual Acuity. *Investig. Ophthalmol. Vis. Sci.* **2016**, *57*, OCT242–OCT246. [CrossRef] [PubMed]
33. Antropoli, A.; Bianco, L.; Arrigo, A.; Bandello, F.; Parodi, M.B. Non-perfusion severity correlates with central macular thickness and microvascular impairment in branch retinal vein occlusions. *Eur. J. Ophthalmol.* **2023**, *34*, 226–232. [CrossRef] [PubMed]
34. De, S.; Saxena, S.; Kaur, A.; Mahdi, A.A.; Misra, A.; Singh, M.; Meyer, C.H.; Akduman, L. Sequential restoration of external limiting membrane and ellipsoid zone after intravitreal anti-VEGF therapy in diabetic macular oedema. *Eye* **2021**, *35*, 1490–1495. [CrossRef] [PubMed]
35. Etheridge, T.; Dobson, E.T.A.; Wiedenmann, M.; Oden, N.; VanVeldhuisen, P.; Scott, I.U.; Ip, M.S.; Eliceiri, K.W.; Blodi, B.A.; Domalpally, A. Ellipsoid Zone Defects in Retinal Vein Occlusion Correlates with Visual Acuity Prognosis: SCORE2 Report 14. *Transl. Vis. Sci. Technol.* **2021**, *10*, 31. [CrossRef] [PubMed]
36. Liu, H.; Li, S.; Zhang, Z.; Shen, J. Predicting the visual acuity for retinal vein occlusion after ranibizumab therapy with an original ranking for macular microstructure. *Exp. Ther. Med.* **2017**, *15*, 890–896. [CrossRef] [PubMed]
37. Parodi, M.B.; Arrigo, A.; Antropoli, A.; Bianco, L.; Saladino, A.; Bandello, F.; Vilela, M.; Mansour, A. Deep Capillary Plexus as Biomarker of Peripheral Capillary Nonperfusion in Central Retinal Vein Occlusion. *Ophthalmol. Sci.* **2023**, *3*, 100267. [CrossRef]
38. Šínová, I.; Řehák, J.; Nekolová, J.; Jirásková, N.; Haluzová, P.; Řeháková, T.; Bábková, B.; Hejsek, L.; Šín, M. Correlation Between Ischemic Index of Retinal Vein Occlusion and Oxygen Saturation in Retinal Vessels. *Arch. Ophthalmol.* **2018**, *188*, 74–80. [CrossRef] [PubMed]
39. Nicholson, L.; Vazquez-Alfageme, C.; Hykin, P.G.; Bainbridge, J.W.; Sivaprasad, S. The Relationship Between Retinal Vessel Oxygenation and Spatial Distribution of Retinal Nonperfusion in Retinal Vascular Diseases. *Investig. Ophthalmol. Vis. Sci.* **2019**, *60*, 2083. [CrossRef] [PubMed]
40. Midena, E.; Toto, L.; Frizziero, L.; Covello, G.; Torresin, T.; Midena, G.; Danieli, L.; Pilotto, E.; Figus, M.; Mariotti, C.; et al. Validation of an Automated Artificial Intelligence Algorithm for the Quantification of Major OCT Parameters in Diabetic Macular Edema. *J. Clin. Med.* **2023**, *12*, 2134. [CrossRef] [PubMed]

Disclaimer/Publisher's Note: The statements, opinions and data contained in all publications are solely those of the individual author(s) and contributor(s) and not of MDPI and/or the editor(s). MDPI and/or the editor(s) disclaim responsibility for any injury to people or property resulting from any ideas, methods, instructions or products referred to in the content.

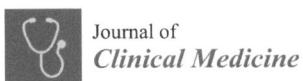

Case Report

Anterior Segment Optical Coherence Tomography for the Tailored Treatment of Mooren's Ulcer: A Case Report

Luca Lucchino, Elvia Mastrogiuseppe, Francesca Giovannetti *, Alice Bruscolini, Marco Marenco and Alessandro Lambiase

Department of Sense Organs, Sapienza University of Rome, Viale del Policlinico 155, 00161 Rome, Italy; luca.lucchino@uniroma1.it (L.L.); elvia.mastrogiuseppe@uniroma1.it (E.M.); alice.bruscolini@uniroma1.it (A.B.); marco.marenco@uniroma1.it (M.M.); alessandro.lambiase@uniroma1.it (A.L.)
* Correspondence: francesca.giovannetti@uniroma1.it

Abstract: Background: Mooren's ulcer (MU) is a rare and debilitating form of peripheral ulcerative keratitis (PUK), characterized by a crescent-shaped ulcer with a distinctive overhanging edge at the corneal periphery. If left untreated, MU can lead to severe complications such as corneal perforation and blindness. Despite various treatment approaches, including anti-inflammatory and cytotoxic drugs, as well as surgical interventions, there is no clear evidence of the most effective treatment due to the lack of randomized controlled trials. AS-OCT is a non-invasive imaging technique that provides high-resolution cross-sectional images of the anterior segment, allowing for accurate evaluation of corneal ulcer characteristics, including depth, extent, and disease progression. **Methods:** We present the case of a 20-year-old male patient with MU managed using a stepladder approach, which included local and systemic corticosteroids, limbal conjunctival resection, and Cyclosporine A 1% eye drops. The patient underwent consecutive AS-OCT examinations and strict follow-up to tailor systemic and topical therapy. **Results:** Complete healing of the corneal ulcer with resolution of the inflammatory process was achieved. There was no recurrence of the disease at the 7-month follow-up. AS-OCT demonstrated progressive reorganization and thickening of the stromal tissue until the complete recovery of stromal thickness. **Conclusions:** The AS-OCT imaging modality allowed for the accurate evaluation of corneal ulcer characteristics, facilitating informed decision-making regarding the use of systemic immunosuppression, surgical interventions, and local immunomodulation and providing detailed and precise assessment of disease progression. This approach enabled a tailored and effective treatment strategy for the patient and played a critical role in guiding the therapeutic approach.

Keywords: Mooren's ulcer; AS-OCT; PUK; cyclosporine A; corneal imaging

Citation: Lucchino, L.; Mastrogiuseppe, E.; Giovannetti, F.; Bruscolini, A.; Marenco, M.; Lambiase, A. Anterior Segment Optical Coherence Tomography for the Tailored Treatment of Mooren's Ulcer: A Case Report. *J. Clin. Med.* 2024, *13*, 5384. https://doi.org/10.3390/jcm13185384

Academic Editor: Jose Ignacio Fernandez-Vigo

Received: 25 July 2024
Revised: 7 September 2024
Accepted: 10 September 2024
Published: 11 September 2024

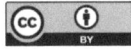

Copyright: © 2024 by the authors. Licensee MDPI, Basel, Switzerland. This article is an open access article distributed under the terms and conditions of the Creative Commons Attribution (CC BY) license (https:// creativecommons.org/licenses/by/ 4.0/).

1. Introduction

Mooren's ulcer (MU) is a rare and debilitating form of peripheral ulcerative keratitis (PUK), prevalent in southern and central Africa as well as the Indian subcontinent, exhibiting a male predilection [1]. Characterized by moderate to severe pain, MU begins with a crescent-shaped ulcer featuring a distinctive overhanging edge at the corneal periphery. It progresses both centrally and circumferentially with minimal scleral involvement [2].

The pathogenesis of MU involves complex interactions between genetic predisposition, altered immune responses, and environmental factors. Despite ongoing research, the exact etiology of MU remains elusive, and it continues to be a diagnosis of exclusion, posing significant challenges in its management [3,4]. It has been hypothesized that the etiology of MU may result from an autoimmune response to calgranulin C, an antigen typically concealed but expressed by stromal keratinocytes [5]. Sensitization to calgranulin C can be triggered by corneal trauma, infection, or aging-related changes, particularly in subjects with specific haplotype expression (HLA-DR17 and DQ2). This may lead to the activation of antigen-presenting cells, likely stimulating T-cell response and subsequently contributing to ulcer formation. Alternatively, helminthic antigens could potentially induce a similar immune response. Furthermore, complement activation and the release of collagenases by neutrophils are implicated in corneal stromal destruction, resulting in progressive corneal damage [3,6].

Different classifications exist for MU, highlighting that while older subjects typically present with a unilateral and indolent form, younger patients often experience bilateral, more severe disease with poorer treatment outcomes [2,7]. MU can lead to severe complications, such as corneal perforation and blindness if not promptly treated. Various treatments are utilized for MU, including anti-inflammatory drugs (steroidal and non-steroidal), cytotoxic drugs (topical and systemic), conjunctivectomy, and cornea debridement (superficial keratectomy) [8]. Despite advances in understanding MU, it still causes significant ocular morbidity, prompting the use of new biological medications to control inflammation in cases unresponsive to conventional therapies such as TNF-α blockers [9], monoclonal antibody targeting CD20 on B cells [10], and interferon alfa-2a [11]. However, due to the absence of randomized controlled trials (RCTs), there is no clear evidence on the most effective treatment. Therefore, a stepladder approach is typically employed based on clinical judgment and patient characteristics [8].

Anterior Segment Optical Coherence Tomography (AS-OCT) is a non-invasive imaging modality that provides high-resolution cross-sectional images of the eye's anterior segment using low-coherence interferometry [12]. In corneal pathologies, AS-OCT plays a pivotal role, adjunct to slit lamp biomicroscopy, in diagnosing and managing various conditions. It aids in evaluating corneal opacities, infections, dystrophies, ulcers, and other disorders by offering precise structural information [13]. AS-OCT assesses corneal thickness, identifies scarring or haze, detects synechiae, and assists in planning surgical interventions like keratoplasty. Moreover, it facilitates monitoring disease progression, grading severity, evaluating treatment response, and providing accurate real-time therapeutic guidance [12].

2. Case Presentation

A 20-year-old male patient of Senegalese descent presented to our clinic in May 2023 complaining of redness and pain in his left eye (LE) for the past few weeks. The patient's ocular and general medical history was unremarkable. Upon initial clinical examination, the best corrected visual acuity (BCVA) was 0 Log MAR in both eyes. The right eye showed no pathological signs, but the LE exhibited an intense perikeratic reaction, more pronounced in the temporal sectors, along with a crescent-shaped peripheral corneal ulcer featuring an epithelial defect with an overhanging edge and stromal thinning in the temporal periphery (Figure 1). Intraocular pressure and the rest of the ocular structures were within normal limits. The ongoing topical antibiotics were discontinued for a 48 h washout period, and corneal scraping was performed to rule out infectious keratitis. Once corneal scraping revealed no pathogenic microorganisms, treatment was adjusted to include topical corticosteroids, dexamethasone 1.5 mg/mL drops, administered six times per day, and topical antibiotic coverage with moxifloxacin 3 mg/mL drops four times daily. To promptly identify and manage potential corticosteroid-related complications, such as infection or intraocular pressure elevation, the patient was closely monitored with almost daily examinations.

Comprehensive laboratory investigations were performed, including complete blood count (CBC) with differential, platelet count, erythrocyte sedimentation rate (ESR), rheumatoid factor (RF), anti-cyclic citrullinated peptide (anti-CCP) antibodies, complement fixation test, antinuclear antibodies (ANA), anti-neutrophil cytoplasmic antibodies (ANCA), circulating immune complexes assay, liver function tests, Venereal Disease Research Laboratory (VDRL) or Fluorescent Treponemal Antibody Absorption (FTA-ABS) test, blood urea nitrogen (BUN) and creatinine levels, serum protein electrophoresis, and urinalysis. Additionally, serological tests for Hepatitis C Virus (HCV), Hepatitis B Virus (HBV), Angiotensin-Converting Enzyme (ACE), and QuantiFERON gold test were conducted, along with chest X-ray and rheumatology consultation. After negative findings from all laboratory and instrumental tests for concurrent systemic diseases, as well as rheumatological evaluation, the diagnosis of Mooren's ulcer was established. Then, after one month, given the patient's stable condition and the healing of the epithelial defect, topical corticosteroids were gradually tapered for three weeks (Figure 1).

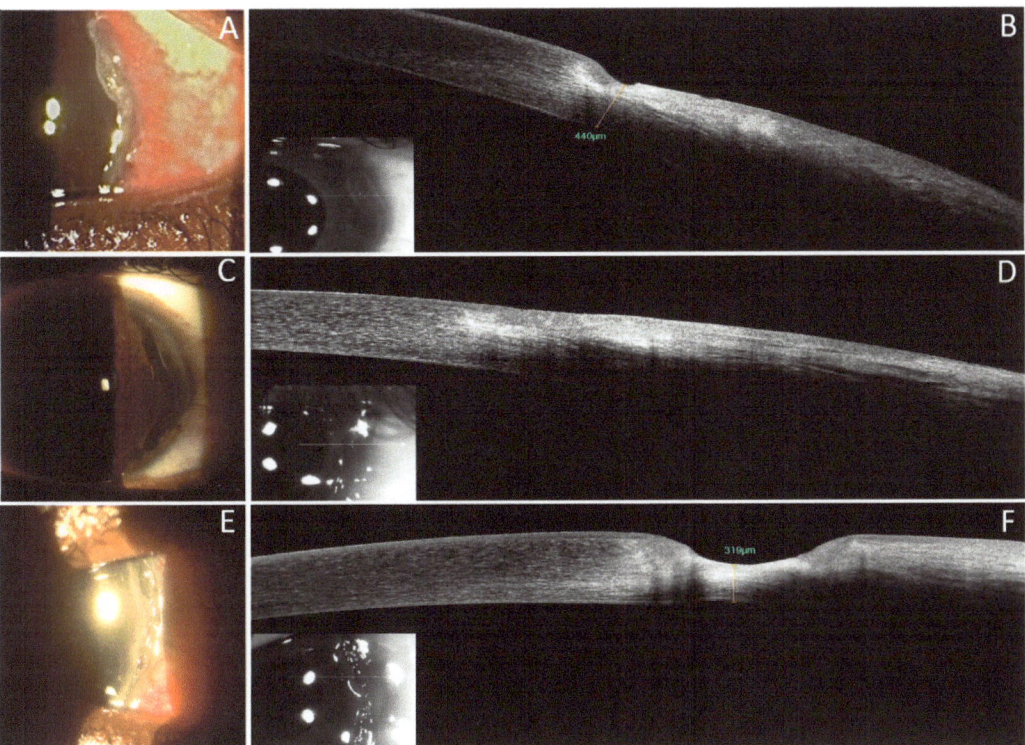

Figure 1. Slit lamp examination and corresponding AS-OCT section pointed out by the line across the area of interest. May (**A**,**B**). Slit lamp biomicroscopy (**A**) shows conjunctival hyperaemia, intense perikeratic reaction, circular paralimbal temporal thinning, and an epithelial defect. AS-OCT scan (**B**) reveals the absence of the epithelium, stromal thinning (residual stromal thickness of 440 µm), and stromal hyper-reflectivity. June 2023 (**C**,**D**): Resolution of the inflammatory condition was observed. The conjunctiva was normoemic with no perikeratic reaction, and the epithelial defect had been repaired (**C**). AS-OCT scan showed that the epithelial layer was irregular and hyporeflective but intact, filling the area of corneal thinning. The underlying stroma was hyper-reflective (**D**). July 2023 (**E**,**F**): Worsening of the clinical condition was observed. Severe perikeratic reaction with temporal ulceration and thinning (**E**). AS-OCT scan revealed the absence of the epithelial layer, significant stromal thinning (319 µm), and stromal hyper-reflectivity (**F**).

The patient was strictly monitored with ocular examinations and AS-OCT imaging, which aided in managing therapy tapering. Corneal thickness measurements were taken using Optovue iVue80 Spectral Domain-OCT (Optovue Inc., Fremont, CA, USA) with the Cornea Anterior Module (CAM), which includes a lens adapter attached to the front of the instrument for imaging the cornea and anterior chamber. AS-OCT scans were performed using the Cornea Angle module, which utilizes a single 5 mm scan line (1 × 1024 A-scans per frame, 16 averaged scans per line) with speckle noise reduction, and a depth resolution of 5 µm. Specifically, linear measurements were recorded at the thinnest point of the cornea with the caliper perpendicular to the endothelium and repeated at the same location during each follow-up visit using the same protocol. The cornea specialist (AL) visually confirmed the measurement location on the infrared images provided by the AS-OCT device to ensure consistency. Unfortunately, at the end of July, the patient returned to our clinic with worsening symptoms, including a severe perikeratic reaction, recurrence of the corneal ulcer, and marked stromal thinning (Figure 1). Therefore, urgent excision of the limbal conjunctiva and tenectomy was performed the next day. Systemic immunosuppression was also started with oral prednisolone, initially 50 mg daily, which was then tapered to 25 mg per day. Local inflammation was managed with peribulbar injections of triamcinolone acetonide (40 mg/mL) and antibiotic coverage was provided with moxifloxacin 3 mg/mL eye drops, administered four times daily in the LE. Despite initial improvement, after two weeks of aggressive therapy, the patient's condition worsened (Figure 2).

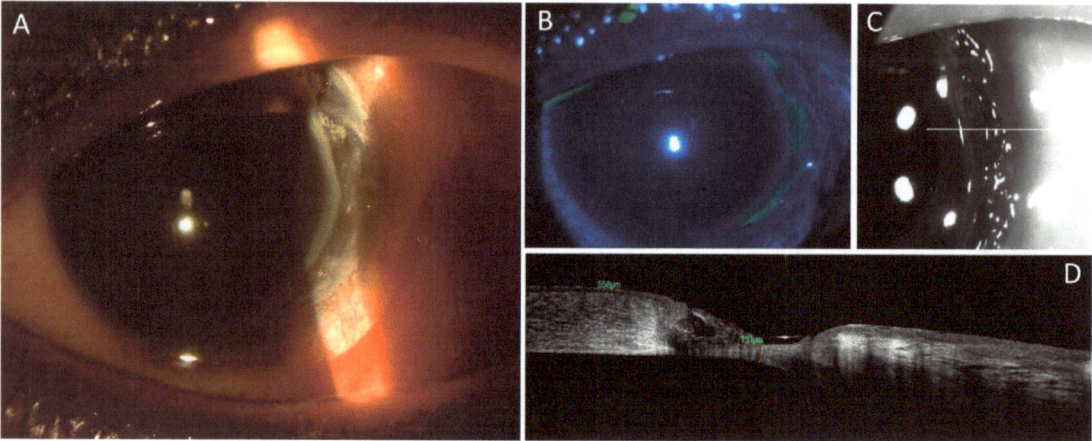

Figure 2. Slit lamp examination (**A,B**) and AS-OCT (**C,D**) in August 2023. Slit lamp biomicroscopy shows (**A**) conjunctival hyperemia, severe perikeratic reaction, significant circular, paralimbal, temporal thinning, and crescent-shaped ulceration. Corneal ulcer positive on fluorescein vital coloration (**B**). AS-OCT images: line across the section of thinning (**C**). Marked thinning (residual stromal thickness 151 µm), absence of epithelium, pronounced stromal disarray, hyporeflective voids amidst hyper-reflective regions.

Therefore, 1% cyclosporine eye drops twice daily were added to the treatment regimen. In September, the resolution of the epithelial defect, with initial conjunctivalization and neovascularization of the tissue, along with early stromal thickening was documented by AS-OCT (Figure 3).

From October to December, oral steroids were slowly tapered while monitoring stromal thickness and continuing topical 1% cyclosporine drops twice daily. AS-OCT revealed progressive reorganization and thickening of the stromal tissue until stromal thickness complete recovery in December (Figure 3). Currently, the patient continues 1% cyclosporine eye drops without recurrence.

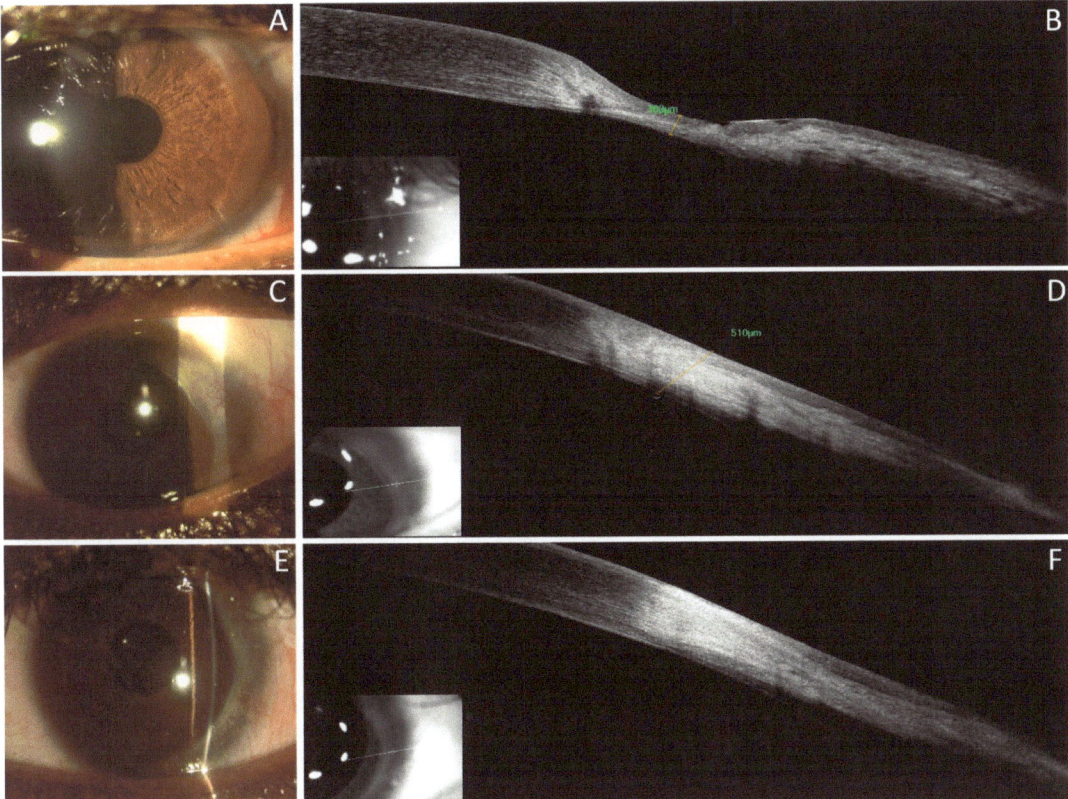

Figure 3. Slit lamp examination and corresponding AS-OCT section pointed out by the line across the area of interest. September (**A**,**B**): At the 1-month follow-up, with topical and systemic therapy, slit lamp biomicroscopy shows reduced conjunctival hyperemia, decreased temporal thinning, and epithelial integrity with initial conjunctivalization (**A**). AS-OCT scans reveal a hyporeflective epithelial layer, significant stromal thinning (residual stromal thickness 163 μm), and diffuse stromal hyper-reflectivity absence of hyporeflective voids. October (**C**,**D**): Resolution of the inflammatory process. Presence of fibrovascular tissue covering the temporal sector (**C**). AS-OCT images demonstrate restored stromal thickness (measured 510 μm) with hyper-reflectivity, indicating substantial stromal remodeling (**D**). December (**E**,**F**). Absence of inflammation (**E**). Enhanced regularity of stromal hyper-reflectivity, suggesting improved alignment of stromal lamellae and overall better tissue organization (**F**).

3. Discussion

PUK can arise from various local or systemic factors, including infectious and non-infectious origins. Accurate identification of the underlying cause is crucial for effective management, necessitating a thorough clinical evaluation, encompassing diverse laboratory and radiological assessments. The diagnosis of MU is a diagnosis of exclusion and requires the absence of an underlying disease [4].

As stated in the introduction, controlling inflammation is crucial to prevent the progression of the condition. There are four prevalent strategies to achieve this: local immunosuppression, systemic immunosuppression, removal of the source (limbus), and removal of the target (keratinocytes) [14].

At present, there is a lack of clear evidence regarding treatment selection due to the absence of randomized clinical trials. However, it is suggested to initiate treatment with topical corticosteroids, followed by limbal conjunctival resection when inflammation remains uncontrolled [8].

The excision of the limbal conjunctiva along with tenectomy aims to distance the limbal blood vessels, removing the source and preventing the delivery of antibodies, immune complexes, and metalloproteinases directed against the cornea [15]. Indeed, initial corneal surgery is generally discouraged, while limbal conjunctival resection, apart from being a more conservative approach compared to keratoplasty, has also demonstrated superior disease control when used alongside keratoplasty [16].

In our case, limbal conjunctival resection and systemic immunosuppression with oral steroids did not achieve complete control of inflammation; therefore, after witnessing the progressive worsening of the condition, detected by AS-OCT images, we added to the treatment regimen topical Cyclosporine A 1 mg/mL for two times a day.

Cyclosporine A (CsA) is a medication used to reduce ocular inflammation. It enters T lymphocytes and forms complexes with intracellular binding proteins. Specifically, this complex inhibits calcineurin phosphatase, disrupting the activation of the NFATc transcription factor and preventing the production of cytokines, including IL-2 and IFN-γ [17]. While primarily studied and used in the treatment of dry eye disease, CsA has also shown efficacy in managing refractory MU [18,19]. In the literature, MU showed a positive response to topical 0.5% cyclosporine in 11 out of 18 cases (61.1%) during long-term follow-up (24–31 months) [18]. Additionally, a reduction in recurrence rates of the condition when combined with keratoplasty at concentrations of 1% and 2% has been demonstrated [16,19].

AS-OCT has proven to be a valuable tool for monitoring the progression and healing of corneal ulcers. Technology has evolved in recent years, enabling detailed assessment of anterior segment structures with finer than slit lamp biomicroscopy [13]. This non-invasive imaging technique allows clinicians to assess various aspects of the ulcer, including the depth of stromal thinning, the extent of the epithelial defect, and the restoration of normal corneal thickness during the healing process. Additionally, AS-OCT provides insights into the structural organization of the cornea, enabling the evaluation of the quality of the scarring and the overall integrity of the tissue [20].

Another great advantage of AS-OCT is the ability to provide reliable and reproducible measurements in case of stromal opacities, whereas corneal topographers, owing to scattered light from corneal opacities, struggle to accurately measure eyes with severe opacities [12]. Yoshihara et al. used three-dimensional AS-OCT to evaluate corneal shape, revealing that in eyes with MU, irregular astigmatism and distortion increase as the lesion moves closer to the center [21]. Our patient maintained 20/20 visual acuity by controlling inflammation and keeping the lesion peripheric.

AS-OCT is recommended for preoperative evaluation in surgical planning before keratoplasty, as it provides precise measurements of the depth of stromal opacities, which is a key determinant for predicting the success of lamellar keratoplasty [22]. Lian et al. performed therapeutic lamellar keratoplasty on six eyes of patients with Mooren's ulcer. The surgical procedure was optimized by AS-OCT precise measurements of stromal thickness beneath areas of fibrovascular tissue that potentially revealed occult perforations during surgical planning. Additionally, AS-OCT enabled postoperative evaluation of the posterior corneal surface to detect any ectatic areas [23].

In the literature, AS-OCT has been utilized for monitoring disease activity and categorizing PUK in patients affected by vasculitis into three stages: (1) acute stage; (2) healing stage; and (3) healed stage. During the acute phase, AS-OCT typically reveals the absence of corneal epithelium and disorganized anterior stroma with focal thinning and heterogeneous stromal reflectivity. In the healing stage, AS-OCT images often exhibit an irregular epithelium with reduced reflectivity and a less heterogeneous stroma. Finally, in the healed stage, AS-OCT reveals a hyporeflective irregular epithelium, a demarcation line between the hyporeflective epithelium, and hyper-reflective stroma [24].

To our knowledge, this represents the first case in the literature of monitoring MU using AS-OCT. Compared to descriptions of PUK secondary to peripheral vasculitis, our case exhibited distinctive characteristics during the three stages. In the acute phases, in addition to the absence of epithelium and irregular appearance of the stroma, pronounced stromal disarray was observed, featuring hyporeflective voids amidst hyper-reflective regions, indicative of stromal edema in the context of significant inflammation. Later, during the healing process, we observed complete restoration of stromal thickness accompanied by stromal tissue reorganization and diminished hyper-reflectivity in the fully healed phase, indicative of significant stromal remodeling. The hyper-reflectivity may indicate variations in refractive indices or reflective properties of the remodeled corneal stroma. This allowed for tailored therapy of the different stages of the corneal ulcer and, finally, for a full restoration of corneal integrity. This case report aims to highlight the importance of AS-OCT guidance in managing patients affected by complex inflammatory processes such as MU, reminding ophthalmologists to incorporate this essential tool in their clinical practice. While a cornea specialist can easily diagnose ulcerative keratitis, AS-OCT is crucial to provide exact micron measurements, teamwork with colleagues with easy follow-up, and accurate detection of signs of disease progression. Diagnostic guidelines are needed to universalize AS-OCT patterns of inflammation.

4. Conclusions

In conclusion, our case underscores the importance of early diagnosis and personalized management in MU. AS-OCT has proven crucial in evaluating disease progression and guiding treatment by accurate detection of disease activity patterns. A tailored therapeutic approach, incorporating systemic immunosuppression with corticosteroids, surgical intervention with limbal conjunctival resection, and local immunomodulation using 1% CsA eye drops, was employed to address inflammation and promote healing, allowing for resolution after four months of treatment.

Funding: This research received no external funding.

Institutional Review Board Statement: This study was conducted in accordance with the Declaration of Helsinki.

Informed Consent Statement: Written informed consent was obtained from the subject to publish this paper.

Data Availability Statement: Data is available upon reasonable request.

Conflicts of Interest: The authors declare no conflicts of interest.

References

1. Tuft, S. Mooren's Ulcer. In *Epidemiology of Eye Disease*; Johnson, G.J., Minassian, D.C., Weale, R.A., West, S.K., Eds.; Arnold: London, UK, 2003; pp. 209–211.
2. Watson, P.G. Management of Mooren's Ulceration. *Eye* **1997**, *11*, 349–356. [CrossRef] [PubMed]
3. Taylor, C.J. HLA and Mooren's Ulceration. *Br. J. Ophthalmol.* **2000**, *84*, 72–75. [CrossRef] [PubMed]
4. Gupta, Y.; Kishore, A.; Kumari, P.; Balakrishnan, N.; Lomi, N.; Gupta, N.; Vanathi, M.; Tandon, R. Peripheral Ulcerative Keratitis. *Surv. Ophthalmol.* **2021**, *66*, 977–998. [CrossRef] [PubMed]
5. Gottsch, J.D.; Li, Q.; Ashraf, F.; O'Brien, T.P.; Stark, W.J.; Liu, S.H. Cytokine-Induced Calgranulin C Expression in Keratocytes. *Clin. Immunol.* **1999**, *91*, 34–40. [CrossRef] [PubMed]
6. Martin, N.F.; Stark, W.J.; Maumenee, A.E. Treatment of Mooren's and Mooren's-like Ulcer by Lamellar Keratectomy: Report of Six Eyes and Literature Review. *Ophthalmic Surg.* **1987**, *18*, 564–569. [CrossRef]
7. Wilhelmus, K.R.; Huang, A.J.; Hwang, D.G.; Parrish, C.M.; Sutphin, J.E.; Whitsett, J.C. External Disease and Cornea. In *Basic and Clinical Science Course for Ophthalmologists Section 8*; Liesegang, T.J., Deutsch, T.A., Grand, M.G., Eds.; American Academy of Ophthalmology: San Francisco, CA, USA, 2001; pp. 217–218.
8. Alhassan, M.B.; Rabiu, M.; Agbabiaka, I.O. Interventions for Mooren's Ulcer. *Cochrane Database Syst. Rev.* **2014**, *2014*, CD006131. [CrossRef]
9. Fontana, L.; Parente, G.; Neri, P.; Reta, M.; Tassinari, G. Favourable Response to Infliximab in a Case of Bilateral Refractory Mooren's Ulcer. *Clin. Exp. Ophthalmol.* **2007**, *35*, 871–873. [CrossRef]
10. Guindolet, D.; Reynaud, C.; Clavel, G.; Belangé, G.; Benmahmed, M.; Doan, S.; Hayem, G.; Cochereau, I.; Gabison, E.E. Management of Severe and Refractory Mooren's Ulcers with Rituximab. *Br. J. Ophthalmol.* **2017**, *101*, 418–422. [CrossRef]

11. Erdem, U.; Kerimoglu, H.; Gundogan, F.C.; Dagli, S. Treatment of Mooren's Ulcer with Topical Administration of Interferon Alfa 2a. *Ophthalmology* **2007**, *114*, 446–449. [CrossRef]
12. Han, S.B.; Liu, Y.-C.; Noriega, K.M.; Mehta, J.S. Applications of Anterior Segment Optical Coherence Tomography in Cornea and Ocular Surface Diseases. *J. Ophthalmol.* **2016**, *2016*, 1–9. [CrossRef]
13. Das, M.; Menda, S.A.; Panigrahi, A.K.; Venkatesh Prajna, N.; Yen, M.; Tsang, B.; Kumar, A.; Rose-Nussbaumer, J.; Acharya, N.R.; McCulloch, C.E.; et al. Repeatability and Reproducibility of Slit Lamp, Optical Coherence Tomography, and Scheimpflug Measurements of Corneal Scars. *Ophthalmic Epidemiol.* **2019**, *26*, 251–256. [CrossRef] [PubMed]
14. Zegans, M.E.; Srinivasan, M. Mooren's Ulcer. *Int. Ophthalmol. Clin.* **1998**, *38*, 81–88. [CrossRef] [PubMed]
15. Brown, S.I. Mooren's Ulcer. Treatment by Conjunctival Excision. *Br. J. Ophthalmol.* **1975**, *59*, 675–682. [CrossRef] [PubMed]
16. Chen, J. Mooren's Ulcer in China: A Study of Clinical Characteristics and Treatment. *Br. J. Ophthalmol.* **2000**, *84*, 1244–1249. [CrossRef]
17. Ames, P.; Galor, A. Cyclosporine Ophthalmic Emulsions for the Treatment of Dry Eye: A Review of the Clinical Evidence. *Clin. Investig.* **2015**, *5*, 267–285. [CrossRef]
18. Zhao, J.; Jin, X. Immunological Analysis and Treatment of Mooren's Ulcer with Cyclosporin A Applied Topically. *Cornea* **1993**, *12*, 481–488. [CrossRef]
19. Tandon, R.; Chawla, B.; Verma, K.; Sharma, N.; Titiyal, J.S. Outcome of Treatment of Mooren Ulcer with Topical Cyclosporine A 2%. *Cornea* **2008**, *27*, 859–861. [CrossRef]
20. Gupta, N.; Varshney, A.; Ramappa, M.; Basu, S.; Romano, V.; Acharya, M.; Gaur, A.; Kapur, N.; Singh, A.; Shah, G.; et al. Role of AS-OCT in Managing Corneal Disorders. *Diagnostics* **2022**, *12*, 918. [CrossRef]
21. Yoshihara, M.; Maeda, N.; Soma, T.; Fuchihata, M.; Hayashi, A.; Koh, S.; Oie, Y.; Nishida, K. Corneal Topographic Analysis of Patients with Mooren Ulcer Using 3-Dimensional Anterior Segment Optical Coherence Tomography. *Cornea* **2015**, *34*, 54–59. [CrossRef]
22. Lucchino, L.; Visioli, G.; Scarinci, F.; Colabelli Gisoldi, R.A.M.; Komaiha, C.; Giovannetti, F.; Marenco, M.; Pocobelli, G.; Lambiase, A.; Pocobelli, A. Influence of Opacity Depth on Big Bubble Formation During Deep Anterior Lamellar Keratoplasty in Corneal Stromal Scars. *Cornea* **2024**. [CrossRef]
23. Lian, X.; Wang, C.; Yang, S.; Zhou, S. Evaluation of Mooren's Corneal Ulcer by Anterior Segment Optical Coherence Tomography. *Photodiagnosis Photodyn. Ther.* **2023**, *44*, 103806. [CrossRef] [PubMed]
24. Bonnet, C.; Debillon, L.; Al-Hashimi, S.; Hoogewoud, F.; Monnet, D.; Bourges, J.-L.; Brézin, A. Anterior Segment Optical Coherence Tomography Imaging in Peripheral Ulcerative Keratitis, a Corneal Structural Description. *BMC Ophthalmol.* **2020**, *20*, 205. [CrossRef] [PubMed]

Disclaimer/Publisher's Note: The statements, opinions and data contained in all publications are solely those of the individual author(s) and contributor(s) and not of MDPI and/or the editor(s). MDPI and/or the editor(s) disclaim responsibility for any injury to people or property resulting from any ideas, methods, instructions or products referred to in the content.

Article

Single-Shot Ultra-Widefield Polarization-Diversity Optical Coherence Tomography for Assessing Retinal and Choroidal Pathologies

Tiffany Tse [1,†], Hoyoung Jung [2,†], Mohammad Shahidul Islam [1], Jun Song [1], Grace Soo [1], Khaldon Abbas [2], Shuibin Ni [3], Fernando Sumita [4], Katherine Paton [4], Yusi Miao [4], Yifan Jian [3], Zaid Mammo [4], Eduardo V. Navajas [4] and Myeong Jin Ju [1,4,*]

1. School of Biomedical Engineering, Faculty of Medicine and Applied Science, University of British Columbia, Vancouver, BC V6T 1Z3, Canada; tse.tiffany@ubc.ca (T.T.); mohammad.islam@ubc.ca (M.S.I.); juns01@student.ubc.ca (J.S.); gracesoo@student.ubc.ca (G.S.)
2. Faculty of Medicine, University of British Columbia, Vancouver, BC V6T 1Z3, Canada; hoyoungj@student.ubc.ca (H.J.); kfabbas@student.ubc.ca (K.A.)
3. Casey Eye Institute, Oregon Health & Science University, Portland, OR 97239, USA; nis@ohsu.edu (S.N.); jian@ohsu.edu (Y.J.)
4. Department of Ophthalmology and Visual Sciences, University of British Columbia, Vancouver, BC V6T 1Z3, Canada; fernando-sumita@hotmail.com (F.S.); katherinepaton@me.com (K.P.); yusi.miao@ubc.ca (Y.M.); zaid.mammo@ubc.ca (Z.M.); eduardo.navajas@ubc.ca (E.V.N.)
* Correspondence: myeongjin.ju@ubc.ca
† These authors contributed equally to this work.

Abstract: Background: Optical coherence tomography (OCT) is a leading ocular imaging modality, known for delivering high-resolution volumetric morphological images. However, conventional OCT systems are limited by their narrow field-of-view (FOV) and their reliance on scattering contrast, lacking molecular specificity. **Methods:** To address these limitations, we developed a custom-built 105° ultra-widefield polarization-diversity OCT (UWF PD-OCT) system for assessing various retinal and choroidal conditions, which is particularly advantageous for visualizing peripheral retinal abnormalities. Patients with peripheral lesions or pigmentary changes were imaged using the UWF PD-OCT to evaluate the system's diagnostic capabilities. Comparisons were made with conventional swept-source OCT and other standard clinical imaging modalities to highlight the benefits of depolarization contrast for identifying pathological changes. **Results:** The molecular-specific contrast offered by UWF PD-OCT enhanced the detection of disease-specific features, particularly in the peripheral retina, by capturing melanin distribution and pigmentary changes in a single shot. This detailed visualization allows clinicians to monitor disease progression with greater precision, offering more accurate insights into retinal and choroidal pathologies. **Conclusions:** Integrating UWF PD-OCT into clinical practice represents a major advancement in ocular imaging, enabling comprehensive views of retinal pathologies that are difficult to capture with current modalities. This technology holds great potential to transform the diagnosis and management of retinal and choroidal diseases by providing unique insights into peripheral retinal abnormalities and melanin-specific changes, critical for early detection and timely intervention.

Keywords: optical coherence tomography; ophthalmology; retinal imaging; wide-field OCT; retinal diseases; polarization

1. Introduction

Optical coherence tomography (OCT) has emerged as a cornerstone in ophthalmic diagnosis and in the ongoing evaluation of treatments for various ocular conditions, given its non-invasive nature and ability to produce high-resolution depth-resolved images [1]. Since its widespread adoption, OCT technology has significantly evolved, achieving notable improvements in acquisition speed, higher-resolution cross-sectional imaging at greater depths [2], and an expansion of the field of view (FOV) [3–6]. Although OCT offers high-resolution three-dimensional images of the retina, it is limited to providing solely structural information based on light scattering properties of tissues and lacks molecular-specific contrast.

Polarization-sensitive OCT (PS-OCT) is a functional extension of OCT that enables non-invasive molecular contrast imaging in the back of the eye by detecting tissue polarization properties [7–9]. Melanin is a pigment molecule found in the iris, ciliary body, and retinal pigment epithelium (RPE) [10], and it is unique because it depolarizes light, which can be detected by the PS-OCT via a measure known as the degree of polarization uniformity (DOPU). By measuring DOPU, which decreases proportionally as melanin concentration increases [11,12], we can quantify and visualize the amount to which light depolarizes after interaction with the sample [8]. Polarization-diversity OCT (PD-OCT) [13,14] is a subset of the PS-OCT that offers a simpler approach for clinical deployment, capable of obtaining both DOPU contrast as well as scattering information from conventional OCT imaging. This integrated approach makes PD-OCT a promising tool for molecular contrast imaging, enabling precise assessment of abnormal melanin distribution within the retina.

According to the International Widefield Imaging Study Group, "widefield" retinal images depict retinal anatomy beyond the posterior pole but posterior to the vortex vein ampulla in all four quadrants, whereas "ultra-widefield" (UWF) images depict retinal anatomic features anterior to the vortex vein ampullae in all four quadrants [15]. Similarly, the Diabetic Retinopathy Clinical Research network (DRCR.net) has established that a threshold FOV greater than 100° is to be considered UWF [16]. As most commercially available OCT systems are generally limited to a FOV of 30° [17], acquisition of a wider view of the retina requires stitching or montaging multiple OCT scans. This approach is time-consuming, computationally expensive, prolongs image acquisition duration, and is susceptible to alignment artifacts [18].

However, despite these inherent complexities associated with UWF and WF imaging, the ability to capture the peripheral retina remains an advantageous diagnostic tool, particularly for patients with conditions involving peripheral retinal or choroidal abnormalities [19]. UWF fundus imaging and angiography have demonstrated increased detection of disease manifestations in the peripheral retina in cases of diabetic retinopathy and retinal vein occlusion [20]. Even in age-related macular degeneration, a pathology known to affect the central retina primarily, UWF imaging has demonstrated peripheral retinal findings distinct from controls. Expanding retinal imaging to include the peripheral retina may thus elucidate different phenotypic presentations of age-related macular degeneration, and the clinical significance of these peripheral findings are an area of ongoing study [21]. The volumetric information provided by UWF OCT imaging has also demonstrated peripheral retinal manifestations in disease processes affecting the peripheral retina such as retinoblastoma, retinitis pigmentosa, and multiple evanescent white dot syndrome [22–24]. Thus, UWF imaging of the retina may provide further insights into the pathophysiology and characterization of various retinal conditions, as well as aid in their diagnosis and clinical monitoring.

In this paper, we introduce our ultra-widefield PD-OCT system which integrates 105° FOV melanin-specific molecular contrast imaging with scattering information from conventional OCT.

2. Methods

2.1. Patient Recruitment and Data Collection

We performed an observational case-series study at three high-volume ophthalmology clinics in the Vancouver General Hospital (Vancouver, BC, Canada). Patients were given dilating eye drops (using 2.5% phenylephrine hydrochloride and 1% tropicamide) and underwent imaging with fundus photography using Topcon TRC-50DX (Topcon Corporation, Tokyo, Japan), scanning laser ophthalmoscopy (SLO) using Optos P200dTx, (Optos

Inc., Marlborough, MA, USA), short-wavelength auto-fluorescence (SW-AF) at 488 nm and 532 nm excitation wavelengths using Optos P200dTx, (Optos Inc., Marlborough, MA, USA) or Heidelberg Spectralis (Heidelberg Engineering Gmbh, Heidelberg, Germany), and a research-prototype PD-OCT. All patients were informed of the purpose and implications of the study, and written informed consent was obtained from each participant prior to participation. This study was approved by the research ethics board at the University of British Columbia (human ethics protocol H19-03110 and H21-01337) and followed the tenets of the Declaration of Helsinki.

2.2. System Configuration and Imaging Protocol

Figure 1 represents the schematic of the PD-OCT system. A vertical-cavity surface-emitting laser (VCSEL, SVM10F-0210; Thorlabs, Inc., Newton, NJ, USA) with 100 nm bandwidth, 400 kHz A-scan rate, and a center wavelength of 1060 nm, is used as a light source. The single-mode optical fiber is used to build the interferometer. The light is split by a 75:25 single-mode optical fiber coupler after passing through the polarization controller, where 25% of the light goes to the reference arm, which consists of a fiber collimator, a dispersion compensation block, and a mirror, after passing through a 50:50 fiber coupler. The remaining 75% of the light from the coupler goes to the sample arm through the 20% of the 80:20 fiber coupler. The sample arm is attached with the custom-built retinal scanner designed and adapted from the 55° FOV handheld OCT scanning head previously published [25], which can image up to 105° FOV. The retinal scanner consists of a dual-axis galvanometer, a scan lens consisting of a paired achromatic doublet, and an ocular lens comprising an advanced double aspheric lens. Together, the scan lens and ocular lens function as a telescope, amplifying the scanning angle to about 105° at the pupil. The distance from the last lens surface to the cornea is approximately 5 mm, which has a shorter working distance than the previous clinical PD-OCT design [14] to secure a larger FOV. The beam diameter at the pupil is measured to be 0.58 mm, with sample power below 2.0 mW at the cornea, which satisfies the safety standard defined by ANSI. The backscattered light from the sample and reference are recoupled to the 80:20 and 50:50 fiber couplers, respectively, where both 80% and 50% light is directed to the polarization diversity detection (PDD) unit followed by another 50:50 fiber coupler. The PDD unit consists of a linear polarizer (LP), two polarizing beam splitters (PBS), one non-polarizing beam splitter (BS), and two 2.5 GHz balanced photodetectors (PDB 482C-AC).

In the PDD unit, the reference and back-scattered light from the eye is combined at the BS, split into horizontal and vertical polarization components by the two PBSs, and finally detected by the balanced photodetectors (BPDs). The detected signal at the BPD is digitized by a 12-bit waveform digitizer (ATS9373, AlazarTech Inc., Pointe-Claire, QC, Canada), allowing for dual-channel acquisition at a rate of 1.8 gigasamples/second in each channel. The sampled interference signal was rescaled to the wavenumber domain using a predefined rescaling parameter obtained via a time-frequency calibration method [26]. The theoretical axial resolution is 7.06 µm in air. Bi-directional high-speed raster scanning centered around the fovea is employed, which results in volume acquisitions consisting of 2304 points per A-scan, 2000 A-lines per B-scan, and 1000 B-scans per volume, yielding a total acquisition time of 5 s per volume. For the patient imaging, a total of 10 volumes were acquired per affected eye, where 5 volumes are acquired with 55° FOV, and 5 volumes are acquired with 105° FOV. The PDD unit implemented in the PD-OCT enables the computation of the degree of polarization uniformity (DOPU) [27] by measuring the orthogonally polarized beam state (horizontal-H and vertical-V channels). The contrast between these channels determines the extent to which the polarization state of the input beam is preserved after interaction with the sample, where 1 indicates full preservation (i.e., no change in polarization state), and 0 indicates no preservation (i.e., completely randomized state).

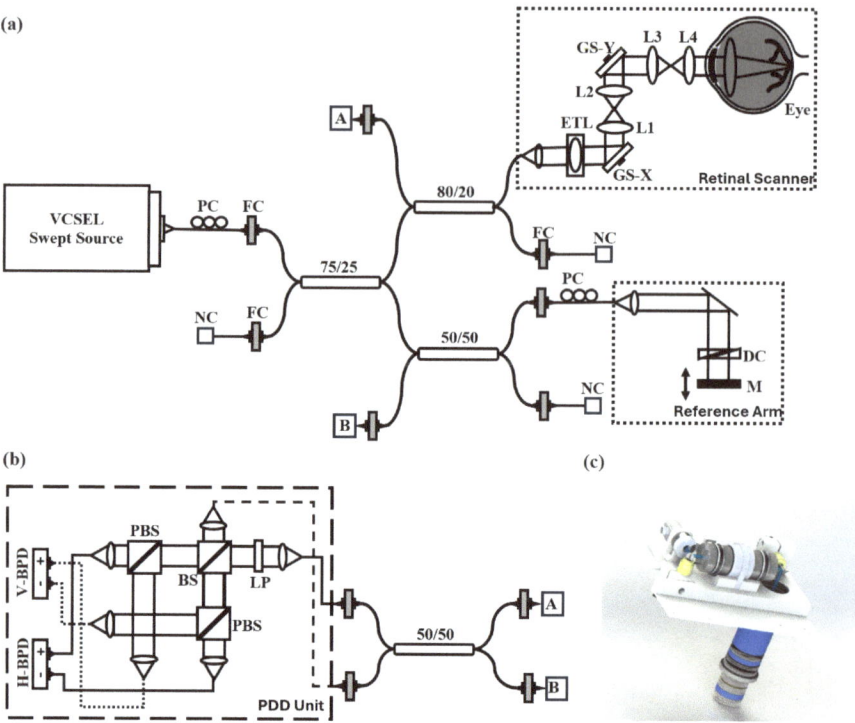

Figure 1. (**a**) Schematic diagram of PD-OCT system. (**b**) Polarization diversity detection unit (PDD). (**c**) SolidWorks design of the ultra-wide-field retinal scanner. L1–4: Lens; LP: linear polarizer; PC: polarization controller; FC: fiber collimator; NC: not connected; M: mirror; GS-X and -Y: galvanometer scanner; DC: dispersion compensation block; ETL: electrically tunable lens; PBS: polarizing beam splitter; BS: beam splitter; H- and V-BPD: balanced photo-detector for horizontally and vertically polarized signals, respectively.

2.3. Field-of-View Characterization

The uniformity, continuity, and absence of irregularities in tissue layers, even at the peripheral sections, serve as qualitative indicators of good ocular health. Figure 2 presents a comparative analysis of the imaging capabilities of our custom-built retinal scanner, emphasizing the differences in FOV of 55° versus 105°. Figure 2a depicts the phantom eye (Rowe Technical Design, Inc., Dana Point, CA, USA) embedded with a resolution target, where the structured concentric circles on the target facilitate the calibration of resolution and provide a visual guide for evaluating the performance of scanner across different FOVs. The green and orange boxes represent the areas covered by the 55° and 105° FOVs, respectively, highlighting the extended imaging capability at the larger FOV. Figure 2b,c show the *en-face* and B-scan images of a healthy control patient's retina, where the green rectangular box marks the area encompassed by the 55° FOV, and the orange box indicates the significantly wider area covered by the 105° FOV. The images clarify how the panoramic FOV can capture a greater extent of the peripheral retinal structure, which is crucial for a thorough retinal examination and for the detection of peripheral retinal pathologies.

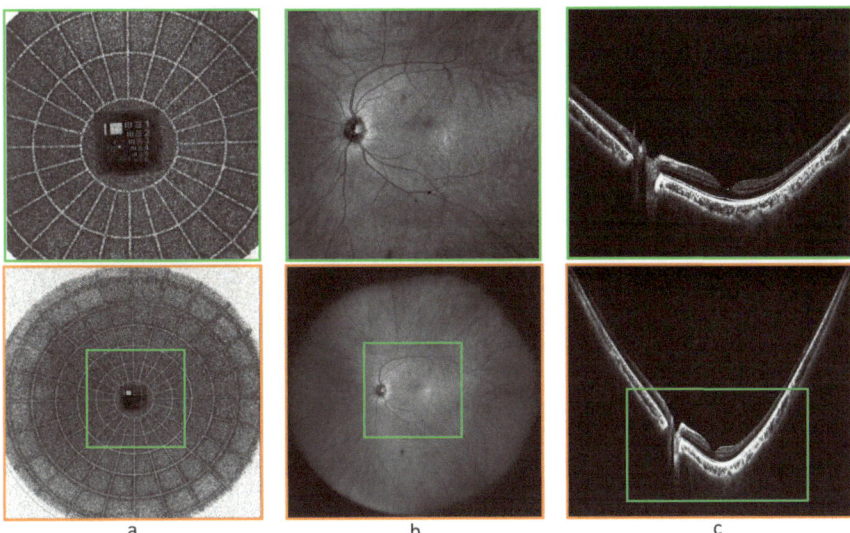

Figure 2. Comparative images of two distinct FOVs (55° and 105°). (**a**) Phantom eye featuring a resolution target with structured concentric circles that serve as a visual guide for FOV and resolution calibration. (**b,c**) OCT en face and B-scan images of healthy control subject where the green rectangular box highlights the 55° FOV and the encompassing orange box designates the 105° FOV.

2.4. Post-Processing and Feature Extraction

Following data acquisition, the post-processing pipeline used for generating multi-contrast images is illustrated by Figure 3. The complex OCT volume (Figure 3a) is derived from the two orthogonally polarized channels using conventional OCT pre-processing steps: Hilbert transform, wavenumber linearization [26], DC subtraction, numerical dispersion compensation [28], and fast Fourier transform. The contrast-enhanced scattering OCT volume is obtained by averaging the complex data (Figure 3b). To account for additive noise inherent in each polarization channel, the noise-induced error is estimated from the PD-OCT signals to obtain noise-error-corrected Stokes parameters [27]. The noise-corrected DOPU is calculated as a measure of the variance in Stokes vectors averaged within a localized area, highlighting variations in polarization state between neighboring pixels (Figure 3c) [11,27,29]. To optimize the contrast and sharpness of DOPU images, a 3×5 pixel averaging kernel is employed. Subsequent thresholding is applied to the DOPU values, which are then smoothed by a three-dimensional median filter ($3 \times 5 \times 3$ pixels) for removal of any remaining background noise. The composite B-scan is created from averaged OCT and DOPU B-scans (Figure 3d) to provide a distribution map of tissue along the retina with polarization-scrambling properties.

For visualization, the RPE layer is manually segmented from each volume based on OCT B-scan images via a segmentation assistant software (ITK-Snap [30]) to distinguish melanin content between the RPE, choroid, and inner retina. The minimum projection of the final DOPU B-scans are taken along the depth axis to generate DOPU en face maps, providing a comprehensive view of the polarization properties across the retinal layers.

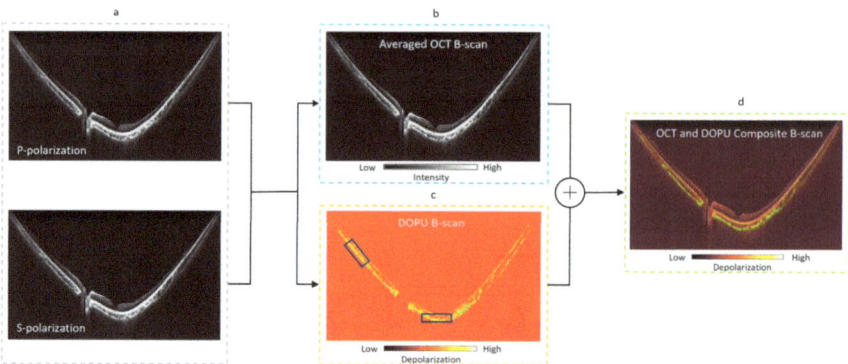

Figure 3. Illustration of post-processing pipeline: (**a**) raw OCT intensity images detected by the PDD unit of P-polarization (horizontal) and S-polarization (vertical) channels; (**b**) scattering OCT B-scan obtained by coherent averaging of P- and S-channels; (**c**) noise-corrected DOPU B-scan kernel averaging [27]; (**d**) OCT and DOPU B-scan composite.

3. Results and Discussion

3.1. Retinitis Pigmentosa

Retinitis pigmentosa (RP) is the most common hereditary retinal dystrophy, with a prevalence of approximately 1 in 4000 individuals [31]. It refers to a heterogenous group of retinal diseases characterized by the degeneration of the RPE, rod photoreceptors, and cone photoreceptors [32,33]. The subsequent visual field losses correlate with the loss of photoreceptor cells, which typically affects the mid-peripheral retina and progresses towards the far periphery and macula [31]. The utilization of fundus photographs, fundus autofluorescence (FAF), and OCT imaging modalities has been the cornerstone of the diagnosis and monitoring of retina disease progression [34]. In RP, OCT assesses retinal thickness, ellipsoid zone (EZ) line width, and the presence of macular edema [31,35]. EZ disruptions correlate with lower visual acuity and other functional impairments [36]. Hyperautofluorescence on SW-AF represents lipofuscin in the RPE, a byproduct of photoreceptor metabolism, marking the transition between healthy and degenerating retinas in RP [12,32,35,37].

Figure 4 shows a case of RP associated with a heterozygous RHO GLu181Lys genetic mutation imaged with UWF PD-OCT. We compared these results with conventional imaging techniques like SLO fundus and SW-AF (Figure 4a,b). Figure 5 is a close-up view of the area marked by the yellow dashed square in Figure 4c. En face projection of the RPE layer (Figure 5b) demonstrated higher depolarization, representing melanin content near the macula, consistent with the region of hyperautofluorescence on FAF (Figure 4b). There was a notable absence of melanin signal in the peripheral RPE, corresponding to the regions with bone spicule pigmentation on fundus photography (Figure 4a). OCT and DOPU B-scans (Figure 5d,e) highlight the absence of melanin signal in the peripheral RPE, whereas melanin signal is still preserved at the macula. The bone spicule pigmentation in Figure 4d appears in the same pattern as in Figure 4a, consistent with the migration of pigment cells from RPE to the inner retina. This pattern is visible in peripheral B-scan locations, marked by areas of high depolarization (Figure 4e,f).

Our findings have demonstrated that ultra-wide FOV allows for the robust evaluation of the central and peripheral retina and choroid while avoiding the need for multiple acquisitions and post-acquisition montaging. This is notable considering that patients with significant peripheral visual field deficits in late-stage disease can have difficulty in identifying fixation targets during multiple serial acquisitions. In the case of RP, the degenerative processes affecting the photoreceptors and RPE typically initiates in the peripheral retina before migrating centrally; thus, ultra-wide FOV imaging can be useful in detecting the early stages of degeneration affecting the peripheral retina. This can be especially beneficial for screening asymptomatic patients with family history of RP. As features such as melanin loss in the RPE and the presence of melanin in the inner retina can be characterized by PD-OCT, melanin may be a potential biomarker in monitoring treatment responses and the efficacy of gene therapy.

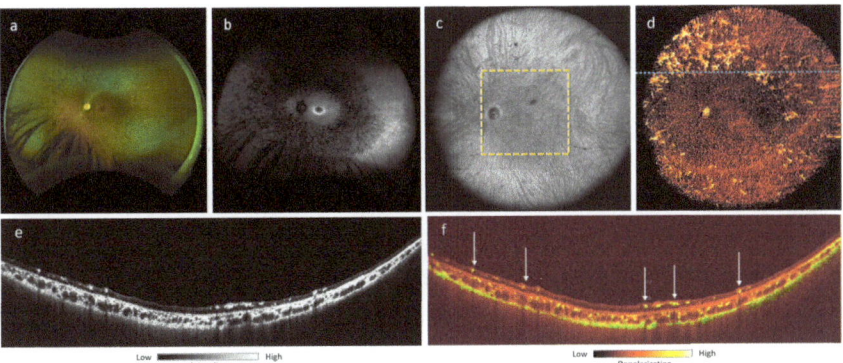

Figure 4. Retinitis pigmentosa patient, a 38-year-old South Asian male with heterozygous RHO GLu181Lys genetic mutation (left eye): (**a**) SLO fundus photograph; (**b**) short-wavelength autofluorescence; (**c**) 105° ultra-wide FOV OCT *en-face* projection image captured by PD-OCT; (**d**) 105° ultr-awide FOV DOPU *en-face* projection image of the inner retina after segmentation; (**e**,**f**) 105° FOV OCT and DOPU B-scans at location marked by dotted blue line in (**d**). Bone spicules in the peripheral retina are highlighted by the white arrows in (**f**).

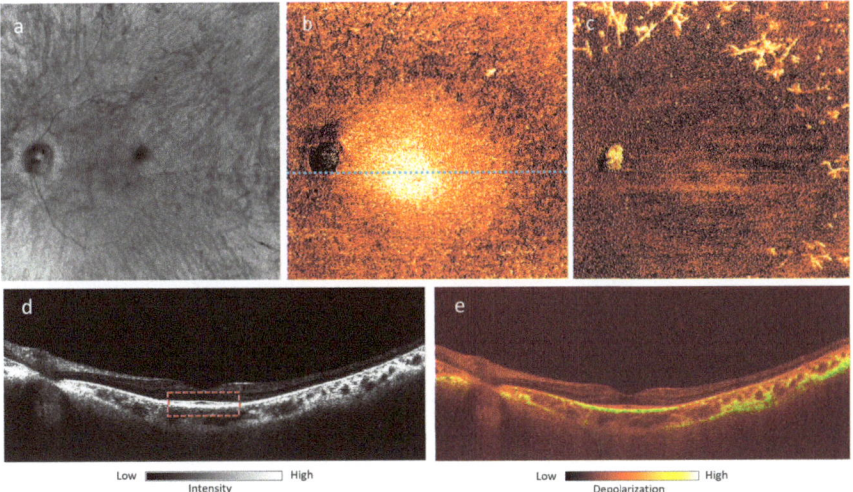

Figure 5. Close-up 55° FOV marked by the yellow dashed square in Figure 4c: (**a**) OCT *en-face* projection image captured by PD-OCT; (**b**) DOPU *en-face* projection image of the RPE after segmentation; (**c**) DOPU en face projection image of the inner retina after segmentation; (**d**,**e**) OCT and DOPU B-scans at location marked by dotted blue line in (**b**). The ellipsoid zone is highlighted by the dotted red rectangle in (**d**).

3.2. Choroidal Nevi

Choroidal nevi represent the most common benign intraocular tumor, with a prevalence of approximately 5%, although this varies by ethnicity [38,39]. Nevi are estimated to have an annual 1 in 8845 risk for malignant transformation into melanoma [40]. Routine monitoring via multimodal imaging via fundus photography, FAF, OCT, and ultrasonography are thus essential in the evaluation of these tumors [41].

In Figure 6, we present a flat melanotic choroidal nevus with a pigmented appearance on the fundus photograph (Figure 6a). The margins of lesion are not readily apparent on OCT en face projection (Figure 6b), whereas DOPU en face and B-scan projections of the lesion demonstrate a well-circumscribed melanotic appearance (Figure 6c,e), consistent with its fundus pigmentation.

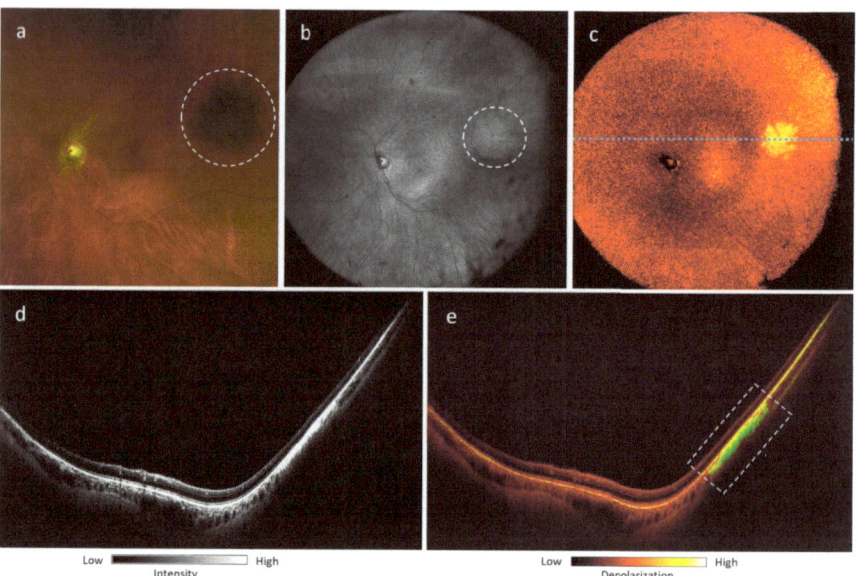

Figure 6. Peripheral flat melanotic choroidal nevus of a 55-year-old Caucasian female (left eye): (**a**) fundus photograph with lesion highlighted by white dotted circle; (**b**) 105° ultra-wide FOV OCT *en-face* projection with lesion highlighted by white dotted circle; (**c**) 105° ultra-wide FOV DOPU *en-face* projection; (**d**,**e**) OCT B-scan and DOPU B-scan of lesion at location marked by blue dotted line in (**c**). The area of depolarization consistent with the melanin-rich area is highlighted by a white dotted rectangle in (**e**).

Figure 7 shows a larger choroidal nevus, for which full margin acquisition with fundus photograph would require montaging (Figure 7a), whereas PD-OCT can acquire full lesion margins in a single acquisition (Figure 7b,c). Retinal elevation due to the mass effect of the lesion can be visualized fully via the B-scan, with clear visualization of subretinal fluid and intraretinal fluid (Figure 7d,e). The lesion appears mostly non-pigmented on the fundus photograph, although the lesion has a mixed melanotic/amelanotic appearance on the DOPU B-scan, showing a focal region of melanin (Figure 7f) with a marked absence of melanin in the RPE and a primarily amelanotic mass body.

We have demonstrated that depth-resolved melanin-specific contrast can provide an additional objective characteristic in the clinical evaluation of choroidal tumors. For melanotic lesions, PD-OCT enables the delineation of axial and longitudinal tumor margins based on melanin signal. PD-OCT also enables the objective assessment of lesion pigmentation. Furthermore, with an expanded FOV of 105°, PD-OCT enables a more comprehensive view of large lesions and can capture its entirety in a single acquisition, thereby enhancing the precision of basal diameter and thickness measurements. This can assist with the serial growth monitoring of nevi and the evaluation of morphologic and melanin-specific changes over time or in response to anti-melanoma treatment.

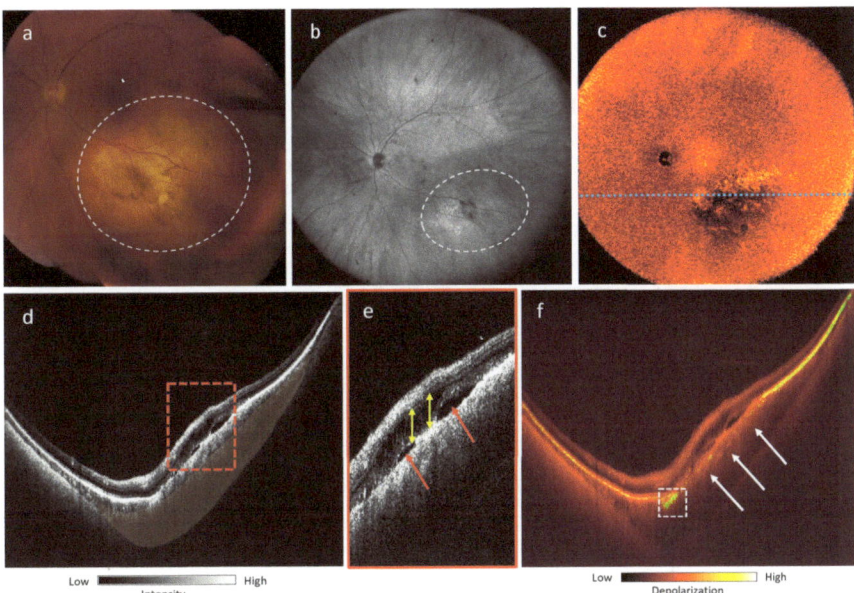

Figure 7. Mixed melanotic/amelanotic choroidal nevus of a 53-year-old Caucasian female (left eye): (**a**) Fundus photograph with lesion highlighted by white dotted circle; (**b**) 105° ultra-wide FOV OCT *en-face* projection with lesion highlighted by white dotted circle; (**c**) 105° ultra-wide FOV DOPU *en-face* projection. (**d**) OCT B-scan of lesion at location marked by dotted blue line in (**c**); Retinal elevation highlighted in orange; (**e**) Magnified view of area highlighted by red dotted rectangle in (**d**), showing subretinal fluid (red arrows) and intraretinal fluid (yellow arrows); (**f**) DOPU B-scan of lesion at location marked by dotted blue line in (**c**). A strong melanin signal at the edge of the lesion is indicated by a dotted white rectangle, and loss of melanin signal at the RPE is indicated by white arrows.

3.3. Multifocal Choroiditis

Multifocal choroiditis (MFC) is a non-infectious, idiopathic disorder that was described by Dreyer and Gass in 1984 [42]. The disease presents with "punched-out" atrophic chorioretinal scars of variable size, typically greater than 250 μm, as well as an anterior chamber and vitreous inflammation. Although MFC is similar to presumed ocular histoplasmosis syndrome, its description includes no evidence of prior histoplasmosis infection. Its incidence is estimated at 0.03 cases per 100,000 people per year [43], and the disease predominantly affects Caucasian women with myopia in their second-to-fourth decade of life [44]. Multimodal analysis findings are well described in the medical literature and include fundus photographs, fluorescein angiography, FAF, and OCT [45]. The lesions are typically at the level of the outer retina, RPE, and choriocapillaris. During the inactive stage of the disease, the lesions demonstrates RPE disruption, and the absence of an ellipsoid zone is common [45]. On FAF, the lesions show a hypoautofluorescence pattern. Active lesions have an hyperautofluorescent halo, which is absent during inactive disease. Symptoms include scotomas, metamorphopsia, floaters, and photopsias. Visual acuity is usually good at presentation. Curvilinear chorioretinal streaks, named Schlaegel lines, might be found in the periphery [46].

Figure 8 shows the findings for a 26-year-old female patient who had myopia and MFC. The patient complained of metamorphopsia on the left eye, with a best corrected visual acuity of 20/60. The fundus photograph (Figure 8a) demonstrates multiple punched-out atrophic chorioretinal scars in the macula and mid-periphery. In the inferotemporal quadrant, the scars group in a curvilinear shape, forming a Schlagel line. FAF demonstrates hypoautofluorescence in the center of the lesions with a hyperautofluorescent halo (Figure 8b), and fluorescein angiography shows hyperfluorescent scars (Figure 8c). Ultra-wide FOV *en-face* OCT projection (Figure 8d) presents an increased reflectivity of the lesions. The 105° ultra-wide FOV DOPU *en-face* images of the RPE (Figure 8e) and of the choroid (Figure 8f) show lesions with absent depolarization in the RPE and increased projection of DOPU in the choroid. The OCT B-scan (Figure 8g) at the level of the lesions shows decreased reflectivity of the RPE at the scars (green arrows), with hypertransmission of the light through the choroid and sclera (red arrows), while the DOPU B-scan (Figure 8h) demonstrates absent depolarization at the level of RPE and choriocapillaris (white arrows).

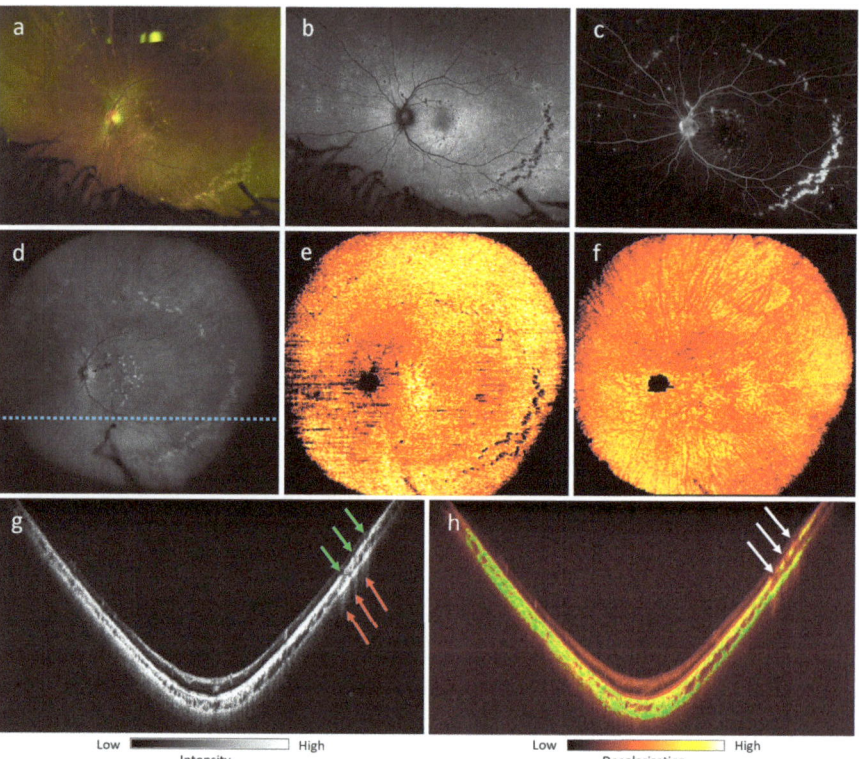

Figure 8. Multifocal choroiditis of a 26-year-old female. Best corrected visual acuity: 20/60. (**a**) Fundus photograph; (**b**) short-wavelength autofluorescence; (**c**) fluorescein angiography; (**d**) 105° ultra-wide FOV OCT *en-face* projection captured by PD-OCT; (**e**) 105° ultra-wide FOV DOPU *en-face* projection of the RPE; (**f**) 105° ultra-wide FOV DOPU *en-face* projection of the choroid; (**g**,**h**) 105° ultra-wide FOV OCT and DOPU B-scans at the location marked by the dotted blue line in (**d**). Green arrows mark decreased RPE reflectivity. Red arrows show increased light transmission through the choroid and sclera at the sites of the scars. White arrows show the absence of depolarization signal at the level of the RPE and choriocapillaris.

These findings demonstrate that UWF PD-OCT DOPU analysis is able to demonstrate depolarization changes in both RPE and choroid in patients with MFC. Moreover, this technology quantifies the degree of increased or decreased polarization in the MFC lesions and surroundings and differentiate the changes that take place in the RPE/choriocapillaris from those that occur in the choroid. As shown in the present case, MFC scars affect the RPE/choriocapillaris complex and results in decreased melanin in that layer, while the choroid remains unchanged. Such differentiation is only possible using UWF PD-OCT.

3.4. Choroideremia

Choroideremia is an X-linked chorioretinal dystrophy caused by a mutation in the CHM gene encoding the Rab escort protein-1 (REP-1). It is characterized by progressive degeneration of the RPE, photoreceptors, and choroid [47]. Clinical manifestations can include impaired night vision in childhood accompanied by progressive peripheral visual field loss. Choroideremia carriers can demonstrate pigmentary mottling on fundus photograph and speckled appearance of hypoautofluorescence and hyperautofluorescence on FAF, even in the absence of obvious fundus changes [48,49].

Figure 9 shows a 41-year-old female choroideremia carrier, visually asymptomatic, with 20/20 visual acuity in both eyes and normal visual fields. The fundus photograph demonstrates subtle pigment mottling throughout the mid and far periphery (Figure 9a). FAF shows a speckled pattern of hypoautofluorescence, primarily affecting the midperipheral retina, sparing the perifovea (Figure 9b). OCT B-scan projection (Figure 9e) demonstrates hyper-reflectivity in the choroid, following a similar pattern to the depolarization signal on the DOPU B-scan (Figure 9f), which shows increased depolarization in the mid and temporal regions. However, increased depolarization in the nasal portion is confined to the inner choroid. This finding may suggest elevated levels of choroidal melanin, although it may also be generally common for Asian patients to exhibit higher melanin content in the choroid.

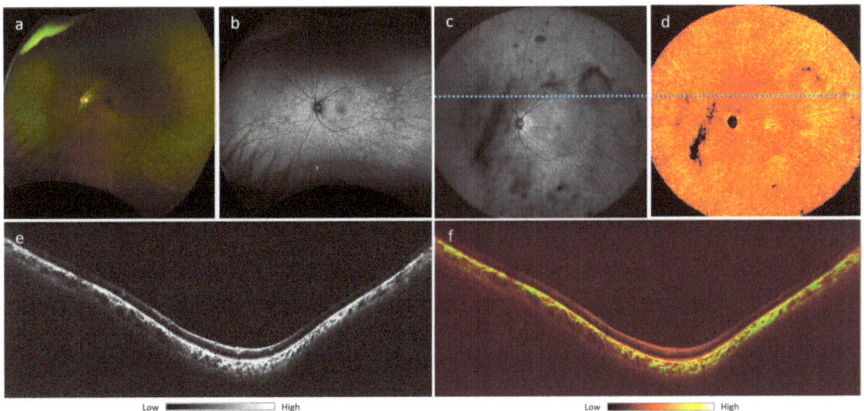

Figure 9. Choroideremia carrier, a 41-year-old Asian female: (**a**) fundus photograph; (**b**) short-wavelength autofluorescence; (**c**) 105° ultra-wide FOV OCT *en-face* projection; (**d**) 105° ultra-wide FOV DOPU *en-face* projection; (**e**) OCT B-scan at location marked by dotted blue line in (**c**); (**f**) PD-OCT B scan projection at location marked by dotted blue line in (**c**).

Previous studies have demonstrated characteristic patterns of fluorescence and RPE mosaic in choroideremia carriers [50]. Melanin-specific contrast imaging using PD-OCT offers an additional contrast modality that can aid in the further investigation of these patterns in both choroideremia and carrier cases, whereas the speckled appearance on FAF is localized and non-specific. This provides additional insight into choroidal involvement that is not evident on fundus photography and FAF. The 105° ultra-wide FOV also allows for the observation of whole-choroidal involvement posterior to the equator. This raises the possibility of a specific choroidal melanin phenotype in carriers that could affect the entire choroid. Further PD-OCT imaging of a larger sample of choroideremia carriers and affected individuals could offer additional insights into the potential association between RPE/choroidal melanin and visual phenotype.

4. Discussion

In this study, we introduced a novel UWF PD-OCT system that provides depth-resolved imaging with depolarization contrast for assessing retinal and choroidal pathologies. This system was evaluated in patients with conditions such as choroidal lesions, multifocal choroiditis, and inherited retinal diseases. Our findings demonstrate the potential of UWF PD-OCT to provide comprehensive imaging of peripheral retinal abnormalities, contributing valuable insights into melanin distribution and pigmentary changes.

We demonstrated several advantages of the PD-OCT over existing imaging modalities. Compared to commercially available wide-field imaging modalities like SLO and FAF, which capture only 2D *en-face* images, PD-OCT provides depth-resolved images that can visualize retinal layers while also offering additional depolarization contrast. This capability enables the detection of melanin distribution abnormalities in ways that other OCT systems currently used in clinics cannot, as conventional OCT primarily relies on scattering contrast. Moreover, PD-OCT acquires a much larger FOV in a single shot, eliminating the need for montaging multiple scans, which not only minimizes patient discomfort and motion artifacts but also reduces computational costs. Furthermore, this technology can be used in conjunction with existing modalities in the clinic to provide complementary information. While conventional tools like fundus photography or standard OCT systems offer valuable structural insights, PD-OCT adds a unique layer of information, which can enhance diagnostic accuracy and offer new perspectives in assessing retinal pathologies. Future development of multi-modal image registration techniques, such as registering fundus images with PD-OCT *en-face* images, would offer a more comprehensive view of retinal health while maintaining consistency with imaging workflows that clinicians are already familiar with. Such multi-modal approaches would also ease the clinical translation of PD-OCT by aligning its functionality with widely accepted practices in ophthalmology.

Despite its advantages, we acknowledge several limitations of our study with the current prototype. First, while the system effectively visualizes melanin distribution through DOPU, it cannot yet quantify melanin concentration, which poses challenges in comparing melanin levels between patients. To address this, future work will focus on implementing a uniform modulation of the input polarization state, allowing us to obtain a quantifiable depolarization index with which to evaluate melanin concentration [51,52]. This enhancement will require multiple volume acquisitions and the development of a sophisticated 3D registration algorithm to align and average these volumes accurately. Second, patient movements such as microsaccades or blinking can introduce significant motion artifacts in the captured volumes, particularly in patients with low visual acuity which affects their ability to fixate, or in those with dry eyes, making it difficult for them to keep their eyes open during the acquisition process. Although 8-10 volumes are acquired per eye during each imaging session, we are developing a feature-based registration algorithm to account for geometric warping of the vasculature and mitigate information loss caused by movement. This will allow us to generate a fully motion-corrected volume, enhancing both the accuracy and reliability of the images. Lastly, it is worth noting that the selection of specific diseases for this study was based on their peripheral abnormalities and the presence of pigmentary changes, which make them suitable for demonstrating the capabilities of the PD-OCT system. However, this focus limits the generalizability of our findings to other retinal conditions that also involve peripheral lesions. In order to explore the application of PD-OCT to a broader range of retinal diseases, future work will expand its functionality to include OCT angiography (OCTA). The integration of OCTA will allow for the visualization of ultra-wide FOV vascular contrast, enabling the exploration of additional conditions such as diabetic retinopathy and glaucoma. Despite these limitations, our prototype has consistently demonstrated its ability to provide detailed morphological and melanin-contrast images with UWF retinal coverage, underscoring its potential to offer novel insights into retinal conditions that are not possible with existing clinical tools.

5. Conclusions

In summary, UWF imaging with PD-OCT enables robust, non-invasive visualization of melanin-specific features in the peripheral retina. Beyond providing melanin-specific contrast, UWF PD-OCT offers detailed visualization of retinal structures comparable to conventional swept-source OCT, while eliminating the need for montaging multiple acquisitions. Our findings establish melanin distribution as a critical marker for assessing retinal health, and future studies will solidify its role as a biomarker in diagnosing and evaluating retinal conditions.

Author Contributions: Conceptualization, T.T., H.J. and M.J.J.; methodology, T.T., J.S., S.N., Y.J., M.S.I. and Y.M.; software, T.T. and Y.M.; validation, T.T., H.J., F.S. and K.A.; formal analysis, T.T., H.J. and K.A.; investigation, M.J.J., Z.M., E.V.N. and K.P.; resources, M.J.J., Z.M., Y.J., S.N., E.V.N. and K.P.; data curation, T.T., H.J., G.S., F.S. and K.A.; writing—original draft preparation, T.T., H.J. and M.S.I.; writing—review and editing, T.T., H.J., M.S.I., J.S., G.S., Y.J., Z.M., E.V.N. and M.J.J. ; visualization, T.T. and H.J.; supervision, M.J.J., Z.M. and E.V.N.; project administration, M.J.J., Z.M. and E.V.N.; funding acquisition, M.J.J., Z.M. and E.V.N. All authors have read and agreed to the published version of the manuscript.

Funding: This research was funded by Canadian Cancer Society (Grant #708165), Natural Sciences and Engineering Research Council of Canada; the Canadian Institutes of Health Research; the Alzheimer Society Research Program; the Canada Foundation for Innovation; the National Institutes of Health (R01 HD107494, R21 EY035816); and the Mohammad H. Mohseni Charitable Foundation.

Institutional Review Board Statement: This study was conducted in accordance with the Declaration of Helsinski and approved by the University of British Columbia Clinical Research Ethics Board (CREB) and the Vancouver Coastal Health Authority, human ethics protocols H19-03110 (approval date: 16 March 2020) and H21-01337 (approval date: 17 November 2021).

Informed Consent Statement: Informed consent was obtained from all subjects involved in the study.

Data Availability Statement: The datasets generated and analyzed during the current study are available from the corresponding author upon request.

Conflicts of Interest: OHSU and Y. Jian have a financial interest in Siloam Vision, a company that may have a commercial interest in the results of this research and technology. This potential conflict of interest has been reviewed and managed by OHSU. All other authors declare no conflicts of interest.

References

1. Huang, D.; Swanson, E.A.; Lin, C.P.; Schuman, J.S.; Stinson, W.G.; Chang, W.; Hee, M.R.; Flotte, T.; Gregory, K.; Puliafito, C.A.; et al. Optical Coherence Tomography. *Science* **1991**, *254*, 1178–1181. [CrossRef]
2. Drexler, W.; Liu, M.; Kumar, A.; Kamali, T.; Unterhuber, A.; Leitgeb, R.A. Optical coherence tomography today: Speed, contrast, and multimodality. *J. Biomed. Opt.* **2014**, *19*, 071412. [CrossRef] [PubMed]
3. Song, S.; Xu, J.; Wang, R.K. Long-range and wide field of view optical coherence tomography for in vivo 3D imaging of large volume object based on akinetic programmable swept source. *Biomed. Opt. Express* **2016**, *7*, 4734–4748. [CrossRef]
4. Ni, S.; Nguyen, T.T.P.; Ng, R.; Khan, S.; Ostmo, S.; Jia, Y.; Chiang, M.F.; Huang, D.; Campbell, J.P.; Jian, Y. 105° field of view non-contact handheld swept-source optical coherence tomography. *Opt. Lett.* **2021**, *46*, 5878–5881. [CrossRef] [PubMed]
5. McNabb, R.P.; Grewal, D.S.; Mehta, R.; Schuman, S.G.; Izatt, J.A.; Mahmoud, T.H.; Jaffe, G.J.; Mruthyunjaya, P.; Kuo, A.N. Wide field of view swept-source optical coherence tomography for peripheral retinal disease. *Br. J. Ophthalmol.* **2016**, *100*, 1377–1382. [CrossRef] [PubMed]
6. Ni, S.; Liang, G.B.; Ng, R.; Ostmo, S.; Jia, Y.; Chiang, M.F.; Huang, D.; Skalet, A.H.; Young, B.K.; Campbell, J.P.; et al. Panretinal handheld OCT angiography for pediatric retinal imaging. *Biomed. Opt. Express* **2024**, *15*, 3412–3424. [CrossRef] [PubMed]
7. de Boer, J.F.; Hitzenberger, C.K.; Yasuno, Y. Polarization sensitive optical coherence tomography—A review [Invited]. *Biomed. Opt. Express* **2017**, *8*, 1838–1873. [CrossRef]
8. Yamanari, M.; Mase, M.; Obata, R.; Matsuzaki, M.; Minami, T.; Takagi, S.; Yamamoto, M.; Miyamoto, N.; Ueda, K.; Koide, N.; et al. Melanin concentration and depolarization metrics measurement by polarization-sensitive optical coherence tomography. *Sci. Rep.* **2020**, *10*, 19513. [CrossRef]
9. Miura, M.; Makita, S.; Yasuno, Y.; Iwasaki, T.; Azuma, S.; Mino, T.; Yamaguchi, T. Evaluation of choroidal melanin-containing tissue in healthy Japanese subjects by polarization-sensitive optical coherence tomography. *Sci. Rep.* **2022**, *12*, 4048. [CrossRef]
10. Hu, D.N.; Simon, J.D.; Sarna, T. Role of Ocular Melanin in Ophthalmic Physiology and Pathology†. *Photochem. Photobiol.* **2008**, *84*, 639–644. [CrossRef]

11. Baumann, B.; Baumann, S.O.; Konegger, T.; Pircher, M.; Götzinger, E.; Schlanitz, F.; Schütze, C.; Sattmann, H.; Litschauer, M.; Schmidt-Erfurth, U.; et al. Polarization sensitive optical coherence tomography of melanin provides intrinsic contrast based on depolarization. *Biomed. Opt. Express* **2012**, *3*, 1670–1683. [CrossRef] [PubMed]
12. Sakai, D.; Takagi, S.; Totani, K.; Yamamoto, M.; Matsuzaki, M.; Yamanari, M.; Sugiyama, S.; Yokota, S.; Maeda, A.; Hirami, Y.; et al. Retinal pigment epithelium melanin imaging using polarization-sensitive optical coherence tomography for patients with retinitis pigmentosa. *Sci. Rep.* **2022**, *12*, 7115. [CrossRef] [PubMed]
13. Hsu, D.; Kwon, J.H.; Ng, R.; Makita, S.; Yasuno, Y.; Sarunic, M.V.; Ju, M.J. Quantitative multi-contrast in vivo mouse imaging with polarization diversity optical coherence tomography and angiography. *Biomed. Opt. Express* **2020**, *11*, 6945–6961. [CrossRef] [PubMed]
14. Miao, Y.; Jung, H.; Hsu, D.; Song, J.; Ni, S.; Ma, D.; Jian, Y.; Makita, S.; Yasuno, Y.; Sarunic, M.V.; et al. Polarization-Diversity Optical Coherence Tomography Assessment of Choroidal Nevi. *Investig. Ophthalmol. Vis. Sci.* **2023**, *64*, 6. [CrossRef] [PubMed]
15. Choudhry, N.; Duker, J.S.; Freund, K.B.; Kiss, S.; Querques, G.; Rosen, R.; Sarraf, D.; Souied, E.H.; Stanga, P.E.; Staurenghi, G.; et al. Classification and Guidelines for Widefield Imaging: Recommendations from the International Widefield Imaging Study Group. *Ophthalmol. Retin.* **2019**, *3*, 843–849. [CrossRef]
16. DRCR Retina Network—Public Site. Available online: https://public.jaeb.org/drcrnet (accessed on 5 September 2024)
17. Nissen, A.H.K.; Vergmann, A.S. Clinical Utilisation of Wide-Field Optical Coherence Tomography and Angiography: A Narrative Review. *Ophthalmol. Ther.* **2024**, *13*, 903–915. [CrossRef]
18. Mori, K.; Kanno, J.; Gehlbach, P.L. Retinochoroidal morphology described By wide-field montage imaging of spectral domain optical coherence tomography. *Retina* **2016**, *36*, 375. [CrossRef]
19. Ripa, M.; Motta, L.; Florit, T.; Sahyoun, J.Y.; Matello, V.; Parolini, B. The Role of Widefield and Ultra Widefield Optical Coherence Tomography in the Diagnosis and Management of Vitreoretinal Diseases. *Diagnostics* **2022**, *12*, 2247. [CrossRef]
20. Patel, S.N.; Shi, A.; Wibbelsman, T.D.; Klufas, M.A. Ultra-widefield retinal imaging: An update on recent advances. *Ther. Adv. Ophthalmol.* **2020**, *12*, 2515841419899495. [CrossRef]
21. Domalpally, A.; Clemons, T.E.; Danis, R.P.; Sadda, S.R.; Cukras, C.A.; Toth, C.A.; Friberg, T.R.; Chew, E.Y. Peripheral Retinal Changes Associated with Age-Related Macular Degeneration in the Age-Related Eye Disease Study 2: Age-Related Eye Disease Study 2 Report Number 12 by the Age-Related Eye Disease Study 2 Optos PEripheral RetinA (OPERA) Study Research Group. *Ophthalmology* **2017**, *124*, 479–487. [CrossRef]
22. Duan, J.; Qi, H.; Shang, Q. Ultrawide-field En face OCT of Multiple Evanescent White Dot Syndrome. *Ophthalmology* **2024**, *131*, 29. [CrossRef] [PubMed]
23. Zheng, F.; He, J.; Fang, X. Ultrawide-field Swept Source-OCT Angiography of Retinitis Pigmentosa. *Ophthalmology* **2023**, *130*, 67. [CrossRef] [PubMed]
24. Skalet, A.H.; Campbell, J.P.; Jian, Y. Ultrawide-field OCT for Retinoblastoma. *Ophthalmology* **2022**, *129*, 718. [CrossRef] [PubMed]
25. Ni, S.; Wei, X.; Ng, R.; Ostmo, S.; Chiang, M.F.; Huang, D.; Jia, Y.; Campbell, J.P.; Jian, Y. High-speed and widefield handheld swept-source OCT angiography with a VCSEL light source. *Biomed. Opt. Express* **2021**, *12*, 3553–3570. [CrossRef]
26. Yasuno, Y.; Madjarova, V.D.; Makita, S.; Akiba, M.; Morosawa, A.; Chong, C.; Sakai, T.; Chan, K.P.; Itoh, M.; Yatagai, T. Three-dimensional and high-speed swept-source optical coherence tomography for in vivo investigation of human anterior eye segments. *Opt. Express* **2005**, *13*, 10652–10664. [CrossRef]
27. Makita, S.; Hong, Y.J.; Miura, M.; Yasuno, Y. Degree of polarization uniformity with high noise immunity using polarization-sensitive optical coherence tomography. *Opt. Lett.* **2014**, *39*, 6783–6786. [CrossRef]
28. Yasuno, Y.; Hong, Y.; Makita, S.; Yamanari, M.; Akiba, M.; Miura, M.; Yatagai, T. In vivo high-contrast imaging of deep posterior eye by 1-µm swept source optical coherence tomography and scattering optical coherence angiography. *Opt. Express* **2007**, *15*, 6121–6139. [CrossRef]
29. Ju, M.J.; Hong, Y.J.; Makita, S.; Lim, Y.; Kurokawa, K.; Duan, L.; Miura, M.; Tang, S.; Yasuno, Y. Advanced multi-contrast Jones matrix optical coherence tomography for Doppler and polarization sensitive imaging. *Opt. Express* **2013**, *21*, 19412–19436. [CrossRef]
30. Yushkevich, P.A.; Piven, J.; Hazlett, H.C.; Smith, R.G.; Ho, S.; Gee, J.C.; Gerig, G. User-guided 3D active contour segmentation of anatomical structures: Significantly improved efficiency and reliability. *NeuroImage* **2006**, *31*, 1116–1128. [CrossRef]
31. Hartong, D.T.; Berson, E.L.; Dryja, T.P. Retinitis pigmentosa. *Lancet* **2006**, *368*, 1795–1809. [CrossRef]
32. Menghini, M.; Cehajic-Kapetanovic, J.; MacLaren, R.E. Monitoring progression of retinitis pigmentosa: Current recommendations and recent advances. *Expert Opin. Orphan Drugs* **2020**, *8*, 67–78. [CrossRef] [PubMed]
33. Milam, A.H.; Li, Z.Y.; Fariss, R.N. Histopathology of the human retina in retinitis pigmentosa. *Prog. Retin. Eye Res.* **1998**, *17*, 175–205. [CrossRef] [PubMed]
34. Sujirakul, T.; Lin, M.K.; Duong, J.; Wei, Y.; Lopez-Pintado, S.; Tsang, S.H. Multimodal Imaging of Central Retinal Disease Progression in a 2-Year Mean Follow-up of Retinitis Pigmentosa. *Am. J. Ophthalmol.* **2015**, *160*, 786–798.e4. [CrossRef] [PubMed]
35. Jauregui, R.; Takahashi, V.K.L.; Park, K.S.; Cui, X.; Takiuti, J.T.; Lima de Carvalho, J.R.; Tsang, S.H. Multimodal structural disease progression of retinitis pigmentosa according to mode of inheritance. *Sci. Rep.* **2019**, *9*, 10712. [CrossRef] [PubMed]
36. Ritter, M.; Zotter, S.; Schmidt, W.M.; Bittner, R.E.; Deak, G.G.; Pircher, M.; Sacu, S.; Hitzenberger, C.K.; Schmidt-Erfurth, U.M. Characterization of Stargardt Disease Using Polarization-Sensitive Optical Coherence Tomography and Fundus Autofluorescence Imaging. *Investig. Ophthalmol. Vis. Sci.* **2013**, *54*, 6416–6425. [CrossRef]

37. Kellner, U.; Kellner, S.; Weber, B.H.F.; Fiebig, B.; Weinitz, S.; Ruether, K. Lipofuscin- and melanin-related fundus autofluorescence visualize different retinal pigment epithelial alterations in patients with retinitis pigmentosa. *Eye* **2009**, *23*, 1349–1359. [CrossRef]
38. Chien, J.L.; Sioufi, K.; Surakiatchanukul, T.; Shields, J.A.; Shields, C.L. Choroidal nevus: A review of prevalence, features, genetics, risks, and outcomes. *Curr. Opin. Ophthalmol.* **2017**, *28*, 228–237. [CrossRef]
39. Greenstein, M.B.; Myers, C.E.; Meuer, S.M.; Klein, B.E.K.; Cotch, M.F.; Wong, T.Y.; Klein, R. Prevalence and Characteristics of Choroidal Nevi: The Multi-Ethnic Study of Atherosclerosis. *Ophthalmology* **2011**, *118*, 2468–2473. [CrossRef]
40. Singh, A.D.; Kalyani, P.; Topham, A. Estimating the risk of malignant transformation of a choroidal nevus. *Ophthalmology* **2005**, *112*, 1784–1789. [CrossRef]
41. Shields, C.L.; Pellegrini, M.; Ferenczy, S.R.; Shields, J.A. Enhanced depth imaging optical coherence tomography of intraocular tumors: From placid to seasick to rock and rolling topography–the 2013 Francesco Orzalesi Lecture. *Retina* **2014**, *34*, 1495–1512. [CrossRef]
42. Dreyer, R.F.; Gass, J.D.M. Multifocal Choroiditis and Panuveitis: A Syndrome That Mimics Ocular Histoplasmosis. *Arch. Ophthalmol.* **1984**, *102*, 1776–1784. [CrossRef] [PubMed]
43. Abu-Yaghi, N.E.; Hartono, S.P.; Hodge, D.O.; Pulido, J.S.; Bakri, S.J. White Dot Syndromes: A 20-year Study of Incidence, Clinical Features, and Outcomes. *Ocul. Immunol. Inflamm.* **2011**, *19*, 426–430. [CrossRef] [PubMed]
44. Tavallali, A.; Yannuzzi, L.A. Idiopathic Multifocal Choroiditis. *J. Ophthalmic Vis. Res.* **2016**, *11*, 429–432. [CrossRef] [PubMed]
45. de Groot, E.L.; Ten Dam-van Loon, N.H.; Kouwenberg, C.V.; de Boer, J.H.; Ossewaarde-van Norel, J. Exploring Imaging Characteristics Associated with Disease Activity in Idiopathic Multifocal Choroiditis: A Multimodal Imaging Approach. *Am. J. Ophthalmol.* **2023**, *252*, 45–58. [CrossRef] [PubMed]
46. Matsumoto, Y.; Francis, J.; Yannuzzi, L. Curvilinear Streaks in Multifocal Choroiditis. *Eur. J. Ophthalmol.* **2007**, *17*, 448–450. [CrossRef]
47. Dimopoulos, I.S.; Radziwon, A.; St Laurent, C.D.; MacDonald, I.M. Choroideremia. *Curr. Opin. Ophthalmol.* **2017**, *28*, 410–415. [CrossRef]
48. Preising, M.N.; Wegscheider, E.; Friedburg, C.; Poloschek, C.M.; Wabbels, B.K.; Lorenz, B. Fundus Autofluorescence in Carriers of Choroideremia and Correlation with Electrophysiologic and Psychophysical Data. *Ophthalmology* **2009**, *116*, 1201–1209.e2. [CrossRef]
49. Dugel, P.U.; Zimmer, C.N.; Shahidi, A.M. A case study of choroideremia carrier – Use of multi-spectral imaging in highlighting clinical features. *Am. J. Ophthalmol. Case Rep.* **2016**, *2*, 18–22. [CrossRef]
50. Aguilera, N.; Liu, T.; Bower, A.J.; Li, J.; Abouassali, S.; Lu, R.; Giannini, J.; Pfau, M.; Bender, C.; Smelkinson, M.G.; et al. Widespread subclinical cellular changes revealed across a neural-epithelial-vascular complex in choroideremia using adaptive optics. *Commun. Biol.* **2022**, *5*, 1–12. [CrossRef]
51. Lippok, N.; Villiger, M.; Bouma, B.E. Degree of polarization (uniformity) and depolarization index: Unambiguous depolarization contrast for optical coherence tomography. *Opt. Lett.* **2015**, *40*, 3954–3957. [CrossRef]
52. Lippok, N.; Braaf, B.; Villiger, M.; Oh, W.Y.; Vakoc, B.J.; Bouma, B.E. Quantitative depolarization measurements for fiber-based polarization-sensitive optical frequency domain imaging of the retinal pigment epithelium. *J. Biophotonics* **2019**, *12*, e201800156. [CrossRef] [PubMed]

Disclaimer/Publisher's Note: The statements, opinions and data contained in all publications are solely those of the individual author(s) and contributor(s) and not of MDPI and/or the editor(s). MDPI and/or the editor(s) disclaim responsibility for any injury to people or property resulting from any ideas, methods, instructions or products referred to in the content.

MDPI AG
Grosspeteranlage 5
4052 Basel
Switzerland
Tel.: +41 61 683 77 34

Journal of Clinical Medicine Editorial Office
E-mail: jcm@mdpi.com
www.mdpi.com/journal/jcm

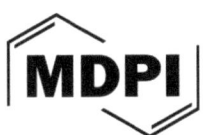

Disclaimer/Publisher's Note: The statements, opinions and data contained in all publications are solely those of the individual author(s) and contributor(s) and not of MDPI and/or the editor(s). MDPI and/or the editor(s) disclaim responsibility for any injury to people or property resulting from any ideas, methods, instructions or products referred to in the content.

www.ingramcontent.com/pod-product-compliance
Lightning Source LLC
LaVergne TN
LVHW072355090526